Swimming Upstream

D0826798

Community & Environmental Studies

Swimming Upstream

Collaborative Approaches to Watershed
Management

edited by Paul A. Sabatier, Will Focht, Mark Lubell,
Zev Trachtenberg, Arnold Vedlitz, and Marty Matlock

The MIT Press
Cambridge, Massachusetts
London, England

© 2005 Massachusetts Institute of Technology

All rights reserved. No part of this book may be reproduced in any form by any electronic or mechanical means (including photocopying, recording, or information storage and retrieval) without permission in writing from the publisher.

MIT Press books may be purchased at special quantity discounts for business or sales promotional use. For information, please e-mail special_sales@mitpress. mit.edu or write to Special Sales Department, The MIT Press, 5 Cambridge Center, Cambridge, MA 02142.

This book was set in Sabon on 3B2 by Asco Typesetters, Hong Kong. Printed and bound in the United States of America.

Library of Congress Cataloging-in-Publication Data

Swimming upstream : collaborative approaches to watershed management / edited by Paul A. Sabatier ... [et al.].
    p.   cm. — (American and comparative environmental policy)
Includes bibliographical references and index.
ISBN 0-262-19520-8 (alk. paper) — ISBN 0-262-69319-4 (pbk. : alk. paper)
1. Watershed management—United States—Decision making. 2. Watershed management—United States—Citizen participation. I. Sabatier, Paul A. II. Series.
TC423.S93   2005
333.91′00973—dc22   2004059577

10   9   8   7   6   5   4   3   2   1

Contents

Series Foreword

For the past century, water quality, urban stormwater runoff, flood control, fish and wildlife habitat, and, to a lesser extent, water supply have been managed by individual, single-function federal and state agencies, each pursuing its own legal mandate. For the most part, decision making has been quite technocratic, with public and private stakeholder involvement usually relegated to public hearings and comment periods that fine-tune agency proposals. The scope of decision making has generally consisted of specific types of pollution sources or specific areas within a watershed (such as a pond or coastal wetlands) rather than the watershed as a whole.

Over the past twenty years, the traditional approach has been subject to increasing criticism and calls for significant reform. In part, this reflects the growing complexity and conflict in water resource and pollution control policymaking. This can be witnessed in increased competition for limited fresh water resources among agriculture, urban and industrial users, and those involved in recreation and fisheries, as well as in the requirement under the Clean Water Act for watershed-based restoration of water quality through the total maximum daily load (TMDL) process. There also has been a general dissatisfaction with leaving important policy decisions largely in the hands of agency experts, many of whom reside far from the local controversy and lack democratic legitimacy. There is no reason to assume, in a situation where each agency seeks to optimize results within its jurisdiction, that the results will be a solution that is optimum overall. Finally, there is increasing skepticism about the ability of highly legalistic agency processes and the accompanying litigation to craft viable, long-term solutions to complex water quality and water resource problems.

A new approach to water management has emerged that explicitly focuses on all sources of a pollutant within the watershed as a whole rather than on types of sources (that is, point and nonpoint sources) or on the arbitrary political boundaries of states, counties, and municipalities. The new decision-making process is collaborative, normally involving face-to-face negotiations among a variety of stakeholders with relatively consensual decision rules. This contrasts with the traditional approach in which each government agency jealously guarded its decision-making authority, with citizens and officials from other agencies largely confined to commenting on proposed standards and regulations. Rather than have each agency single-mindedly pursue its legal mandate, the new approach seeks win-win solutions to an interrelated set of social, economic, and environmental issues confronting the watershed. The end result is a collaborative process involving interrelated negotiations over a number of years rather than a series of standardized rule-making decisions in which an agency proposes a rule, receives comments, revises the rule, and then awaits litigation by one or more dissatisfied stakeholders. The new, collaborative approach represents a significant shift from a top-down, agency-dominated approach with some provision for citizen comment to a much more collaborative bottom-up strategy involving negotiations and problem solving among a variety of governmental and nongovernmental stakeholders.

Collaborative watershed management approaches have the potential to bring together and foster cooperation among current, highly adversarial stakeholders in the management of different types of water bodies. Such an effort will require careful consideration of the institutions and deliberative processes necessary to reach acceptable decisions concerning how to manage water resources most cost-effectively. In addition to enlarging the focus on particular polluters and individual municipalities to encompass an entire watershed, state and federal policymakers must consider providing more policymaking autonomy to stakeholders at the grassroots level.

The development of institutions and processes to control storm-water pollution will require, among other things, the integration of politics and policymaking theory. Specifically, theories concerning political participation, agenda building, conflict resolution, and organizational development must be connected to procedures to identify pollutants, geographical conditions, emerging technological approaches, and best management practices. *Swimming Upstream: Collaborative Approaches to Watershed Management*, edited by Paul A. Sabatier and his colleagues, demonstrates the potential value of doing this by addressing the overall viability of collaborative approaches to watershed management in different areas of the United States. Using the shift from a top-down, agency-dominated approach to a far more collaborative bottom-up approach as a springboard, this study analyzes the contexts and processes conducive to the development of collaborative efforts and to their success; who participates in these efforts, why, and in what ways; the extent to which such efforts increase trust among participants; the extent to which trust increases the likelihood of reaching agreements; the level of success of collaborations in reaching agreements on management plans, implementing those agreements, and improving outcomes; the principal contextual and process-related variables that contribute to success; the extent to which these efforts are viewed as procedurally and substantively legitimate by stakeholders and related parties; and the prospects for sustaining such efforts.

The authors of *Swimming Upstream* present original research and report findings that have important implications for collaborative watershed management. Their work makes a significant contribution to the literature on environmental policy in two ways. First, the study presents and later refines a fairly broad and elaborate conceptual framework for understanding collaborative watershed management. Operating within this framework, the authors integrate and test a number of specific theories concerning the role of socioeconomic and ecological conditions, government institutions, human and social capital, political efficacy, trust, legitimacy, and collective action beliefs. Second, the study analyzes a variety of collaborative watershed planning projects across the country using qualitative and quantitative approaches. The work is therefore an important addition to the literature because of its theoretical and analytical contributions to our understanding of collaborative mechanisms.

Instructors, academic researchers, and practitioners should find this book valuable in their work. The investigations presented here are new and add to our knowledge of theory and policy application. Furthermore, the book is clearly written and is suitable for adoption in undergraduate and graduate courses on environmental studies, environmental politics and policy, natural resource management, conflict resolution, and public administration. Although some of the data analyses in later chapters are fairly advanced for undergraduates, care is taken to explain different statistical and methodological techniques in the text and in the notes.

The analyses represented in this collection illustrate well our purpose in the MIT Press series in American and Comparative Environmental Policy. We encourage work that examines a broad range of environmental policy issues. We are particularly interested in books that incorporate interdisciplinary research and focus on the linkages between public policy and environmental problems and issues both within the United States and in cross-national settings. We welcome contributions that analyze the policy dimensions of relationships between humans and the environment from either a theoretical or empirical perspective. At a time when environmental policies are increasingly seen as controversial and new approaches are being implemented widely, we especially encourage studies that assess policy successes and failures, evaluate new institutional arrangements and policy tools, and clarify new directions for environmental politics and policy. The books in this series are written for a wide audience that includes academics, policymakers, environmental scientists and professionals, business and labor leaders, environmental activists, and students concerned with environmental issues. We hope they contribute to public understanding of the most important environmental problems, issues, and policies that society now faces and with which it must deal.

Sheldon Kamieniecki, University of Southern California
Michael E. Kraft, University of Wisconsin–Green Bay
American and Comparative Environmental Policy Series Editors

Preface

The idea for this broad-ranged, comparative examination of stakeholder participation in decision making on watershed policies began in 1999 when two of our authors, Will Focht and Marty Matlock, and one of their colleagues, Tom Webler, approached Barbara Levinson, then water and watersheds program coordinator at the U.S. Environmental Protection Agency. She was interested in bringing together the findings of a number of STAR (Science to Achieve Results) grants funded by the EPA that involved stakeholder participation in watershed decision making. Levinson asked them to synthesize the information about stakeholder participation in decision making from these and other studies, and make it available to other interested scholars and practitioners. To support this effort, the EPA provided a supplemental grant of $29,873 to the Texas A&M STAR grant to provide funding for travel, working conferences, and other support to facilitate the book project and bring it to completion. A guiding consideration behind this effort was the belief that in difficult, conflict-prone policy areas such as this one, stakeholder participation in debating and selecting policy options would probably be crucial to building acceptable, workable policy solutions. This belief led to questions about how this participation should best be structured, how scientific information should be incorporated into the process, what personal and interpersonal attributes facilitate cooperation, how representative this participation should be, and ultimately what difference this participation makes for community welfare and environmental quality.

To examine these questions, Levinson asked Focht, Matlock, and Webler to pull together a team of researchers from around the country who were working on these issues and weld them into a team to write a state-of-the art book on this topic. From this nucleus, first Arnold

Vedlitz and Zev Trachtenberg were added to the team. With their help, Paul Sabatier and Mark Lubell were recruited. As the project ideas developed, Tom Webler withdrew, leaving the core team of Sabatier, Focht, Lubell, Matlock, Trachtenberg, and Vedlitz.

Each of these scholars brought a specific set of experiences and qualifications to the team. Focht and Trachtenberg had hands-on experience with a specific watershed stakeholder decision-making process in Oklahoma. Matlock and Vedlitz had hands-on experience linking science information to watershed decision making in two stakeholder watershed planning processes in San Antonio. Sabatier had systematically gathered detailed stakeholder information on dozens of stakeholder watershed processes in Washington State and California. And Lubell had gathered national data on stakeholder participation in twelve National Estuary Program (NEP) sites and ten comparable non-NEP sites.

For more than three years, this team of six project leaders engaged in joint creativity, debate, and compromise to determine this book's outline, goals, interconnections, and conceptual framework. A key event in this process was a two-day workshop at Texas A&M in October 2000 in which initial drafts were discussed and advice sought from a group of knowledgeable practitioners. A second workshop was held in October 2002 at the University of California, Davis, in which subsequent drafts were reviewed and the concluding chapter was written. While only chapters 1 and 9 were written by all six authors in concert, the remaining chapters were evaluated and encouraged by the whole team.

The project leaders' joint efforts at guiding and framing this book have been complemented by their individual efforts on the chapters for which they are lead authors. And their work has been enhanced by the invaluable contributions of other scholars on their research teams. These authors and additional coauthors are credited on their respective chapters.

This book is an unusual blend of team collaboration and individual expertise, very much like the collaborations necessary to address the complex watershed management problems facing our society.

The project leaders dedicate this book to Barbara Levinson, for many years the program director of the Water and Watersheds Program, funded primarily by the U.S. EPA with assistance from the National Science Foundation and the U.S. Department of Agriculture. Levinson was critical in getting the project started, providing the funding for the two workshops, and "encouraging" us to complete the project.

We thank the practitioners who participated in the Texas A&M workshop and provided us with a wealth of very useful advice about how to frame the book and the individual chapters so that they would be accessible—and perhaps even attractive—to practitioners:

• Michael R. Bira, environmental scientist, Environmental Protection Agency Region 6
• Shannon Phillips, senior technical writer/water quality analyst, Oklahoma Conservation Commission
• Gail Rothe, environmental planner, Texas Commission on Environmental Quality (formerly Texas Natural Resource Conservation Commission)
• Mark P. Smith, director of water policy, Massachusetts Executive Office of Environmental Affairs

We thank Michael Kraft, Sheldon Kamieniecki, and Clay Morgan of The MIT Press, who have been very supportive of this project since we first approached them with a prospectus in July 2001, as well as the three anonymous reviewers for The MIT Press, who have been highly supportive overall as well as making a number of very helpful suggestions for improvement. Thanks are due as well to Ruth Schemmer for her editorial assistance. We give our strongest thanks to Nell Frazer Lindquist, of the Institute for Science, Technology and Public Policy at the George Bush School of Government and Public Service at Texas A&M, who herded our ménage of cats to completion of this project. Her organization of our team effort, her role as the center of our communications network, and her thorough review, editing, and formatting of the book were essential to its completion and accuracy. Additional thanks are also due to current and former staff members at the Institute for Science, Technology and Public Policy, particularly Michelle Krohn.

At the end of the day, all of these folks have helped us produce what we promised Barbara Levinson several years ago: a state-of-the-art analysis of collaborative watershed processes in the United States.

Contributors

Letitia T. Alston
Associate Director, Institute for
Science, Technology and Public Policy
George Bush School of Government
and Public Service
Texas A&M University
College Station, TX

Jared Ficker
M.S. candidate
Department of Environmental Science
Policy
University of California, Davis
Davis, CA

Will Focht
Assistant Professor of Political Science
Oklahoma State University
Stillwater, OK

Susan J. Gilbertz
Director of Environmental Studies
Assistant Professor of Geography
Montana State University—Billings
Billings, MT

William D. Leach
Research Director
Center for Collaborative Policy
Sacramento, CA

Mark Lubell
Assistant Professor
Department of Environmental Science
and Policy
University of California, Davis
Davis, CA

Marty Matlock
Assistant Professor
Department of Biological and
Agricultural Engineering
University of Arkansas
Fayetteville, AR

Neil W. Pelkey
Assistant Professor
Environmental Science and Studies
and Information Technology
Juniata College
Huntingdon, PA

Tarla Rai Peterson
Associate Professor
Department of Communication
University of Utah
Salt Lake City, UT

Paul A. Sabatier
Professor
Department of Environmental Science
and Policy
University of California, Davis
Davis, CA

Charles D. Samuelson
Associate Professor
Department of Psychology
Texas A&M University
College Station, TX

Zev Trachtenberg
Associate Professor
Department of Philosophy
University of Oklahoma
Norman, OK

xvi   _Contributors_

Arnold Vedlitz
Director
Institute for Science, Technology, and
Public Policy
George Bush School of Government
and Public Service
Texas A&M University
College Station, TX

Chris Weible
Ph.D. candidate
Center for Environmental Conflict
Analysis
Department of Environmental Science
and Policy
University of California, Davis
Davis, CA

Guy D. Whitten
Associate Professor
Department of Political Science
Texas A&M University
College Station, TX

I

Watershed Management Approaches in the United States

1

Collaborative Approaches to Watershed Management

Paul A. Sabatier, Will Focht, Mark Lubell, Zev Trachtenberg, Arnold Vedlitz, and Marty Matlock

A quiet revolution is occurring in water management institutions in the United States (Born and Genskow 1999, 2001; John 1994; Kenney 1999; National Research Council Committee on Watershed Management 1999). For the past century, water quality, flood control, fish and wildlife habitat, and, to a lesser extent, water supply have been managed by single-function federal and state agencies, each pursuing its own legal mandate. For the most part, decision making has been quite technocratic, with public involvement usually relegated to public hearings and comment periods that fine-tune agency proposals. The scope of decision making has generally consisted of specific types of pollution sources or specific areas within a watershed (such as the coastal wetlands) rather than the watershed as a whole.

Over the past twenty years, the traditional approach has come under increasing criticism. In part, this reflects the increasing complexity and conflict in water resource issues. The most important have been increased competition for limited fresh water resources among agriculture, urban and industrial users, recreationists and fisheries, as well as the requirement under the Clean Water Act for watershed-based restoration of water quality through the Total Maximum Daily Load (TMDL) process. There has also been a general dissatisfaction with leaving important policy decisions largely in the hands of agency experts, who often reside far from the local controversy and lack democratic legitimacy. Finally, there is increasing skepticism of the ability of highly legalistic agency processes and the accompanying litigation to craft viable, long-term solutions to complex water resources problems.

A new approach to water management has emerged. It has explicitly focused on all sources of a pollutant within the watershed as a whole (or distinct subwatersheds) rather than on types of sources (such as point sources) and is not confined to the arbitrary political boundaries represented by states and counties.[1] The new decision-making process is collaborative: it involves face-to-face negotiations among a variety of stakeholders with relatively consensual decision rules.[2] This contrasts with the traditional approach in which each agency jealously guarded its decision-making prerogatives, with private citizens and personnel from other agencies largely confined to commenting on proposed regulations. Rather than have each agency single-mindedly pursuing its legal mandate, the new approach seeks win-win solutions to an interrelated set of social, economic, and environmental issues confronting the watershed. The end result is a collaborative process involving interrelated negotiations over a number of years rather than a series of standardized rule-making decisions in which an agency proposes a rule, receives comments, amends the rule, and then awaits litigation by one or more dissatisfied stakeholders.

This represents a shift from a top-down, agency-dominated approach with some provision for public comment to a much more collaborative bottom-up approach involving negotiations and problem solving among a variety of governmental and nongovernmental stakeholders. This shift needs to be seen in the context of efforts since the mid-1960s to increase meaningful public participation in water resources decisions (Beierle and Cayford 2002, Mazmanian and Clarke 1979, Pierce and Doerksen 1976).

It brings a number of important themes and issues into the foreground:

• What contexts and processes are conducive to the formation of collaborative efforts and to their success?

• Who participates in these collaborative efforts, and why? In what ways do different actors participate?

• To what extent do these collaborative efforts enhance trust among previously warring participants, and to what extent does trust increase the prospects of reaching and implementing agreements? Is enhanced trust an end in itself, quite apart from its contribution to reaching and implementing agreements?

• How successful are collaboratives in reaching agreements on management plans, implementing those agreements with restoration projects, and actually improving environmental and socioeconomic outcomes in the watershed?

• What are the principal contextual and process-related factors that contribute to success?

• To what extent are collaborative efforts viewed as procedurally and substantively legitimate by stakeholders and interested observers?

• What are the prospects for survival of collaborative efforts? Will they simply be swallowed up by preexisting local governments? To what extent does survival depend on procedural and substantive legitimacy?

These are some of the main questions this book seeks to answer.

The Collaborative Approach to Watershed Management

The new governmental approach to watershed decision making emerged because of dissatisfaction with the traditional strategy's inability to deal with a variety of problems, including nonpoint source pollution, the protection of coastal estuaries, water quality planning under the TMDL provisions of the Clean Water Act, protection of aquatic species under the Endangered Species Act, and the development of management plans under the National Forest Management Act.[3] These problems require detailed knowledge of local situations and the coordination of multiple agencies, which proved extraordinarily difficult to accomplish under the old top-down, dominant-agency strategy. The traditional strategy also resulted in policy decisions that left many actors dissatisfied, and they, in turn, looked to the courts for redress. In addition to its ineffectiveness at handling numerous water management issues, the old paradigm suffered from problems of legitimacy because citizens perceived decisions as being made by far-off, faceless bureaucrats with little knowledge of or concern for how those decisions affected local conditions. The emergence of the "wise use" movement in the West is the most visible sign of this legitimacy crisis (Gottlieb 1989). (This is discussed in greater detail in chapters 2 and 3.)

In contrast, the more recent collaborative approach involves face-to-face information exchange and problem solving among all the relevant stakeholders, usually under fairly strict civility guidelines and some form of consensus rule (Weber 1998, 2003). This method emphasizes finding creative, win-win solutions to a variety of problems facing different stakeholders. Admittedly this takes time. However, proponents argue, such a process is likely to generate mutual understanding and trust, rather than animosity and suspicion, among stakeholders. Over time, this should facilitate decision making, enhancing the collaborative's efforts to deal with a whole series of interrelated problems. In addition, since any solutions developed will have the support (or at least the acquiescence) of all parties, implementation should be less problematic than under the traditional approach and less plagued by endless litigation. Finally, because collaborative partnerships seek to involve all the major affected stakeholders and usually operate under some form of consensus rule, they should have greater legitimacy than traditional approaches that rely on the legal authority provided bureaucracies by legislatures (Bingham 1986, Born and Genskow 2001, John 1994, O'Leary and Bingham 2003).

The collaborative watershed management approach is not a detailed blueprint, but rather a broad strategy for solving very complex sets of interrelated problems. It includes several variants:[4]

Collaborative engagement processes.   These are techniques for conflict resolution among diverse stakeholders, developed by outside actors, then applied to specific planning exercises of relatively limited duration (but still longer than the public participation procedures under the old approach). The techniques include environmental mediation (Bingham 1986), collaborative learning (Daniels and Walker 2001), and the analysis and deliberation framework developed by the National Research Council (Stern, Fineberg, and NRC Committee on Risk Characterization 1996).

Collaborative watershed partnerships.   These are relatively informal organizations involving a wide variety of governmental and nongovernmental stakeholders seeking to develop a management plan for the watershed and then implementing it through specific restoration projects, changes in land use practices, water quality regulations, and other ways. Partnerships are intended to be rather long-term affairs (five to ten years). The partnership itself holds little formal legal authority to carry out projects or prescribe regulations. Rather, it provides a forum in which management plans and implementing actions are negotiated, then turned over to member agencies for formal legal actions. Thus, partnerships complement and, it is hoped, transform, rather than replace, traditional agencies. Such partnerships are quite widespread. In 1999, for example, Leach and Pelkey (2001) counted approximately 150 in California and

60 in Washington. Multistakeholder partnerships receive financial support from state agencies in at least six states: Massachusetts, Oregon, Washington, Wisconsin, Pennsylvania, and California.

Collaborative superagencies. These are formalized partnerships that both negotiate management plans and implement actions. They are still quite rare, with the foremost example probably being the CALFED superagency in California. It began as an interagency committee to recommend provisions for implementing the 1994 water quality standards for the San Francisco Bay/Delta and has evolved into an agency with a $900 million annual budget, charged with overall water management and restoration throughout the Sacramento and San Joaquin River watersheds of the Central Valley. Its Policy Council includes representatives of twenty-one federal and state agencies, as well as several private (or quasi-private) stakeholder groups.

As an indicator of the popularity of the new approach, nine federal agencies and departments have endorsed the Clean Water Action Plan (U.S. Environmental Protection Agency and U.S. Department of Agriculture 1998) calling for a new cooperative approach to watershed protection in which state, tribal, federal and local governments, and the public first identify the watersheds with the most critical water quality problems and then work together to focus resources and implement effective strategies to solve those problems.[5]

Concerns about the Collaborative Approach

Despite its recent popularity, the collaborative watershed approach is not without critics concerned about both its procedural and substantive legitimacy.

Representation

One set of criticisms focuses on problems of representation within partnerships. Leaders of several national environmental groups are concerned that they cannot possibly place representatives in the huge number of partnerships and planning processes throughout the country (Kenney et al. 2000, McCloskey 1996). This procedural criticism is then linked to substantive concerns that nonlocal environmental interests will be sacrificed (Sagoff 1999). Similarly, landowner and property rights groups that take the position that only landowners should be involved in decisions affecting their land criticize the inclusiveness of partnerships and worry about the threats to property rights they entail (Gottlieb 1989). Others worry that stakeholder processes take enormous amounts of time and thus effectively exclude the general public or all but the most interested actors with substantial resources (Coglianese 2001). They certainly include very few elected officials, and thus one can legitimately worry about the extent to which they represent the distribution of views within the watershed.[6]

In a democracy, citizens and officials alike must be sensitive to questions about how, and if, political decision-making processes reflect democratic values. Representation is the core democratic value associated with procedural legitimacy, where representation refers to whether all relevant ideas and interests are included in collective choice. When adequate representation is not achieved, democratic processes at best fail to meet normative criteria and at worst lead to ineffective policies that do not affect the attitudes and behaviors of excluded stakeholders. Yet, as we will discuss in chapters 3, 4 and 5, achieving representation in collaborative policy is not an easy task conceptually or in practice.

Building Trust and Civic Community

Studies of democratic participation over the past 200 years also indicate the importance of democratic processes, and citizen participation in them, for building the trust and cooperation needed to hold democratic communities together (Putnam 2000, Verba and Nie 1972). Through accepted forms of participation, even if one's own side does not win, one feels that the outcome should be supported and obeyed. This sense of fairness in the process is one of the foundational elements of a successful democratic nation. The experience of working together on decisions, as a political community, builds the trust, structures, and patterns of behavior needed to address future problems successfully. The issue of trust is particularly important to the actions of collaborative processes, and this study considers some new approaches to trust in this evolving form of joint, democratic participation.

In more traditional forms of political participation (such as voting and contacting officials), trust is positively related to levels of participation: the more trust one has, the more likely one is to vote or contact. Evidence presented in chapter 4 suggests this may not be the case for the very specialized form of direct stakeholder participation. Long-term stakeholder participation requires significant effort and dedication. For those who have high levels of trust in other participants of the process, direct participation may not be necessary. For those who are distrustful of other participants, direct participation may seem necessary to protect their group's interests. In long-term stakeholder decision processes, then, it may be that greater levels of trust lead to less participation and greater levels of mistrust lead to increased participation. Empirical tests of these important considerations appear in chapters 4 and 5.

An important challenge to building trust is the self-interested behavior of involved stakeholders. Throughout this book, we assume most stakeholders pursue their own self-interest most of the time, but must also deal with a variety of cognitive constraints and perceptual biases, many of them linked to well-developed systems of political values. One advantage of collaborative processes is that repeated interaction within the context of a partnership allows for the development of norms of reciprocal cooperation, which are completely congruent with the self-interest of the stakeholders.

Yet, the perceptual biases that stakeholders bring into collaborative processes often act as barriers to reciprocal cooperation and trust. For example, environmentalists are likely to view trends in environmental outcomes as indicators of a serious problem and see economic interests as less trustworthy than they really are. Economic interests often have the opposite biases, and the biases of both sides can infect the applied science brought into collaborative processes. Chapter 7 discusses these biases in more detail and investigates whether collaborative processes can mitigate this type of biased information processing, thereby enhancing the possibility of long-term cooperation that offers benefits to all stakeholders.

Effectiveness
Process is only part of the picture, however. The trust, legitimacy, compliance, and community decision-making skills that collaboration arguably builds are important, but another, and significant, set of questions looms. This third set of concerns regards the effectiveness of collaborative processes and partnerships in developing and implementing solutions to watershed problems. These are among the important issues

discussed in chapters 6, 7, and 8. A major issue is whether the collaborative stakeholder decision process encourages agreement on, and the implementation of, policy solutions that actually improve the environmental and socioeconomic conditions of the watershed. While solutions reached in collaborative, community decision-making settings clearly offer the hope of real, implementable solutions with improvements one can eventually see, they are also a potential recipe for delay and for avoiding the most complex and difficult problems (Coglianese 1999).

Two questions are important: Are the decisions good ones from an environmental and socioeconomic perspective? And can they be implemented from a political and legal perspective? Many of the "solutions" reached in collaborative stakeholder settings may be good political compromises, but they may not really solve the environmental or socioeconomic problems plaguing a watershed. Conversely, many negotiated solutions may be appropriate from a physical environmental standpoint, but they may leave out key stakeholders who will pursue other avenues of blocking implementation. Many collaborative efforts create policies that rely on voluntary cooperation without any formal legal enforcement mechanisms, which often creates considerable doubt about the likelihood of policy implementation. Because agencies and private interests find it necessary to resort to traditional enforcement mechanisms, such as the Endangered Species Act, the evidence is mixed about whether collaborative processes are more successful in avoiding litigation than more traditional single agency rule making (Bingham 1986, Coglianese 1997).

Finally, critics of collaborative processes worry about their effectiveness in comparison to the traditional regulatory approaches embodied in the Clean Water Act and other relevant laws. Clearly, existing environmental laws have successfully addressed some environmental problems, most notably point source water pollution, in a reasonably successful (if not optimally efficient) fashion. Critics of collaboration believe these coercive approaches should be extended to the complex problems now being addressed by collaborative processes. Indeed, collaborative processes are often criticized as symbolic policies designed to deflect political attention from ongoing water management problems and maintain the status quo pattern of water use. The main counterargument is that collaborative processes address problems that are just too complex for coercive approaches—problems that span entire watersheds. In addition, there is a fairly widespread perception that traditional and collaborative approaches complement each other. Traditional approaches, such as TMDL, are the "hammer" that encourages stakeholders to negotiate seriously (Born and Genskow 2001). These effectiveness themes run throughout this book.

Survival

A final set of threats to the viability of the new approach involves the ability of collaborative processes and partnerships to find a permanent niche in a landscape dominated by single-function agencies that often depend on legal boundaries with little relationship to watersheds. Collaborative processes may threaten agency autonomy and thus create an incentive for traditional agencies to usurp control of collaborative outcomes. For example, there is some anecdotal evidence that Law 2514 in Washington State puts multistakeholder partnerships clearly under the thumb of general-purpose local governments, whose boundaries typically split watersheds into conflicting fiefdoms. To the extent a single agency controls a given collaborative project, other agencies and private interests will often seek alternative venues to pursue their policy goals.

In order for the new approach to succeed, it must demonstrate its superiority to traditional approaches on both procedural and effectiveness criteria, as well as win its fair share of turf battles with traditional agencies. None of this is given. Like the salmon swimming upstream to spawn in home waters, only the fittest collaborative projects are likely to survive in any institutionally complex political system—hence, the title of this volume.

Previous Studies of Collaborative Management

Unfortunately, the literature on collaborative watershed planning is dominated by studies of one or two cases that rely on very subjective methods of data acquisition and analysis and are usually not well grounded in a body of theory (Leach and Pelkey 2001). Such studies are useful for gathering descriptive information about partnerships and generating hypotheses about the factors contributing to partnership success. The latter contribution is now fully realized. As of 2000, such studies had produced a set of 210 "lessons learned," which can be grouped into over twenty general themes.[7] However, this literature has a number of important limitations:

Interpretive methods.   Studies relying on subjective methods of data acquisition and analysis may provide intriguing insights, but an outsider has virtually no way of knowing if they are valid. Different people observing the same phenomena can "see" different things unless they are given relatively detailed categories in which to standardize perceptions. The fundamental dictum of science is that methods be public enough that they can be replicated (King, Keohane, and Verba 1994).

Sampling bias.   Since different people in a partnership observe different things, it is crucial to gather data from a variety of participants and even knowledgeable outsiders. For example, there is now solid evidence that partnership coordinators perceive partnerships as more trust generating and more successful than do most of their members (Leach 2002). This renders problematic data from several surveys of large numbers of collaborative groups that rely heavily on the views of one to two people (often the coordinator) per partnership (Kenney et al. 2000, Yaffee et al. 1996).

A multivariate world.   If, as the literature suggests, there are up to 25 variables affecting partnership success and the study involves only one to two partnerships, the author cannot possibly ascertain the relative importance of each of the explanatory variables. Determining the relative importance of each of the 25 requires at least 150 cases. In short, studies with only a small number of cases have some very serious problems with internal validity. In addition to this statistical problem, the literature deals largely with factors under the control of participants, and this tends to ignore the broader socioeconomic, legal, and political context in which they operate.

Generalizability of conclusions.   Studies of collaborative processes involving data collected systematically from numerous participants potentially have high internal validity. But, if they involve only one or two partnerships or processes, their results cannot generalize to cases in different settings. For example, if the case studied involves relatively low conflict, the results may not be generalizable to situations involving high conflict.[8]

Explicit theories.   Theories are very useful for guiding empirical research because they clarify concepts and relationships, remind the researcher of possibly interesting relationships that have not occurred to participants, and provide a means for relating findings from different studies that share the same theoretical framework.[9] Ideally, researchers should compare competing theories so as not to become inappropriately wedded to any of them (Allison 1969, Platt 1964). In the literature on collaborative watershed processes, only about 25 percent make reference to any body of theory and only one or two test multiple theories.

In Riechenbach's (1938) terms, studies of collaborative watershed approaches have been largely conducted in the "context of discovery," where the generation of hypotheses is the focus and the use of rigorous scientific methods is secondary. The emphasis is on generating intriguing ideas. In the "context of verification," however, the emphasis is on determining the internal and external validity of posited relationships (hypotheses). This requires classic scientific methods, including intersubjectively reliable methods of data acquisition and analysis, explicit attention to the uncertainty arising from measurement and sampling error, and testing propositions developed from one or more bodies of theory (King, Keohane, and Verba 1994).

A principal objective of this book is to set a new standard for studies of collaborative management approaches. In our view, second-generation studies should be based on explicit frameworks of presumed causal relationships. They should, where possible, use intersubjectively reliable methods of data acquisition and analysis. And they should, where feasible, use multivariate methods—those that examine the relative importance of several causal factors simultaneously. Thus, this book is addressed to scholars and others interested in understanding the processes and driving principles affecting the procedural and substantive legitimacy of collaborative management approaches.

But we also wish to make the book accessible to policy practitioners who are responsible for planning and implementing stakeholder processes. Toward this end, approximately a half-dozen practitioners participated actively in an October 2000 workshop at which the first drafts of the chapters were discussed.[10] They provided useful comments concerning technical jargon, the types of analyses they found most useful, and the appropriate weight to be given to general conceptualization versus very specific examples. Being academics, we have almost certainly violated their counsel on the last point. But we listened conscientiously to their advice on the first two and hope that our conceptualizations are straightforward enough to help improve readers' understanding of the very specific cases we discuss.

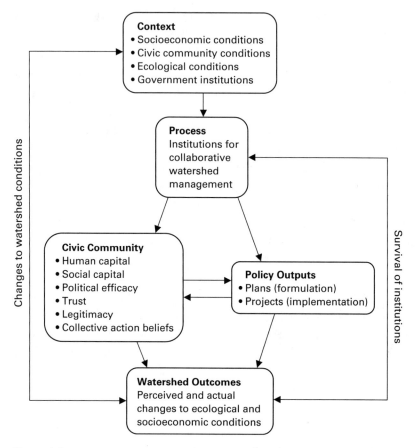

Figure 1.1
A dynamic framework for watershed management

A Conceptual Framework for Understanding Collaborative Watershed Management

Figure 1.1 lays out a relatively simple conceptual framework for understanding the factors affecting collaborative watershed management.

Causally prior factors (at the top) are the socioeconomic, ecological, civic, and institutional conditions predating partnership formation. These include the economic and social structure of a community, preexisting social networks, the seriousness of various environmental and socioeconomic problems, and the set of governmental institutions.

This context heavily constrains the type of collaborative watershed management approach that will emerge, as well as its probability of success. For example, communities composed of widely dispersed, relatively transient populations with wide ideological differences are less likely to be successful than smaller, more stable, and more homogeneous communities. Communities facing difficult situations are likely to be very distrustful and thus insist on a wide variety of procedural rules to protect each group's interests. Conversely, more promising communities are more likely to have substantial reservoirs of trust and social capital (networks) to build on, and thus require less elaborate procedural rules.

Following Ostrom (1990, 1999), we conceptualize a collaborative process as essentially a set of rules regarding the types of participants, their entry and exit from the process, their authority to undertake tasks, and how their actions lead to policy outcomes. Context variables then interact with processes to produce both civic community and policy outputs. Civic community and policy outputs interact to affect real and perceived conditions, both environmental (e.g., water quality) and socioeconomic (e.g., unemployment rates).

One causal pathway leads from process and context to "civic community," which includes human capital (e.g., knowledge about watershed conditions), social capital (e.g., networks of reciprocity), trust of others, legitimacy concerns, and attitudes toward collective action. These civic community variables are conceived as both an end in themselves and a means to better policy outputs. This book assumes that increasing trust and networks of reciprocity in a community is desirable, even if it does not result in water quality improvements. But we also hypothesize that a watershed collaborative effort that increases trust and social reciprocity is more likely to result in watershed management plans and specific restoration projects than one that does not. The framework also hypothesizes that agreeing on a plan or restoration project feeds back into enhanced trust because it indicates that people resolve many of their differences if they take the time to listen carefully to others' concerns, propose solutions compatible with others' interests, and honor agreements.

The last set of variables, watershed outcomes, is probably the most important but also the most difficult to measure. For example, ascertaining the impact of a watershed partnership's restoration projects on water quality (e.g., fencing a stream to keep out cattle) requires both baseline and postproject monitoring. It also requires long time-series data to account for changes in precipitation and other background factors. Unfortunately, very few collaborative partnerships possess this sort of monitoring data, making it extremely difficult to ascertain their actual impacts. Instead, most studies, including ours, rely primarily on perceived impacts. But as we shall see in chapter 8, perceived impacts are susceptible to systematic distortion.

Finally, the model contains two feedback loops from watershed outcomes—first to background context and, second, to the survival of collaborative efforts as institutions with different rules than, for example, local water districts or state pollution control agencies.

In this book we evaluate and test aspects of this general theoretical framework with these systematic studies:

• A collaborative planning exercise on the Illinois River watershed in Oklahoma (chapter 4)
• A collaborative planning process involving two watersheds in San Antonio, Texas (chapter 5)
• A comparative analysis of perceptions regarding collaborative planning in a nationwide sample of twenty coastal watersheds in the National Estuary Program and a control group of ten relatively similar watersheds not in the NEP (chapter 7)
• An analysis of the factors affecting trust and partnership success in a random sample of seventy-six watershed partnerships in California and Washington (chapter 8)

Most of the case study chapters involve analyses of the effects of process rules on some aspects of civic community, whether that be participation rates, trust, or attitudes toward the desirability of participating in collaborative efforts. Chapters 4 and 8 investigate the reciprocal effect of trust on process rules and participation rates. Chapter 8 also examines the effect of context, process, and civic culture on policy outputs and on perceived outcomes.

In short, while this book provides extensive evidence on the interactive effects of trust and process—and some analysis of context, outputs, and perceived outcomes—it does not provide a comprehensive analysis of all of the variables in our general model. What it does provide are continuing reference to a particular theoretical framework; systematic methods of data acquisition, usually involving surveys; systematic methods of multifactor data analysis, generally utilizing multiple regression; and explicit indications of the extent to which the relationships in our data may be due to random chance. In short, this represents an innovative second-generation research on collaborative watershed processes. We trust these results will be useful to practitioners and will encourage other scholars to investigate the relationships in Figure 1.1 in a variety of empirical settings, with a particular emphasis on the factors affecting policy outputs and real-world policy outcomes.

Organization of the Book

The book is divided into four parts. Part I, "Watershed Management Approaches in the United States," contains three chapters that provide an overview of watershed management in the United States, setting the stage for the chapters that follow. This introductory chapter informs the reader of the topic of the book, the questions to be addressed, and the methods used. Chapter 2 provides a history of water management in the United States, with a particular focus on the extent to which various aspects of the collaborative approach were present in previous periods. Chapter 3 presents a normative theoretical framework that proposes criteria for the evaluation of procedural and substantive policy legitimacy relevant to collaborative approaches. This framework is central to the book because we hold that the collaborative approach will survive largely to the extent that it is perceived as procedurally and substantively superior to alternative approaches, such as command-and-control regulation or strong deference to private property owners.

Part II, "Collaborative Engagement Processes in Watersheds," extends the arguments presented in part I in two chapters that consider, both theoretically and empirically, the application of collaborative stakeholder involvement strategies in watersheds in Oklahoma and Texas. Based on the level of trust that private stakeholders have of other policy actors, chapter 4 tests a prescriptive framework for the selection of stakeholder participation processes that seeks to satisfy the policy legitimacy criteria discussed in chapter 3. Chapter 5 considers the elements affecting the willingness of stakeholders to participate in collaborative watershed planning processes in San Antonio. It also examines the extent to which those who participate in the planning process mirror the beliefs and preferences of the public they supposedly represent.

Part III, "Measuring and Explaining the Success of Watershed Partnerships," addresses the factors affecting the formation and success of collaborative watershed partnerships. Recall that watershed partnerships differ from the relatively short-term planning processes discussed in chapters 4 and 5 in that they are expected to develop and implement watershed management plans over several years, if not decades. As we shall see in chapter 8, this normally takes at least four years. Chapter 6 outlines several theories of collective action and policymaking relevant to such partnerships: the social capital framework of Putnam et al. (1993, 2000), the institutional rational choice framework of Ostrom (1990, 1999), and the advocacy coalition framework of Sabatier and Jenkins-Smith (1988, 1993, 1999), supplemented by hypotheses from alternative dispute resolution (Carpenter and Kennedy 1988; Susskind, McKearnan, and Thomas-Larmer 1999) These frameworks are generally broader and more detailed than the relatively simple one presented earlier in this chapter. Chapter 7 tests several hypotheses from these frameworks on participants in a sample of twenty partnerships in the NEP compared to a sample of policy activists in ten watersheds not involved in the NEP. Chapter 8 examines the effects of a variety of contextual and process-related variables on the development of trust and, in turn, the development and implementation of management plans, on a sample of seventy-six watershed partnerships in California and Washington.

Part IV, "Conclusions," presents our findings on the six major topics introduced earlier in this chapter, as well as our lessons learned for both practitioners and academics.

Throughout this book, the focus is on collaborative watershed approaches in the United States. We are mindful that collaborative stakeholder processes are also an important institutional innovation in Australia (Margerum 1999), Canada (Cormick et al. 1996; Fisheries and Oceans Canada, and Western Europe (United Kingdom, 2000; European Community 2001; Harrison et al. 2001; United Nations Economic Commission for Europe 1998, 1999; United Nations Economic Commission for Europe ECE/UNEP Network of Experts, 2000). But the topic is new enough, and the situation in the United States complex enough, that for purely practical reasons, we have limited our inquiry to a single country. In the future, we certainly hope that other scholars (and perhaps some of us) will apply the basic features of our second-generation approach to the analysis of collaborative watershed approaches in other countries.

Collaborative institutions are really an experiment in democratic governance within the context of American federalism. The heart of democratic governance is groups of people coming together to make collective decisions about solutions to common problems, then adhering to the behavioral prescriptions that emerge from the process. This is precisely what happens when watershed stakeholders come together to form a management plan. Democratic governance is often thought of only in terms of voting for representatives, and then letting representatives make policy decisions about common problems. But forums for democratic decision making are much more widespread than conventional electoral politics, and they often appear in the context of citizens participating directly in policy decisions (John 1994, Weber 2003). Collaborative watershed institutions represent one such forum, and collaborative institutions in general can be found in many other policy arenas. These less visible forums must be evaluated according to the same criteria applied to democratic governance more generally, which is precisely why the studies in this book cover legitimacy, representation, and effectiveness.

Finally, it is important to appreciate how collaborative processes symbolize the adaptive qualities of democratic systems as a whole. Democratic systems should combine old and new ideas into fresh institutions designed to address lingering problems like nonpoint source pollution and habitat destruction. Collaborative institutions emerge in the face of declining social capital in other forms (Putnam 2000; Putnam, Leonardi, and Nanetti 1993). In fact, they truly represent a new kind of social capital. As an experiment, they may fail, but we certainly think these experiments merit the highest quality of analysis that we can bring to bear on them.

Notes

1. Sources of water pollution are divided into two types: in point sources, pollutants come out of a pipe; in nonpoint sources, the discharge is spread over a much wider area, such as pesticides draining from all over a field.

2. We acknowledge that the term *stakeholder* is notoriously ambiguous. It includes policymakers, agency implementers, experts both within and outside government who participate in policymaking and policy implementation, private sector businesses that are economically affected by policies, members of the general public who are economically or otherwise affected by policies, and environmental interest groups that purport to represent nonhuman values, among other groups. Perhaps this is one reason that the National Research Council adopted the term *interested and affected party* in lieu of *stakeholder* (Stern, Fineberg, and NRC Committee on Risk Characterization 1996). In this book, we distinguish between governmental stakeholders, who have a role in policymaking by virtue of their legal authority or technical expertise, and nongovernmental stakeholders, who have an interest (or stake) in the resource at issue but no legally mandated role in formulating and implementing policy. Of course, a given individual might be both a governmental and a nongovernmental stakeholder: a public official who happens to be a resident of the watershed would have both sorts of interests. Nonetheless, we can distinguish between the two roles that such an individual would play.

3. Total Maximum Daily Loads (TMDLs) arise from section 303 of the Clean Water Act designed to deal with "residual" pollution sources—those not subject to technology-based standards. Most, but not all, deal with nonpoint sources. States must first determine reaches of water bodies that are impaired (i.e., do not meet water quality standards). For impaired water bodies and their associated pollutants, the state must issue a TMDL for each pollutant and water body that includes an assessment of all pollution sources, a total load for the water body, and an allocation of pollution reduction among the sources. TMDLs provide a substantial incentive for pollution sources to negotiate a TMDL rather than wait for the state or U.S. EPA to impose one on them. Leach, Pelkey, and Sabatier (2001) found that TMDLs were by far the most important stimulus to the formation of partnerships in California.

4. Though we discuss only three variants of collaboration here, two dimensions distinguish them: duration (short term versus long term) and decision power or influence (informal advisory versus formal authoritative). This suggests that four variants can be identified: collaborative partnerships (long-term, informal advisory collaboratives), collaborative superagencies (long-term, formal authoritative collaboratives), collaborative engagements (short-term, informal advisory) and collaborative panels (short-term, formal authoritative). We did not encounter collaborative panels in our studies of watershed partnerships and therefore do not discuss them in this book.

5. Several federal agencies have issued guidebooks that advocate decentralized, consensus-oriented policymaking. Examples include the U.S. Department of Housing and Urban Development's Community-Building Coming of Age (Kingsley, McNeely, and Gibson 1997), the U.S. Environmental Protection Agency's Community-Based Environmental Protection, the National Oceanic and Atmospheric Administration's Watershed Restoration (Kier 1995), and the U.S. Forest Service's Guidelines for a Watershed Approach (2000). State and federal programs have recently channeled millions of dollars through watershed partner-

ships. Examples include the EPA's section 104(b)(3), 205 and 319 grants; the Department of Agriculture's EQIP program; California's CALFED program and propositions 12, 13, and 204; Washington State's Watershed Planning Act of 1998 (about $4.5 million annually); and the Massachusetts Watershed Initiative, which funds full-time partnership coordinators in each of the state's twenty-seven watersheds. Following Sommarstrom (1998) and Cook (2000), we think it important to distinguish watershed partnerships, which are composed of actors with diverse views, from watershed groups, which are composed of like-minded individuals (usually landowners or environmentalists).

6. In their survey of 76 watershed partnerships in California and Washington, Sabatier, Weible, and Leach (2001) found that while 25 percent of partnership members were from local governments and agencies, only 3 percent were elected officials from cities and counties.

7. Following are the themes relating to partnership success (Leach and Pelkey 2001): (1) funding, (2) broad and inclusive versus limited membership, (3) cooperative, committed participants, (4) effective leader/coordinator/facilitator, (5) bottom-up initiation/leadership versus balanced local/state/federal participants, (6) trust, (7) low or medium level of conflict versus conflict unimportant, (8) geographic scope, (9) limited versus broad scope of activities, (10) adequate time, (11) well-defined process rules versus flexibility/informality, (12) consensus rules: yes versus no, (13) formal enforcement mechanisms, (14) effective communication, (15) adequate scientific and technical information, (16) monitoring outcomes, (17) training in collaborative skills, (18) agency support and participation, (19) legislative encouragement, (20) community resources, and (21) other.

8. Given limited resources, there is an inherent conflict between internal and external validity. Getting high scores on both requires both large numbers of systematic observations within each collaborative process (internal validity) and large numbers of collaborative processes (external validity). In the existing literature, we know of only two studies that combine both (beyond work by authors of this book): Susskind, Wansem, and Ciccarelli (2000) and Beierle and Cayford (2002). In contrast, two of the four empirical studies in this book (chapters 7 and 8) have this desirable combination.

9. As we shall see in chapter 8, one of the most important factors explaining the success of watershed partnerships is the (lack of) an alternative decision-making venue, taken from from the literature on alternative dispute resolution (Carpenter and Kennedy 1988, Ury 1993). It is barely mentioned in the 210 "lessons learned" identified by Leach and Pelkey (2001).

10. Michael R. Bira, environmental scientist, U.S. EPA Region 6; Shannon Phillips, technical writer/water quality analyst, Oklahoma Conservation Commission; Gail Rothe, environmental planner, Texas Commission on Environmental Quality (formerly Texas Natural Resource Conservation Commission); and Mark P. Smith, director of water policy, Massachusetts Executive Office of Environmental Affairs.

2

Eras of Water Management in the United States: Implications for Collaborative Watershed Approaches

Paul A. Sabatier, Chris Weible, and Jared Ficker

In the hundred years following the Civil War, water resources management in the United States evolved from a single-minded pursuit of largely ad hoc development projects in the nineteenth century to a considerable degree of management by large federal and state bureaucracies through the 1960s. Subsequent decades have witnessed repeated calls for greater public involvement in this process, first by environmental groups in the 1970s and then by local property owners in the 1990s.

This chapter briefly reviews 150 years of water management in the United States in an effort to answer the question: In each era, which features resemble aspects of the collaborative management processes that have become popular since the 1990s? Conversely, which features in an era are not shared by the collaborative paradigm?

As we saw in chapter 1, following are the most salient features of collaborative watershed approaches (Born and Genskow 2000, 2001; Kenney 1999; Weber 1998):

• They use a hydrographic watershed as the jurisdictional boundary rather than county or state lines.
• They involve a wide variety of stakeholder groups (interest groups, agencies from multiple levels of government, scientists, and, where relevant, Native Americans) operating under norms of rough equality. This is in contrast to the traditional format, in which one agency has principal jurisdiction, with other agencies and interest groups acting as supplicants.
• The principal negotiations involve face-to-face interactions among representatives of the major stakeholders under agreed-on process rules designed to ensure civility and engender trust.
• The goal of the process is to reach win-win solutions on a set of interrelated social, economic, and environmental problems so that no one

goes away from the process seriously displeased. Again, this is in contrast to the more traditional approach, in which the primary agency was principally concerned with fulfilling its statutory mandate—for example, flood control and navigation for the Corps of Engineers, water quality for the U.S. EPA—with other values relegated to secondary status.

• The process entails a fairly extensive fact-finding phase designed to promote understanding of the magnitude and causes of various problems. Typically, this involves a mixture of standard scientific techniques and a respect for "local knowledge" (Ostrom 1990), with the result that local stakeholders are often involved in the formulation of research questions and the collection of data (Stern, Fineberg, and NRC Committee on Risk Characterization 1996).

This chapter seeks to assess the extent to which each of these features characterized water management in the United States during five periods: (1) the Manifest Destiny Era (pre-1890), (2) the Progressive Era (1890–1924), (3) the Federal/New Deal Era (1925–1964), (4) the Environmental Era (1965–1986) and (5) the Collaborative Era (1987–present).[1] For each era, we describe these facets:

The geographic scope of management. Is it based on hydrographic units or traditional political boundaries?

The mixture of public and private authority in making water management decisions. Are most decisions left to private market transactions? To the extent that government is involved, is it largely through relatively intrusive policy instruments such as ownership or command-and-control regulation?

The principal actors participating in water management decisions. Are decisions largely left to technical experts, or do nonexperts also play critical roles? Is participation largely limited to governmental officials, or are interest groups and ordinary citizens also involved in important ways? What levels of government are involved: local, state, or federal, or some combination? In sum, does meaningful participation extend to virtually all governmental and nongovernmental stakeholders, or is it considerably narrower than that?

The extent to which the decision process is consultative as opposed to collaborative. Does it involve a clear decision maker who consults with other stakeholders largely at his or her discretion? Or are most stakeholders involved in a collaborative process in which most important parties are represented and involved in structuring the ground rules for face-to-face discussions?

The principal purposes or goals of water management, such as water supply, quality, flood control, navigation, hydropower, and habitat protection. What is the balance between resource (environmental) protection versus resource use for economic development?

As we shall see, a watershed focus, public-private partnerships, the involvement of experts (and some nonexperts), representation from multiple levels of government, a fairly active governmental role, and some efforts to balance multiple water uses and goals are fairly common after 1890. The more distinguishing features of the Collaborative Era are the use of collaborative rather than consultative decision-making processes and the large range of governmental and nongovernmental, expert and nonexpert, actors involved.

The Manifest Destiny Era (pre-1890)

Such quantities of land to waste as we please ... to the hundredth and thousandth generation.
—Thomas Jefferson (Cortner and Moote 1999, 12–13)

Watershed management was essentially absent in the Manifest Destiny Era. The period after the Civil War was a time of unprecedented growth and expansion in the United States, fueled by immigration from Europe and Asia and the industrial revolution in eastern and midwestern cities. Water was for drinking, waste disposal, power, and navigation. Rivers and lakes were the highways of commerce. In the East, the population of cities like New York and Philadelphia reached over 1 million, creating serious problems of water supply and the disposal of human and industrial wastes. In the West, the federal government was promoting settlement with programs to dispose of public land to homesteaders. Mining and logging on federal lands were essentially free. An area was exploited for its natural resources, and then the companies moved on to another site without worrying about the denuded hillsides, depleted soils, and slag heaps left behind. Natural resources were perceived as bountiful and thus in no need of conservation (Loomis 1993, Petulla 1977).

America's "manifest destiny" required that land be carved up so as to provide clear title, with no particular concern for local conditions. Hence, most of the land in the Midwest and West was broken up into 640-acre sections, giving rise to the familiar checkerboard pattern. Rivers were perceived as convenient boundaries for major political units, such as territories, states, and counties, with the result that watersheds were divided among multiple legal jurisdictions. By the time that John Wesley Powell made his famous plea in 1890 for making local government boundaries coincide with hydrographic units, the jurisdictional decisions had long been made, and he was ignored (Adler 1995).

Throughout this period, decisions about how to use (and misuse) natural resources were made by private entrepreneurs, largely unfettered by government regulation. The English common law provided doctrines of riparian use of water and protection from nuisances linked to clearly identifiable sources, but the nuisance doctrine was virtually useless in situations involving multiple sources (Sax 1968). In the West, the concepts of "prior appropriation" and "reasonable use" were developed (Pisani 1992). Note that while the riparian use doctrine is consistent with watershed-scale thinking, the prior appropriation doctrines in the West were often used by water companies to transport water from one watershed to another in order to benefit miners and farmers.[2]

Water was used almost exclusively to fuel economic development. Water quality and habitat protection were on virtually no one's radar screen. As Pisani (1992, 31) has noted, "The welfare of the community became the product of a multitude of discrete decisions made in the marketplace, with no sense of planning and little of collective responsibility." This period provided no precursors to collaborative watershed management.

The Progressive Era (1890–1924)

The greatest good of the greatest number in the long run.
—Gifford Pinchot, 1905 (Adler 1995, 14)

During the Progressive Era, the watershed concept emerged and gained fairly widespread acceptance.[3] John Wesley Powell's understanding of interrelationships within a watershed led him to urge Congress to divide the West into "natural districts" that corresponded to natural drainage basins and would have the authority to allocate and regulate water resources. In 1908, President Theodore Roosevelt observed that "every river system, from its headwaters in the forest to its mouth at the coast, is a single unit and should be managed as such" (U.S. Inland Waterways

Commission 1908). The establishment of forest reserves, which became national forests in 1905, generally followed watershed boundaries and were often a response to public concern about the impacts of upstream mining and timber harvesting on downstream water supplies (Culhane 1981, Hays 1959).

During this period, several western cities, including San Francisco, Oakland, and Los Angeles, created aqueducts hundreds of miles long to transport water from relatively pristine mountain watersheds to coastal cities. The Newlands Act of 1917 authorized the Army Corps of Engineers to prepare comprehensive river basin plans, with an emphasis on flood control, for the Mississippi and Sacramento rivers. At the same time, watershed science was still in its infancy. In 1912, the National Waterways Commission recommended that upstream management of land impacts was uncertain to provide flood prevention benefits and thus existing engineering practices should continue (Adler 1995).

The Progressive movement was a coalition of reformers—populists, civil service reformers, middle-class professionals, social workers, and some small businessmen—who were convinced that the American dream had been distorted (Cortner and Moote 1999). Jeffersonian democracy envisaged a land populated with prosperous and independent small farmers that would avoid the European pattern of wealthy landlords and impoverished peasants. Unfortunately, the assumption that natural resources were inexhaustible produced a land wracked by soil depletion (particularly in the South), destructive timber harvesting, and miners oblivious to the destruction they were causing, such as, hydraulic gold mining in California and immense slag heaps throughout Appalachia and the West. Large monopolistic corporations exercised enormous economic and political power. The subsidies offered the railroads as part of Manifest Destiny had populated the West, but also created corporations such as Southern Pacific that held immense power (Kolko 1965). The Jacksonian model of political parties had created a corrupt spoils system in which governmental offices and contracts went not to the competent but to the politically well connected (Knott and Miller 1987).

To rectify these evils, the Progressives proposed reforms in a number of areas. The most dramatic was an effort to correct market flaws through vigorous efforts to break up monopolies and substantially increase governmental regulation of many economic sectors, including the railroads (the Interstate Commerce Act of 1887), food and drug companies (Food and Drug Act of 1906) and child labor (DeWitt 1915). To benefit small farmers in the West, the Reclamation Act of 1902 envisaged the creation of dams and irrigation districts through the West, with membership limited to those farming fewer than 160 acres (Berkman and Viscusi 1973).

To address the issue of governmental corruption, the Progressives proposed a clear separation of "politics" from "administration." Administration would involve the creation of governmental bureaucracies in which entrance would be governed by technical competence (not political connections), coordination and control would be ensured by a hierarchical structure, and decisions would be based on the impartial application of written rules designed to maximize net social welfare. The Progressives sought to put as much of government as possible in the hands of politically neutral civil servants, who would use their expertise to help administer a system of legal rules in an impartial manner (Knott and Miller 1987).

In the domain of natural resources, the Progressives proposed a set of conservation principles (Nash 1968). First, the overarching goal would be to create "the greatest good for the greatest number in the long run" rather than the greatest wealth for entrepreneurs in the short run. And, second, governmental programs would be administered by technically trained neutral bureaucrats, not local cronies of the dominant political party.

These principles led to a number of strategies. The first, and probably most important, was to place much of the public lands in national forests and national and state parks (Nash 1968). Yosemite National Park was created in 1890. The forest reserve system, created in 1891, became the National Forest System in 1905. The Weeks Act of 1911 authorized the Forest Service to purchase forested land at the headwaters of navigable streams, thus permitting the establishment of national forests in the East. Second, there were some less successful efforts to regulate the behavior of economic actors as it affected water and other natural resources. The Rivers and Harbors Act of 1899 authorized the Army Corps of Engineers to regulate water quality, particularly as it affected navigation. The Mineral Leasing Act of 1920 made some effort to regulate mining on federal lands. The Federal Water Power Act of 1920 authorized the Federal Power Commission (now the Federal Energy Regulatory Commission) to regulate water projects on navigable waters for hydroelectric power or navigation.

Most of the good and bad aspects of the Progressive Era can be illustrated by two of its enduring legacies. The first is the U.S. Forest Service, the product of the preeminent Progressive conservationist, Gifford Pinchot. During the Progressive Era, it took jurisdiction over 165 million acres of the public domain and acquired 20 million more under the Weeks Act, representing about 10 percent of the total land area of the forty-eight states. Many of the forests follow watershed boundaries (Culhane 1981). Its officials are all well-trained professionals in forestry, hydrology, wildlife biology, and other relevant areas. It has a clear hierarchical structure from the district to the forest to the region to the National Office. It has developed a set of control procedures (including periodic rotation of personnel and formal appeals processes) to ensure that district and forest officials are not "captured" by local interests (Kaufman 1960). It has long subscribed to the balancing of multiple uses (timber, livestock, recreation, water supply, habitat) toward the goal of providing the greatest good for the greatest number over the long term.

The second illustration of Progressive principles is the Owens Valley Project in California (Hundley 1992, Kahrl 1982, Reisner 1986). In the beginning of the twentieth century, Los Angeles was the largest city on the West Coast. At the same time, the city's aqueduct was in decline, and city officials claimed that the Los Angeles River could not support the city's growth rate. Los Angeles sought supplemental water supplies from the Owens Valley, a sparsely populated, high-desert ranching region about 400 miles to the northeast. In particular, Los Angeles sought to purchase virtually all of the land in the Owens Valley watershed, evict the existing residents, and send virtually the entire snow melt via the Los Angeles Aqueduct to the City of Angels. In order not to arouse suspicions and to keep land prices from escalating, the Los Angeles Department of Water and Power bought up the ranches in great secrecy, involving local government and business leaders only when absolutely necessary. The funds to purchase the land and build the aqueduct were paid for by city bonds. As one might expect, the Owens Valley ranchers were not pleased, and the construction of the aqueduct was periodically interrupted by violence.

The Owens Valley Project characterizes the dark side of several aspects of the Progressive Era, while also highlighting several important differences between the Progressive Era and the Watershed Era. First, Los Angeles pursued a watershed approach by seeking to capture high-quality water from an entire mountain watershed, but gave very little concern to the ecological and social consequences of its strategy. Second, the project was conceived by a very innovative civil engineer, Robert Mulholland, and carried out by a bureaucracy dominated by engineers. The decision-making process was typified by closed-door, top-down decision making and a strong reliance on bureaucratic experts. Local actors, particularly in the Owens Valley, played virtually no role at all. Third, there is no doubt that the decision represented the greatest good for the greatest number over time. The economic benefits from using the Owens Valley water in Los Angeles dwarf those from ranching and recreation in the area of origin. The problem is that a focus on net benefits to society completely overlooks the destruction of many people's lives. Despite these problems in procedure (excessive secrecy and reliance on experts, very limited participation) and in distributional impacts, the executive order granting permission to build the aqueduct over federal lands was signed by the epitome of the Progressive Era, President Theodore Roosevelt.[4] The Owens Valley episode illustrates many of the problems of procedural legitimacy, substantive welfare, and distributive justice, addressed more systematically in chapter 3.

Thinking back to the criteria for characterizing water management in different epochs, the Progressive Era was marked by (1) a fairly strong adherence to the watershed or river basin as the appropriate scope of management, particularly considering the infant state of watershed science at the time; (2) a recognition that in many cases, markets could not be trusted to manage water resources and thus that a strong governmental role was needed; (3) a decision-making process that was dominated by bureaucratic experts, with relatively little consultation with affected stakeholders; and (4) a multiple use approach that sought to balance economic and environmental objectives, although water supply, flood control, and navigation were the primary concerns.

The Federal/New Deal Era (1925–1964)

The Tennessee Valley Authority ... should be charged with the broadest duty of planning for the proper use, conservation, and development of the natural resources of the Tennessee River drainage basin.
—Franklin Roosevelt (Lilienthal 1944, 36)

In many respects, the Federal Era represented a continuation and refinement of approaches developed during the Progressive Era in terms of managing at a watershed scale, an active governmental role in decision-making processes dominated by the bureaucratic expert, and efforts to balance multiple objectives. These trends were strongly affected by two sets of events: major floods on the Miami River in 1913 and the Mississippi River in 1927, and "hard times" (the Great Depression, Dust Bowl, and later World War II). They resulted in three innovative water management features that characterized the Federal Era: (1) multipurpose dams by the Corps of Engineers and Bureau of Reclamation; (2) multipurpose and region-wide planning, as illustrated by the Tennessee Valley Authority; and (3) intergovernmental coordination in erosion control as embodied in the Soil Conservation Service.

The Miami Valley flood of 1913 and the Lower Mississippi Valley floods of 1927 demonstrated the limitations of a levees-only approach to flood control and led to a multipronged engineering approach employing both upstream reservoirs and downstream levees (Morgan 1951, White 1969). This often required a basin-wide strategy spanning several states, and thus particularly appropriate for the federal government. These were reflected in 1925 and 1928 legislation charging the Army Corps of Engineers and the Bureau of Reclamation with preparing a series of comprehensive river basin plans (the "308 Reports"). The Mississippi floods, together with technological advances in dam construction and electrical transmission lines and the multiple-use thinking encouraged in the 308 Reports, made possible the advent of multiple use dams for flood control, hydropower, irrigation, and navigation. These were first incorporated into the 1928 Hoover Dam project and became a nationwide program in the Flood Control Act of 1936. It should be noted that while the principal flood control agencies—the Army Corps of Engineers and the Bureau of Reclamation—adopted a basin-wide approach, they remained committed to engineering solutions and quite hostile to the incorporation of controls on land use and agricultural practices as a means to limit sedimentation and runoff (White 1969).

The Great Depression led to the 1932 election of Franklin Roosevelt and a Democratic Congress, ushering in the New Deal. It involved greatly increased support for an activist government committed to the use of public works projects and other measures to provide jobs, electricity, education, and health services to poverty-stricken regions. This was embodied in the Tennessee Valley Authority Act of 1933.

The TVA was an extremely ambitious attempt to use natural resource planning to improve the socioeconomic welfare of communities in a large river basin covering several southeastern states. It involved the construction of multiple dams to provide flood control, water supply, and hydroelectric power. For perhaps the first time in the nation's history, there was an explicit effort to link land and water. In the words of David Lilienthal, one of the initial directors of the TVA (1944), "Through the long years there has been a continued disregard of nature's truth: that in any valley of the world what happens on the river is largely determined by what happens on the *land*—by the kind of crops that farmers plant, by the types of machines that they use, by the number of trees they cut down. The full benefits of stream and soil cannot be realized by the people if the water and the land are not developed in harmony" (50).

However successful it may have been, the TVA as a model of comprehensive, basin-wide natural resources planning has not been exportable. Explicit attempts to extend the TVA model to the Columbia and the Missouri basins failed because of regional rivalries, public versus private power controversies, and a variety of other reasons (Richardson 1973). More modest attempts at basin-wide planning, often involving interstate compacts, have been more successful. The Colorado River Compact of 1922 was purely concerned with allocating water diversions, first between the Upper and Lower Basins and then between California and Arizona (Hundley 1975, Sax 1968). Similar allocation compacts were established on many other river basins, mostly during the New Deal. The Delaware River Basin Commission was created in 1961 and has reasonably broad authority for water management, but is still less ambitious than the TVA (Barton 1967). Arguably the most important interstate compact dealing with water management (after the Colorado Compact) has been the compact establishing the Port of New York Authority (approved in 1921). It has been enormously successful in building and operating a host of facilities, but it involved only two states (Caro 1975, Leach and Sugg 1959).

Another illustration of the dawning realization of the integration of land and water was the creation of the Soil Conservation Service (SCS) in 1935. Created primarily as a response to the Dust Bowl in the Midwest, the SCS sought to control erosion on agricultural and forested lands and adjacent to streams through encouraging changes in cultivation, land use practices, and engineering solutions (Adler 1995, Clarke and McCool 1985). In general, the SCS sought to foster demonstration projects on private and public lands and then to use voluntary grants programs to promote the diffusion of effective practices. The SCS's focus on upstream land protection controls brought it periodically into conflict with the Corps of Engineers, which continued to favor downstream dams and levees (White 1969, 38). The situation was partially clarified when the Watershed Protection Act of 1954 gave the SCS authority to develop flood control solutions in upstream areas, but these frequently involved stream channelization projects, which turned out to be a mixed blessing (Anderson and Daniels 1973).

The Army Corps of Engineers, TVA, and SCS were all federal agencies whose legitimacy derived from their congressional authorizations and their expertise. They differed, however, in the involvement of external actors in their decision making. The Flood Control Act of 1936 institutionalized the corps and the Bureau of Reclamation as pork barrel agencies. The corps and bureau used their expertise to evaluate the benefits and costs of alternative solutions to flood control and navigation problems, but the choice of projects (and often the framing of alternatives) involved heavy deference to congressional public works committees. These operated in classic pork barrel fashion: every "worthy" member of Congress would periodically get a project in his or her district—as long they did not object to each other's projects and recognized that members of the relevant committees were likely to get more than nonmembers. Members, in turn, relied heavily on local constituents, primarily economic development groups, to identify problems and rank alternatives. In evaluating alternatives, the corps was required to consult with relevant agencies, particularly the U.S. Fish and Wildlife Service and often the SCS, but these consultations were purely advisory (Andrews 1976, Ferejohn 1974, Maass 1951, Mazmanian and Clarke 1979).

The TVA was officially governed by a board of directors appointed by the president. Its leaders espoused an ideology of "democratic planning" involving heavy involvement of local governments and constituencies in its decision making (Lilienthal 1944). They also recognized that a crude top-down federal presence in the rural South would be poorly received. Thus, there evolved a decision-making process in which locally based TVA experts would consult with local constituencies about specific projects. In the process, the TVA wound up skewing its programs toward politically powerful farmers rather than poorer farmers and sharecroppers (Selznick 1949).

The SCS was the most decentralized of the federal resource agencies. The agency initially adopted a technical adviser role in funding demonstration projects. Because diffusion of results was slow, the agency developed a strategy of creating soil conservation districts around the country. By 1949, there were over 2,000 districts covering about 60 percent of the nation's farm and ranch land. Each district was created by a referendum of local landowners and was governed by a board composed of their representatives. They receive funding and technical assistance from both state agencies and the SCS, but specific projects generally were required to have a local cost share. This pattern of locally based organizations receiving nonlocal support was reinforced by the 1954 Watershed Protection Act, which required that every SCS project be supported by local sponsoring organizations (Andrews 1976, Clarke and McCool 1985).

Of all the organizations discussed thus far, the Soil Conservation Districts (now termed Natural Resource Conservation Districts in many states) most resemble collaborative watershed partnerships. They focus on land and water interactions at a small watershed scale. They have been dominated by local landowners, but also include a few state and federal agencies (largely as technical advisers). They have relied heavily on small, largely voluntary projects.

They differ from 2000-style collaborative efforts, however, in at least two important ways. First, while most Soil Conservation Districts espouse both resource conservation and development objectives, they have been dominated by landowners within the district. Landowners can certainly be dedicated conservationists, but seldom have environmental activists explicitly been involved. Second, Soil Conservation Districts are units of government, created by and responsible to landowners within the district through formal elections. In contrast, most watershed partnerships are not themselves units of government, have members who are largely self-selected, and have only informal ties to local residents. In short, Soil Conservation Districts typically involve a narrower range of both governmental and nongovernmental actors than do watershed partnerships. They also involve more formal selection processes. As we shall see in later chapters, Soil Conservation Districts (and their successors) are often one of the critical members of watershed partnerships because of their legitimacy among local landowners, their access to project funding, their experience with erosion control, their ability (as a formal organization) to administer governmental grants, and their history of bottom-up intergovernmental partnerships.[5]

Most of the New Deal legislation dealt with resource use and conservation in the Progressive sense of the term. The focus was on efficient, nonwasteful use of natural resources. By the early 1960s, however, more protectionist legislation began to emerge, particularly dealing with public lands. The Multiple Use Act of 1960 largely codified the principles that the Forest Service had been using for decades, but it also clearly authorized nonconsumptive uses, such as recreation, habitat protection, and clean water supply. The 1964 Wilderness Act helped protect upper watersheds on federal lands. The 1965 Water Resources Planning Act authorized the establishment of several federal and state river planning teams (similar to the previous 308 Reports), but these were too expert dominated and insufficiently environmental to have an impact on the shifting tides of the late 1960s (Gregg 1989, White 1969).

Throughout the Federal/New Deal Era, there was relatively little concern by the federal government with resource protection on private lands. For example, water quality was almost exclusively a local concern, and most localities were perfectly content to use waterways for waste disposal ("the solution to pollution is dilution"). The emphasis in federal policy was to help localities build sewage treatment plants (Davies 1970), which began as a component of New Deal public works programs. The first explicit federal water pollution control legislation was the Water Pollution Control Act of 1948, which authorized the federal government to conduct research on water pollution problems and provide loans to municipalities for sewage treatment plants. The loan program was strengthened by the 1956 Amendments, which also created a cumbersome mechanism—interstate conferences—to deal with interstate problems. The 1949 and 1956 legislation was quite explicit, however, that states had primary responsibility for water pollution control.

Thinking back to our criteria for characterizing water management in different epochs, the Federal/New Deal Era was characterized by continued development of the watershed concept to include multistate basins for flood control purposes. There was increasing recognition of the effect of upstream cultivation and land use practices on water quality and flooding, but this linkage received only reluctant recognition by the Corps of Engineers and downstream residents (who continued to put their faith in levees and reservoirs). The ideology of the times was explicitly multiple use, although in a period of economic difficulty (the Great Depression, then World War II), the emphasis was more on economic development than on resource protection. This began to change slowly, particularly in the late 1950s and early 1960s. This period witnessed an expansion of the role of government in water pollution control. Decision-making processes continued to emphasize the role of experts (particularly engineers), but state and local actors and other federal agencies were given more of a consultative role than in the Progressive Era. The Soil Conservation Districts, composed of local landowners relying on federal and state agencies for funding and technical assistance, represented a partial precursor to watershed partnerships.

The Environmental Era (1965–1986)

One of our most urgent needs is the creation of an independent watchdog agency, uninvolved with the operating programs of the government, and dedicated solely to the protection and enhancement of environmental quality. We cannot afford to vest the duty to enforce environmental standards in the very agencies involved in the development of those resources for public use.... The Atomic Energy Commission should not set water pollution control standards for nuclear power plants.
—Senator Edmund Muskie (Davies 1970, Introduction)

The Environmental Era began in the mid-1960s, reached a crescendo in the early 1970s, and then began to shift its focus in the 1980s. It was marked by several important changes in the attitudes of the general public and policy elites: (1) an increased priority to environmental values (versus economic development values), (2) a growing distrust of bureaucratic experts in federal agencies, and (3) a distrust of state and local governments as too susceptible to influence by economic interest groups. The end result was a flood of legislation, most of which enhanced environmental values and the federal role but subjected federal agencies to greater congressional direction and expanded public participation. There was also a conscious strategy to enhance the technical and financial capabilities of state and local agencies, particularly in water pollution control.

Rising public and elite concern for the environment was a function of many factors. Increasing income and educational levels during the 1950s and 1960s intensified demand for outdoor recreation and gave people greater awareness of environmental problems. The development of ecosystem science enhanced the capacity to detect minute concentrations of chemical residues and provided evidence that ecological systems are interrelated—for example, that using DDT for malaria control in Southeast Asia affects penguin reproduction in Antarctica (Carson 1962, Odum 1969). The Hubbard Brook watershed studies provided strong evidence that upstream logging practices affect sedimentation and downstream water quality (Likens et al. 1970). There were numerous examples of environmental disasters, including repeated closures of beaches and shellfish beds, the 1969 fire on the Cuyahoga River, the 1969 San Barbara oil spill, and the discovery of toxic chemicals at Love Canal. These resulted in substantial increases in public concern with environmental problems, peaking in Earth Day 1970 but remaining strong throughout the 1970s and 1980s (Dunlap and Mertig 1992, Hays and Hays 1987, Rosenbaum 2002).

Accompanying this rising concern with environmental values was a growing distrust of the ability of governmental agencies at all levels to address these concerns. Part of this reflected the recognition that state and local pollution control agencies had neither the financial resources nor the legal authority to address many water quality problems adequately. They were too dependent on regulated industries for critical information and were under constant political pressure not to impose damaging costs on industry (Nader and Esposito 1970, Zwick and Benstock 1972).

There was, however, a more general argument in both the academic literature and the various Nader reports that federal regulatory agencies, including those in natural resource management, were "captured" by economic interest groups—that supposedly "independent" and professionalized agencies were too dependent for legal and financial resources on the most powerful interest groups in their policy subsystem (Berkman and Viscusi 1973, Lowi 1969, McConnell 1966, Sabatier 1975, Zwick and Benstock 1972). The Forest Service was portrayed as "captured" by timber harvesting firms, the Army Corps of Engineers by local chambers of commerce interested in flood control and navigation, the Bureau of Reclamation by agricultural water districts, and water pollution control agencies by industrial and municipal polluters. Perhaps most damaging was evidence that agencies manipulated their technical analyses to fit the interests of their dominant clientele. For example, a number of studies suggested that the Corps of Engineers and the Bureau of Reclamation manipulated their benefit-cost analyses by, for example, double-counting recreation benefits and ignoring adverse environmental impacts from their projects (Berkman and Viscusi 1973, Drew 1970, Hannon and Cannon 1971, Stratton and Sirotkin 1959). These revelations tarnished the Progressive Era image of the impartial, expert civil servant.

From this critique of existing resource management emerged a fivefold set of reforms (Clarke and McCool 1985, Davies 1970, Lowi 1969, Zwick and Benstock 1972). First, use federal grants to improve the financial and technical capabilities of state and local resource agencies at the same time that such agencies should be subjected to more stringent oversight by federal authorities. Second, environmental groups should be granted enhanced access to bureaucratic decision making by ensuring procedural access early in the decision process, as well as by granting citizen access to challenge agency decisions in the courts (Sax 1971). Third, a new federal pollution control agency should be created that would integrate pollution control programs, be unencumbered with other responsibilities (see the Muskie quotation at the start of this section), and be an effective spokesperson for environmental protection. Fourth, the discretion of federal and state agency officials should be tightly constrained by detailed procedural and substantive rules. Fifth, the relative priority of environmental values in existing statutes should be increased and new legislation passed to fill the many gaps.

With respect to intergovernmental relations, both the 1965 Water Quality Act and the 1972 Water Pollution Control Act Amendments established a system involving (1) federal mandates to state agencies to set water quality standards and adopt implementation plans, subject to federal agency (EPA) review; (2) states that performed well were then subject to less federal review; and (3) state capacity was enhanced through a variety of federal grant programs, as well as incentives to increase state funding of their own pollution control programs. There is no doubt that state (and local) capacity has increased substantially over time. State expenditures on water quality went from $52 million in 1972 to $976 million in 1986 and to $1.9 billion in 1994. In constant 1992 dollars, water quality expenditures increased from $155 million in 1972 to $1.8 billion in 1994. However, wide variations remained among states. For example, total state environmental expenditures per capita in 1994 ranged from $338 in Alaska to $66 in California to lows of $20 in Michigan and $18 in Ohio. In terms of performance, EPA had granted authority to thirty-eight of the fifty states by 1994 to issue their own water discharge permits. This increasing capacity led many states to resent continued EPA review of their programs—one of the features leading to state support for more collaborative approaches (Davies and Mazurek 1998).

The second strategy of the environmental movement, best represented by the National Environmental Policy Act (NEPA), was to increase its access to the decision-making process by requiring agencies to consider environmental impacts early in the process and increasing environmental groups' legal standing to intervene in agency processes and appeal agency decisions to the courts. However, there is also substantial evidence that agency responsiveness to NEPA varied widely across and within agencies. In general, the Corps of Engineers and Forest Service made a more concerted effort to comply than did, for example, the Soil Conservation Service or the Bureau of Reclamation. But there was also wide variation among districts and regions in the two model agencies (Andrews 1976, Clarke and McCool 1985, Hill and Ortolano 1978, Mazmanian and Clarke 1979). In addition, the citizen suit provisions in the 1972 Water Pollution Control Act Amendments, the 1974 Pesticide Act, and the 1976 National Forest Management Act clearly gave environmental groups greater standing to sue than they had previously enjoyed.

Senator Muskie's dream of an independent pollution control agency unencumbered with conflicting responsibilities was realized in 1970 when President Nixon, by executive order, created the U.S. Environmental Protection Agency. To it were transferred responsibilities for water pollution control (from the Department of Interior), air pollution control (from the Department of Health, Education and Welfare), and pesticide regulation (from the Department of Agriculture).

The fourth basic strategy—increasingly detailed legislation to limit agency discretion—will be illustrated in two areas: management of the national forests and water pollution control.

Prior to the 1970s, the Forest Service was governed largely by its Organic Act and by the two-page Multiple Use Act of 1960, which simply listed six permitted uses of the national forests and required the Forest Service to adopt a multiple-use strategy. In 1974, Congress passed the sixteen-page Resource Planning Act (RPA), which mandated Congress to establish annual output targets (e.g., for timber, recreation, and grazing) for the national forests as a whole, which the Forest Service would then allocate among the several forests.

This represented a rather substantial transfer of authority from the Forest Service to Congress. This was followed two years later by passage of the fifteen-page National Forest Management Act (NFMA), which established more of a bottom-up planning process in which each forest would develop a plan for selecting a mix of output levels that optimized net present value. The end result was a planning process in which virtually every major Forest Service decision was appealed by environmental or timber harvesting groups. The Forest Service went from an agency with virtually unlimited discretion to one that was buffeted by conflicting demands from Congress, the courts, local governments, and competing interest groups (Davis 1997; Mohai 1995; Sabatier, Loomis, and McCarthy 1995).

Federal water pollution legislation prior to 1965 consisted almost entirely of a few small grant programs for technical assistance and the construction of sewage treatment works, plus a very cumbersome process of interstate conferences for dealing with interstate problems. The Water Quality Act of 1965 strengthened the various grant programs (which generally required state matching funds for 30 to 70 percent of total costs) and added a new one providing 50 percent matching grants for water quality planning. The planning and administration grants required the states to establish water quality standards and implementation plans for various reaches of streams, but the federal government had only very limited authority to review the proposed state programs. In many respects, the 1965 Water Quality Act represented transition legislation whose basic approach was still rooted in the New Deal Era.

All of this changed dramatically with passage of the 1972 Federal Water Pollution Control Act Amendments. First, federal legislation grew from twenty-two pages in the 1965 Act to eighty-nine pages in the 1972 Amendments. Second, the 1972 Amendments represented a massive transfer of authority from states to the federal government, as it became clear that the financial incentives in the 1965 act were not producing water quality standards and implementation plans sufficiently stringent to satisfy federal agency officials (Ingram 1977, Quarles 1976, Udall 1967). This transfer was politically feasible only because of the enormous rise in public concern with air and water quality, combined with the massive subsidies for sewage treatment plants in the 1972 Amendments (Mann 1975).[6] Third, the 1972 Amendments remained rather schizophrenic in their strategy. On the one hand, sections 201, 208, and 303 continued the traditional water quality planning approach in which the beneficial uses for a particular stream segment were first designated, followed by the requisite water quality standards and implementation plans (effluent controls) needed to meet those beneficial uses. On the other hand, the 1972 Amendments also adopted a completely new technology-based approach involving uniform nationwide effluent standards for industrial pollutants and a huge sewage treatment grant program to essentially provide secondary effluent standards for all urban areas. The basic logic was that national effluent standards and subsidies were needed to overcome the reluctance of state and local water quality agencies to impose stringent standards on local industries and municipalities (U.S. Senate 1971). During most of the 1970s and 1980s, EPA focused its attention on the incredibly complex task of developing technology-based standards for every industry and pollutant (Magat,

Krupnick, and Harrington 1986). By the mid-1980s, however, it was clear that while technology-based standards might be an adequate (if inefficient) means of dealing with point sources, a completely different strategy was needed to deal with nonpoint sources.

Several other federal statutes passed in the Environmental Era had implications for water and watershed management: the 1968 Wild and Scenic Rivers Act, the 1972 Coastal Zone Management Act, the 1973 Pesticide Act, the 1973 Endangered Species Act, the 1974 Clean Drinking Water Act, the 1976 Toxic Substances Control Act, the 1976 "Organic Statute" for the BLM, and the 1980 Superfund legislation. Of these, the most important for watershed management, at least in the West, has been the Endangered Species Act. The listing of aquatic species—whether it be snail darters on the Tennessee River, salmon throughout the Pacific Northwest, delta smelt and salmon in the San Francisco Bay/Delta, or squawfish on the Colorado River—have created massive potential disruptions throughout entire river basins. As we shall see in the next section, the plethora of federal agencies and statutes, combined with the difficulties of translating legislation into effective on-the-ground activities, was one of the major rationales for the development of collaborative watershed approaches in the late 1980s.

Thinking back to our criteria for characterizing the principles of water management in each epoch, the Environmental Era represents some significant backsliding on the use of watershed, rather than political, boundaries. In particular, the 1972 Amendments' focus on national effluent standards and subsidized secondary treatment for all urban effluent was oblivious to watershed boundaries. Similarly, the Endangered Species Act's focus on protecting populations of specific species, rather than large habitats for multiple species, has not encouraged watershed thinking. With respect to the second principle, expanded participation, the Environmental Era certainly increased the access of environmental interests to agencies and courts. In particular, NEPA (and similar state statutes) gave interest groups and agencies with technical expertise an excellent vehicle to influence agency decisions. However, the setting of national effluent standards was a technical and time-consuming process that restricted effective participation to industry and agency engineers (Magat, Krupnick, and Harrington 1986). As for the third principle, collaborative decision-making processes, the Environmental Era probably had a net negative impact. The federalization of authority and heavy re-liance on litigation as a strategy in both water pollution control and for-est planning fostered confrontation and competition concerning general principles rather than the innovative search for win-win solutions in spe-cific decision situations. At the same time, the detailed nature of most legislation substantially weakened any agency's discretionary authority to cut innovative deals. This combination was a recipe for gridlock.

In many respects, the Collaborative Era can be interpreted as a reac-tion to some of the Environmental Era's excesses in terms of the federal-ization of authority, tight constraints on agency discretion, reliance on litigation as a major strategy,[7] fostering of environmental interests at the expense of property rights, and a general confrontational cloud over water management (Weber 1998, 2003).

Nevertheless, the Environmental Era provided several positive seeds for the growth of collaboration. First, the growth of environmental groups and their success in litigation encouraged their opponents in the property rights community to do the same. Second, NEPA and similar state legis-lation acclimatized agency officials to interacting with stakeholders. The traditional practice of backroom planning was becoming increasingly untenable. Finally, the capacity-building strategy targeted at state and lo-cal agencies meant that by the mid-1980s, state agencies and local water districts had the expertise to participate in collaborative negotiations with their federal counterparts.

The Watershed Collaboration Era (1987–Present)

EPA's Office of Wetlands, Oceans and Watersheds recognizes that it must involve everyone—other governmental agencies, businesses, communities, and individuals—to meet its environmental goals.
—U.S. Environmental Protection Agency (2001, 25)

The Watershed Collaboration Era emerged in the late 1980s and devel-oped throughout the 1990s. It grew out of a number of factors, including (1) the emergence of environmental mediation and alternative dispute resolution (ADR) as alternatives to litigation; (2) dissatisfaction with the implementation of the Federal 1972 Water Pollution Control Act Amendments, particularly regarding nonpoint sources and TMDLs; and (3) a growing sense that much of environmental policy, particularly regarding the Endangered Species Act, was neither democratically legitimate nor effective at solving environmental problems (Born and Genskow 2001, Kenney 1999, Tobin 1990).

As the volume of case law spawned by environmental legislation piled up, it became increasingly obvious to many people that litigation as a strategy had major limitations (Bingham 1986, Rabe 1988). First and foremost, it seldom solved real-world problems. Courts tended to rule on procedural issues and remanded the case back to the offending agency, which usually fixed the procedural problem and then reissued a slightly modified substantive decision. Litigation usually had its greatest substantive impacts when the delays it spawned allowed polluters to postpone costly controls for a few more years or convinced proponents of large capital projects to abandon their plans. Litigation also made agencies exceedingly cautious and preoccupied with procedure, rather than with finding creative solutions to complex problems. Second, parties in litigation tend to be preoccupied with winning rather than with finding mutually beneficial "win-win" solutions. In such a zero-sum atmosphere, today's losers in one venue simply search for another venue to continue the fight. Third, as environmental controversies became increasing complex—in both the number of actors and the technical uncertainties involved—litigation became less useful. In response to these limitations, a new strategy for resolving conflict emerged under the rubric of "alternative dispute resolution" (ADR) or "environmental mediation" (Bingham 1986; Blackburn 1988; Carpenter and Kennedy 1988; Fisher, Ury, and Patton 1991; O'Leary and Bingham 2003; Susskind, McKearman, Thoney-Larner 1999). It involved face-to-face negotiations among all affected parties in an effort to find a solution acceptable to everyone (as enforced by a consensus rule). It stressed detailed process rules, leadership by a trained mediator or facilitator, and a focus on interests rather than preferences. Environmental mediation began in the mid-1970s with the assistance of funding from the Ford and Hewlett Foundations and had 161 documented cases by 1984, of which about 75 percent reached some sort of agreement (Bingham 1986). Whether environmental mediation has been cheaper or prone to less delay than litigation remains a subject of dispute (Bingham 1986; Coglianese 1997, 2001).

The second major stimulus to a collaborative watershed approach was dissatisfaction with the implementation of the 1972 Federal Water Pollution Control Act Amendments. By the mid-1980s, it was reasonably clear that discharges from point sources (industries and municipal treatment plants) had declined and that water quality in affected areas had improved—even though economists and others were critical of the inefficiencies of those programs (Davies and Mazurek 1998, Randall 1981, Tietenberg 1984). It was also clear, however, that little progress had been made in reducing pollution (largely sediment, fertilizers, and oils) from nonpoint sources (e.g., farms, forests, urban streets with no storm sewers), even though it was estimated that nonpoint sources contributed over 60 percent of the pollution levels in streams that violated water quality standards. The 1972 Amendments anticipated this problem. Section 303(d) required that

"each State shall identify those waters within its boundaries for which the [point source] effluent limitations are not stringent enough to implement any water quality standard applicable to such waters.... Each State shall establish, for [those] waters, the total maximum daily load for those pollutants which the [EPA] Administrator identifies as suitable for such calculation. Such load shall be established at a level necessary to implement the applicable water quality standards with seasonal variation and a margin of safety which take into account any lack of knowledge concerning the relationship between the effluent limitations and water quality."

EPA did very little to implement this section until the mid-1980s. The reasons included the technical difficulty of determining pollutant discharges from farms, road cuts, and timber harvesting practices, for example; a desire to focus resources on the easier point source problems; and, probably, a reluctance to take on the politically potent agricultural lobby. The hope was that the voluntary conservation programs in farm legislation and best management practices (BMPs) in section 319 would solve the problem, but it gradually became clear that those would not be sufficient.

The nonpoint problem was recognized as sufficiently serious that the 1987 Clean Water Act Amendments made the control of nonpoint sources a specific national goal (section 101). Congress could not, however, agree on any major new programs to realize this goal, except for a new section 319 grants program. The statute also reaffirmed that water pollution control was primarily a state and local responsibility (Rosenbaum 2002). Out of this vague "mandate," EPA crafted a strategy based on section 303(d): nonpoint source control would be done on a watershed basis. Impaired waters (those that did not meet water quality standards) would be identified by state officials, and then TMDLs would be required for each major pollutant on those stream reaches. Most important for our purposes, EPA recognized that it should be only a minor partner in this enterprise. For it to impose uniform national standards on extremely varied and complex local situations would be suicidal. So the EPA encouraged the formation of watershed partnerships composed of the relevant agencies and private stakeholders to develop TMDLs. Unfortunately, it took five years to develop the relevant regulations, and the TMDL process did not kick into high gear until a number of lawsuits in the 1990s (many brought by the Sierra Club Legal Defense Fund) forced EPA to devote significant resources to this program.[8]

A third factor contributing to the Watershed Collaboration Era was widespread dissatisfaction, particularly in the West, with both the democratic legitimacy and the substantive effectiveness of environmental regulation (see chapter 3). Several sources of discontent can be identified. First, resource users—ranchers, farmers, timber harvesters, miners—felt that too many decisions were being made by distant federal bureaucrats and that their property rights were being violated. Under the guise of "the Sagebrush Rebellion" and "the Wise Use movement," it helped elect Ronald Reagan as president in 1980 and was rewarded when one of their leaders, James Watt, was named secretary of the interior (Gottlieb 1989). While the Reagan Revolution was probably less successful than is often thought (Durant 1992), the Wise Use movement certainly reminded everyone of the dangers of top-down regulation by federal and state bureaucrats that did not involve extensive local participation and neglected economic impacts on local communities and on property rights. The second major source of discontent involved environmental scientists and policy analysts in universities, consulting firms, and federal and state agencies upset with the tendency of federal environmental legislation to focus on one medium or problem (e.g., air pollution, water pollution, erosion, endangered species) at a time, to impede interagency coordination, to get bogged down in endless litigation, and to neglect social and economic impacts. They wanted a more holistic approach that would treat ecological systems as an integrated unit composed of biotic and abiotic elements, with human communities included in the system (Cortner and Moote 1999; Montgomery, Grant, and Sullivan 1995; Ruhl 1999; Yaffee et al. 1996). The third source of discontent involved advocates of "place-based management" (Snyder 1990; Woolley and McGinnis 1999, 2000). Their focus was on people's commitment to their local area and to finding solutions to the interrelated set of environmental, social, and economic problems in their locale. They shared the Wise Use movement's objection to regulation by distant bureaucrats that ignored many of the social and economic impacts on local communities. They shared the scientists' concern with integrated management within geographically based systems, but also insisted on the need for local knowledge to supplement scientific knowledge in local management decisions. The final source of discontent was Native Americans. Over the past twenty-five years, a century of injustice has periodically been reversed by the federal courts. The most important case involved 1974 and 1979 federal court rulings that revolutionized fishery management in the State of Washington by essentially entitling Native Americans to 50 percent of the total catch bound for their traditional fishing grounds (Singleton 2000, 2002).[9] While the dust has not yet settled on that and similar cases (e.g., on the Colorado), it is clear that Native Americans are increasingly important stakeholders, particularly in many western states.

The result has been a fairly widespread commitment to—or at least interest in—collaborative, place-based management. Its scale is geographically based and usually relatively small—watersheds, subwatersheds, and bioregions, but not entire river basins. It is quite democratic: anyone can be involved, and decisions are made by consensus, thus respecting everyone's interests and rights. The group seeks to solve an interrelated set of environmental, economic, and social problems. Agencies are involved—but as technical advisers and stakeholders, not as ultimate decision makers. The process is collaborative, involving extensive face-to-face negotiations with stakeholders who are treated more or less as equals. The process is often run by a professional facilitator or mediator skilled in conflict-resolution techniques.

Interest in this new paradigm grew in the 1990s. Kenney et al. (2000) identified 346 watershed partnerships west of the Mississippi River, but

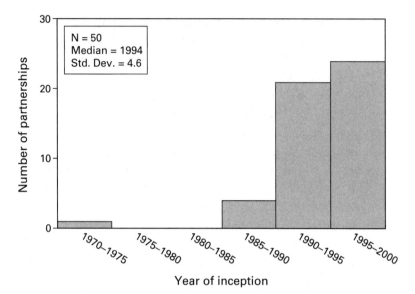

Figure 2.1
Year of inception for sample of fifty watershed partnerships in California and Washington

this is almost certainly an undercount, as we have found 150 in California alone. Figure 2.1 indicates that the vast majority emerged in the mid- to late 1990s. Watershed partnerships are also common in the eastern United States, as well as Canada and Australia (Leach and Pelkey 2001). Nine federal agencies have endorsed the Clean Water Action Plan (U.S. Environmental Protection Agency and U.S. Department of Agriculture 1998), which calls for a new cooperative approach to watershed protection in which state, tribal, federal, and local governments, and the public, first identify the watersheds with the most critical water quality problems and then work together to focus resources and implement effective strategies to solve those problems Several states—Massachusetts, Oregon, Washington, Wisconsin, Pennsylvania, and California—have established programs to encourage watershed partnerships. There are a wide variety of state and federal grant programs to fund watershed planning and restoration projects in which sponsorship by a broad-based partnership is either required or a major advantage.[10]

Of course, the watershed collaborative paradigm is not universally endorsed. National environmental groups remain skeptical of local control (Kenney 1999, McCloskey 1996). Stakeholder satisfaction does not necessarily produce better environmental or social outcomes (Coglianese 2002; chapter 8, this book). The Bush-Cheney administration has been much less supportive than the Clinton-Gore administration had been.[11] Within EPA, the funds and personnel devoted to watershed management are dwarfed by those assigned to the traditional industrial discharge permit and municipal waste treatment programs. Resource users and tribes remain cautious, if not skeptical. In fact, the most supportive partnership participants are generally federal and state agency officials (Sabatier and Leach 2002).

Conclusions

This book analyzes collaborative approaches to watershed management over the past ten years. As we have seen in this chapter and the previous one, collaborative watershed institutions are marked by (1) the use of hydrographic watersheds as the principal jurisdictional boundary, (2) the involvement of a wide variety of stakeholders (including interest groups, experts, and agency officials from multiple levels of government), treated more or less as equals; (3) a reliance on face-to-face negotiations with agreed-on procedural rules (and often a professional facilitator) designed to ensure civility and engender trust; (4) a goal of seeking win-win solutions to a variety of interrelated environmental and socioeconomic problems; and (5) a fairly extensive fact-finding phase designed to develop a common understanding of the seriousness and causes of relevant problems.

In order to understand this phenomenon, we first need to see it in its historical context: Which features of collaborative watershed approaches utilized in the past ten years are novel to this period, and which are essentially continuations of approaches developed over the past 150 years? That has been the purpose of this chapter.

With respect to scale, we have seen that management at the watershed scale has been sought since the beginning of the twentieth century, with particular emphasis during the Federal/New Deal Era and some backsliding during the Environmental Era. Thus, today's preference to manage at a watershed scale is more of a continuation of past practices than a recent innovation.

Similarly, managing watersheds in order to accomplish multiple purposes—water supply, water quality, flood control, water power and hydropower, wildlife habitat—has been common since the Progressive Era. What has changed is the relative influence of economic development goals versus environmental protection goals. Prior to 1890, the emphasis was almost exclusively on economic development. During the Progressive and New Deal Eras, a rough balance was sought, with some tilting toward economic development. During the Environmental Era, the emphasis shifted to water quality and habitat protection, and the Collaborative Era has seen an attempt to restore the traditional equilibrium. But the search for win-win solutions to address a multitude of conflicting goals and purposes is nothing new. Nor is the recognition that addressing almost any of these goals will involve both governmental and market institutions.

The most novel feature of the Collaborative Era is the involvement of multiple stakeholders representing diverse interests who treat each other more or less as equals. Most agencies have recognized that their traditional strategy of a single-minded focus on implementing their statutory mandate is much more likely to result in multiple lawsuits than solutions to problems of concern to them. Rather than each agency treating other stakeholders as supplicants, there is now an increased recognition that agencies are stakeholders with interests and resources but no monopoly of authority. In an era when every stakeholder has the option of initiating litigation that will frustrate departures from the status quo, all stakeholders are forced to deal with each other as equals and as necessary components of an overall solution. That is the effect of a consensus rule. The inclusion of multiple stakeholders has also meant that decision making has included experts and nonexperts, this bridging of scientific knowledge with local knowledge is another novel feature of the Collaborative Era. The Progressive ideal of government by neutral, expert bureaucrats is dead. It is not unusual to find local governments coordinating with federal or state agencies to implement watershed restoration projects initiated by a watershed partnership.

In sum, the most novel features of the Collaborative Era are (1) the replacement of traditional consultative agency practices with much more collaborative and consensus-based approaches, (2) the large range of governmental and nongovernmental actors involved, and (3) the recognition that decision making should not be left to bureaucratic experts. Scientific knowledge needs to be integrated with local knowledge, and the concerns of a wide range of stakeholders need to be incorporated into decision-making processes.

Notes

We thank Don Pisani, Steve Born, Larry O'Toole, and Doug Kenney for their helpful comments on previous drafts of the manuscript for this chapter.

1. These epochs are generally consistent with those used by Goldfarb (1994), Adler (1995), and Kenney (1999). In principle, each epoch should be relatively homogeneous with respect to the salient features of watershed management. For a similar analysis of regulatory regimes, see Eisner (1993).

2. The riparian use doctrine essentially limits use to riparians (landowners along the stream), subject to some "reasonable use" restrictions. In contrast, "prior appropriation" allocates water rights on a first come, first served basis. It was developed in mining communities in the West to allow large diversions of water from far-away streams to specific sites. Prior appropriation was codified into state law in California in 1872 and Colorado in 1876. It was subsequently applied to large water projects to benefit agriculture and, later, cities.

3. The extent to which watershed thinking permeated the Progressive Era is contested by Pisani (2002).

4. A similar story could be told about the efforts of San Francisco to acquire water rights in the beautiful Hetch Hetchy Valley in the Sierra Nevada (Nash 1967).

5. For example, in the study of 76 watershed partnerships in California and Washington discussed in chapter 7, 15 percent of respondents named the Natural Resource Conservation Service or the Resource Conservation District (or both) as being one of the three most influential participants, and 25 percent mentioned them as being one of the three best sources of information and advice.

6. In short, the 1972 Amendments represented a mixture of stringent regulation and class pork barrel (grants for sewage treatment plants).

7. The Environmental Era fostered a litigation strategy in several ways. First, and most obvious, were the citizen suit provisions of the Water Pollution Amendments, NFMA, and ESA, among others (Sax 1971). If interest group attorneys are given standing to sue, they are likely to find a reason to sue. Second, the more detailed the legislation is, the more opportunities the agency had to commit sins of omission or commission. Third, some of the mandates were either internally inconsistent or politically infeasible (e.g., the 1972 Water Amendments' goal of zero discharges by 1985). Impossible goals and deadlines invite litigation because the agency has no feasible means of meeting them.

8. Sources for this section include various EPA reports (e.g., U.S. EPA, 2001) and, most of all, conversations with the relevant EPA officials (notably, Tom Brady and Carol Campbell) at an EPA workshop, November 5–6, 2001.

9. The specific cases were a district court decision in *U.S.* v. *Washington,* 384 F. Supp. 312 (1974), which was reaffirmed by the U.S. Supreme Court in *State of Washington* v. *Washington State Commercial Passenger Fishing Vessel Association et al.,* 443 U.S. 658 (1979).

10. Examples include Oregon's Save the Salmon Program, California's CALFED program, Washington's Watershed Planning Act of 1998 (about $4.5 million annually), EPA's 104(b)(3), 205, and 319 grant programs, and USDA's EQIP Program.

11. This is based on July 2002 conversation with several U.S. EPA officials.

3

Legitimacy and Watershed Collaborations: The Role of Public Participation

Zev Trachtenberg and Will Focht

In this chapter, we examine watershed policymaking from an explicitly moral point of view. Our intention is to provide a normative outlook on the descriptive framework presented in chapter 1, to allow for a moral evaluation of collaborative watershed management. Because watersheds typically are public resources under the jurisdiction of governmental agencies, this evaluation enlists the values that justify our political system at large. Thus, this chapter invokes the idea of political legitimacy: the condition whereby a government's use of power is morally right. Our subject therefore is how public participation in watershed policymaking contributes to political legitimacy.

By focusing on legitimacy, we emphasize a different question from other chapters in this book. Other chapters (notably chapters 7 and 8) emphasize effectiveness: what makes collaboratives successful at formulating policies.[1] Of course effectiveness can be elusive. But in this chapter we take it as granted, in order to examine something else. For we hold that effectiveness is not the whole normative story: while it is obviously a good thing for policy to be effective, other moral considerations—typically, the fairness of the procedure that produced it—might give participants and outside observers alike qualms about an effective policy. Thus, in this chapter, we place policy effectiveness in a broader normative context that encompasses additional moral values.

The values we discuss are those used to legitimate the American system of government generally. Legitimation involves morally justifying a political system by showing its consistency with a set of accepted moral principles (Barker 1990). The fundamental values we take to justify the U.S. political system are autonomy, welfare, and justice.[2] We assume a consensus across American society on the centrality of these values, and hence take them to be an important element of the social context for watershed collaboratives. This chapter explains how they figure in the justification of watershed policymaking.

Let us briefly characterize each value now, and elaborate them later in this chapter:

- *Autonomy*: People ought to choose the rules under which they live.
- *Welfare*: Government ought to improve the conditions of life.

Note that the value of justice relates to welfare—it concerns how welfare is distributed.

- *Justice*: Even if total welfare rises, improvements for some people ought not come at the expense of worse conditions for others.[3]

In the watershed context, autonomy legitimates watershed residents' participation in the process of creating water quality regulations because they must live under these rules. But although a policy that improves water quality thereby increases welfare, the policy, to be legitimate, must distribute the costs of this improvement fairly. If no group bears an unfair share of the costs, the policy is rightful because it increases welfare justly.

How can we know if a collaborative watershed management process in fact implements the values of autonomy, welfare, and justice? We propose a set of criteria to serve as tests for evaluating the legitimacy of collaborative institutions.[4] Insofar as complete political legitimacy is an ideal moral standard, never fully attained, the criteria can each be met to varying degrees. Further, although the concept of legitimacy is typically applied to a political system as a whole, here we apply it at a much smaller scale: actions at a local or regional level by particular subunits of government. Although the operations of the subunits of a legitimate government are presumptively legitimate (assuming they follow legal mandates), it is useful to show how local public participation conforms directly to deeply held political values.[5]

The criteria are presented in two groups, corresponding to the distinction between procedural and substantive legitimacy. This distinction captures the commonsense notion that both the way decisions are made (the procedure) and what they actually propose (the substance) are morally relevant. Thus, the first set of criteria we discuss addresses procedural legitimacy; they articulate how public participation in policymaking must be structured for that procedure to be justified, primarily in terms of the value of autonomy. The second set of criteria addresses substantive legitimacy; they articulate a general description of what the goals of policy must be in order for the policy to be justified, primarily in terms of the values of welfare and justice.

Note that our claim is not that procedural legitimacy outweighs substantive legitimacy. It is clearly the case that a collaborative process might illegitimately sacrifice effectiveness on the altar of procedure. Actual situations typically require an appropriate trade-off between these requirements. However, our goal here is simply to explain why substantive considerations do not exhaust the question of legitimacy, but rather must be paired with procedural ones.[6]

Procedural Legitimacy

The idea of procedural legitimacy is that there are moral standards governing how watershed policy should be made. If produced by a dictator's fiat or coercion of policymakers, few would regard it as legitimate, even if it were effective. Rather, policy must be formulated in the right way, and our procedural criteria are meant to provide relevant standards of rightness.[7] To help explain the criteria, we begin with an abstract picture of collaborative watershed management.

The Parties to the Policymaking Process

To frame the issue that public participation raises, we take up the distinction, introduced in chapter 1, between governmental stakeholders and nongovernmental stakeholders. Recall that governmental stakeholders have a role in policymaking in virtue of their legal authority (governmental officials) or technical expertise (scientists, engineers, and economists, among others); nongovernmental stakeholders have an interest (or stake) in the resource at issue but no legally mandated role in formulating and implementing policy.[8] Let us now consider in more detail the justifications that legitimize the participation of these different parties.

Governmental Stakeholders: Public Officials and Experts   In general, participation by governmental stakeholders is justified in terms of welfare.

The case of experts is easiest to see: the participation of experts in policy discussions is legitimated precisely by their expertise, which (we shall assume) improves welfare by helping improve conditions in the watershed. The case of public officials, such as elected officials and agency personnel, is a bit more complex.[9] On the one hand, they participate in the policymaking process as a matter of the legal requirements of their positions. But in this respect, public officials' participation in policymaking does not raise a problem we need to address: we assume their participation is procedurally legitimate. On the other hand, a main theme of this book is the movement to bring together officials from different agencies with overlapping jurisdictions to formulate a single coherent policy for a given watershed.[10] A central goal of this movement is to make policy more effective; it assumes that involving many agencies will foster policy that is based on a more comprehensive understanding of the watershed as well as better cooperation among agencies in policy implementation. Thus, the participation of public officials in broad watershed collaborations is legitimated in the same way as the participation of experts: it will improve conditions in the watershed, thereby enhancing welfare.

Nongovernmental Stakeholders: Members of the Public   Our main focus, however, is not on governmental stakeholders. Rather, we ask why members of the public ought to have a role in watershed policymaking. To put the question starkly, why is it morally right for ordinary residents of a watershed to participate in policymaking, even if they have no particular expertise they can contribute to policy deliberations, or there is no law that mandates their participation?[11]

A cornerstone of Western moral philosophy is the notion that the ability to choose one's actions for oneself—autonomy—is essential to a good human life; it is the absence of autonomy that makes even a comfortable slavery dehumanizing (Kant 1981, Riley 1982). In politics, autonomy means helping to determine the structure of law under which one lives (Rousseau 1987, Cohen 1997). Thus, appeals to autonomy help explain the legitimacy of democracies: representation allows citizens to take part in legislation. Conversely, political systems that severely limit political participation are illegitimate precisely because they compromise their citizens' autonomy—even if they happen to enhance welfare.[12] Procedural legitimacy embodies precisely these considerations of autonomy.

Now the claim that the value of autonomy justifies participation by nongovernmental stakeholders in policymaking raises this question: When speaking of the broad public, precisely whose participation is required? Who counts as a nongovernmental stakeholder? The idea of autonomy directs us to those individuals who will be affected by, or otherwise have an interest in, the policies under consideration (Crowfoot and Wondolleck 1990; Stern, Fineberg, and NRC Committee on Risk Characterization 1996). For example, say that water quality in a river that serves as a town's water supply has deteriorated due to phosphorus run-off from fertilizer applied to farms in the local watershed, and water quality standards are proposed to address this problem. Then the residents of the town who seek better water, the farmers whose fertilizer application will be regulated, and environmentalists concerned about ecological diversity and habitat preservation all ought to participate in the drafting of the rules. All count as stakeholders because each has an interest, or stake, in the way the watershed is managed.

Criteria of Procedural Legitimacy

Let us now restate our conception of procedural legitimacy: nongovernmental stakeholders ought to have a voice in policymaking because participation implements the value of autonomy. What does this mean in practical terms? In most cases there are so many nongovernmental stakeholders that it is impossible for each individual to participate directly in policymaking. What must a procedure therefore be like to fulfill the moral requirements of autonomy? Our criteria of procedural legitimacy (P1–P3) are designed to address these questions:

P1: Participants in watershed collaborations must appropriately represent the full range of nongovernmental stakeholders.

P2: Participants in watershed collaborations must fairly consider the concerns of the full range of nongovernmental stakeholders.

P3: Participants in watershed collaborations must genuinely consent to the policy decision.

These criteria obviously rely on the notions of appropriate representation, fair consideration, and genuine consent, which will be explained shortly. Let us first emphasize that the criteria together reflect the ideal that the nongovernmental stakeholders as a whole must consent to the decision that results from the policymaking procedure. Consent has an obvious tie to autonomy, based on the deep intuition that an action must be voluntary to have moral value; this is why consent is seen as a necessary element of political legitimacy (Riley 1982). In our view, the requirement of consent operationalizes the value of autonomy.

However, obtaining the consent of all nongovernmental stakeholders for every policy decision is virtually impossible. Instead of actual consent, therefore, we ground procedural legitimacy on the notion of hypothetical consent—the notion that if given the opportunity, a majority of nongovernmental stakeholders would agree to a given policy.[13] What supports the belief that they would consent to a particular policy decision if they were asked? Our criteria explain how the procedures of watershed collaboratives should be structured in order to increase the likelihood of stakeholder consent.[14] Imagine, then, that in our watershed example, a Watershed Council has been created to determine water quality standards. The membership of the council includes governmental stakeholders, such as elected officials and agency personnel, and nongovernmental stakeholders, such as farmers, townspeople, and environmentalists.[15] The criteria reflect conditions that make it likely that nongovernmental stakeholders as a whole would consent to rules produced by the council.

Criterion P1: Appropriate Stakeholder Representation Obviously the membership of the Watershed Council must be limited; it is impractical to include every stakeholder. Hence some nongovernmental stakeholders have more influence over policy than others: the participants in the policymaking process, compared to those who do not participate. On its face, this might seem unfair. Why is it right, in our example, for Farmer Brown, who happens to be on the Watershed Council, to have a vote on water quality standards that will affect everyone in the watershed?

To maintain procedural legitimacy, the fact that Farmer Brown has a vote when other stakeholders do not must be consistent with the fact that other stakeholders' autonomy is nonetheless not violated. This requirement would be met if Farmer Brown were to be a representative.[16]

What would make someone appropriately representative of the non-governmental stakeholders? Election in a fair system of representation is an obvious example. Thus, Farmer Brown might win a vote held among all nongovernmental stakeholders. Or nongovernmental stakeholders might be divided into groups, so that Farmer Brown is chosen by other farmers and other groups choose their own representatives. The legitimacy of a nongovernmental stakeholder who was elected to participate in policymaking would thus be on a par with the legitimacy of governmental stakeholders, whose own authority ultimately rests on a democratic foundation.

However, for the kinds of policymaking procedures studied here, it is highly unusual for the participants to be elected. More typically, individuals volunteer, based on their own personal interest in a policy question or their position with some organized interest group.[17] In some cases, organizers of collaborative institutions actively solicit volunteers. Self-selection is an appropriate form of representation on the condition that the policymaking procedure remains open to all stakeholders. If participation is limited—for example, by the need to maintain a manageable number of participants—no stakeholder group may be denied representation unfairly, and the number of representatives from each group should be in rough proportion to the group's size and the intensity of its interests in the policy outcome.[18] When volunteers are solicited, it may require strong efforts by organizers to obtain the proper balance of group members—most frequently by encouraging members of under-represented groups to participate.[19]

Two other conditions contribute to our conception of appropriate representation of nongovernmental stakeholders. First, the participants should be in active communication with those they represent. When participants inform nonparticipants about the process and solicit and respond to their views, their representative function is enhanced, especially if participants convey to nonparticipants the deeper understanding of the issues they have learned from their participation. Second, other things being equal, if the participants reflect the range of interests, values, and relevant demographic characteristics of the nongovernmental stakeholders whom they represent, then their representativeness is improved. If participants were drawn from only some groups among the nongovernmental stakeholders, members of other groups might feel that their interests were not considered by the policymaking process, and hence might reject its results.[20] But if the participants are representative of the nonparticipants in these two ways, it is plausible that the consent of the former functions as evidence of the latter's (hypothetical) consent to a policy decision.

Criterion P2: Fair Consideration of Stakeholders' Concerns   Representation is important to collaboration because it helps collaborative institutions take account of the beliefs and interests of those their decisions will affect. When collaboratives collect and consider stakeholders' concerns and when the rules they propose fairly reflect the views, values, and interests of many individuals, these rules will, plausibly, garner the (hypothetical) consent of nongovernmental stakeholders, that is, they will be procedurally legitimate.

As chapter 2 showed, earlier eras of watershed management were marked by top-down management models, in which agency officials made the final decision. Stakeholders often were dissatisfied by this system, thinking that any testimony they might give at public hearings came after the real decision had been made. The belief that their concerns were not being treated fairly led them to call for a greater role in decision making, and thus provided an impetus to the collaborative movement. What then is involved in fair consideration of stakeholder concerns?

Continuing our example, criterion P2 requires that the Watershed Council consider all points of view on the question of whether and how to regulate phosphorus. Fair consideration can be achieved in a variety of ways, from having a membership that represents the full range of views, to conducting survey research, to soliciting testimony, among others. (For convenience, we will use the term *testimony* to refer to expressions of stakeholder concerns, however obtained.)

Obviously, fairness demands that no stakeholder's testimony be arbitrarily refused or devalued. The Watershed Council must accept testimony from as many stakeholders as is feasible and must provide a forum in which stakeholders are able to express their views fully and candidly.[21] The requirement for fair consideration has two dimensions, stemming from two aspects of stakeholders' testimony: empirical descriptions of the watershed and normative claims about how the watershed ought to be—in other words, facts and values. As we shall see, an important connection exists between both dimensions of fairness and the value of autonomy.

First, in considering stakeholder testimony, the Watershed Council will evaluate the accuracy of the picture of the watershed that testimony embodies. One important reason for soliciting information from nongovernmental stakeholders is that they frequently provide quite accurate, indeed expert, information: their local knowledge of the workings of their watershed (Lindblom and Cohen 1979, Ostrom 1990). Note that in this case, their participation contributes to policy effectiveness and is a matter of substantive legitimacy. The underlying justification of their participation derives from the value of welfare (the benefits it provides to all) rather than autonomy (their own interest in self-rule).

But what if the testimony provided by nongovernmental stakeholders is mistaken? In this case, acting on the testimony could lead to an ineffective or harmful policy outcome. In order to improve the watershed, that is, the Watershed Council must discount the testimony of misinformed stakeholders. While discounting incorrect testimony protects welfare, it seems also to diminish the stakeholders' autonomy. To respect autonomy, therefore, the council must provide adequate reasons for its rejection of mistaken testimony, by explaining the error and providing the correct account. Where the situation involves profound scientific uncertainty, the council should accept alternative accounts, including those provided by the stakeholders themselves, and then provide its reasons for acting on one account over any other.[22] Autonomy is preserved by such measures because the council expresses respect for the stakeholders as rational people who wish to make decisions and act based on the most accurate information available. Where stakeholders are treated in this way, they have good reason, and are more likely, to consent to the resulting decisions.

The second dimension of fairness deals with the way the Watershed Council treats the values that stakeholders express in their testimony. Obviously, if the council arbitrarily dismisses stakeholders' values, its decision is not likely to generate consent, especially if it uses its authority to impose its members' own personal values arbitrarily. But the more likely difficulty here stems from the fact that collaborative institutions operate within a legal context that carries a mandate to enforce laws and regulations that themselves reflect value positions. For example, laws such as the Clean Water Act generally give higher priority to environmental protection than to other values. Where a policy outcome goes against nongovernmental stakeholders' values, fairness demands a compelling explanation that might include a reference to the broader legal mandate, but also offers a justification showing that what the mandate calls for is a good thing. In this way, a council would address nongovernmental stakeholders as rational people capable of examining and revising their values in the light of good reasons (Sagoff 1988).

An especially difficult problem for a Watershed Council would be that nongovernmental stakeholders hold conflicting value positions; some think that a watershed should be managed to promote economic growth, for example, while others think it should be preserved in its natural condition.[23] In this case, minimum standards of fair procedure are crucial: the council can demonstrate its impartiality between value positions by accepting testimony from all sides and giving all positions due consideration. That is, the council must explain and justify the weight given to different groups' value positions in its ultimate decision. Such explanations, as with the case of facts discussed above, express respect for autonomy by offering a reason for consenting to the policy to the people who must live under it.

Criterion P3: Genuine Stakeholder Consent   So far, the consent of participants in the Watershed Council has served as a stand-in for the consent of nongovernmental stakeholders as a whole. Now suppose that the participants' consent was given improperly, because they were somehow deceived or coerced into agreeing with a policy. In this case, the participants' consent would not have the appropriate moral force; it would not provide a reason for the nongovernmental stakeholders at large to consent to the given policy, if they were asked. Criterion P3 therefore requires that participant consent be genuine. We suggest three standards of genuineness: the first two derive from the common law understanding that responsibility for fulfilling an agreement depends on free and informed consent; the third deals with the breadth of consent.

According to the first standard, an agreement that is coerced is not binding; consent has moral force only if it is truly voluntary (Beran 1987). This standard follows directly from the value of autonomy: obviously people have not freely chosen to live under rules if they are forced to accept them. Coercion can range from gross to subtle. For example, gross coercion could involve a threat by one participant against another—say, a governmental official threatening a citizen (or vice versa). Subtle coercion could involve domineering participants who induce others to vote a particular way simply to avoid conflict.[24] Anything that makes nongovernmental participants feel constrained to endorse a decision that goes against their wills violates criterion P3.

The second condition holds that genuine consent relies on being fully informed. Again, this condition follows from autonomy: self-imposed rules are chosen freely only if they are truly understood. Thus, the condition that consent must be fully informed overlaps the condition that it be free. To illustrate the connection, an insidious form of coercion involves control over technical information in policymaking (Webler 1995). In our example, if governmental stakeholders withheld a report relevant to a proposed policy from nongovernmental participants who then voted for the proposal, their consent should be considered invalid.[25] Likewise, if experts argue for a proposal using arcane technical language, it seems clear that lay participants cannot give the proposal their informed consent. Therefore, criterion P3 requires that participants have complete and comprehensible information about the policy problem at hand.[26]

The third condition is somewhat different from the first two: it has to do with the distribution of opinions among nongovernmental participants. Say that all nongovernmental participants in the Watershed Council freely and in an informed way agree with a proposed policy. Their unanimity would make the group's consent genuine. Thus, part of the appeal of consensus is that such decisions are supported by the full moral force of consent.[27] However, in the absence of unanimity, we might wonder how the minority can be said to consent to the majority's decision and how their autonomy would be respected if the decision goes into effect.[28]

Now if the majority is much larger than the minority, one may reasonably determine that the group's consent is genuine enough—since sometimes it is simply necessary to get things done, hence, to trade off some autonomy for some welfare. However, if the minority is substantial, it makes less sense to say that the group as a whole has genuinely consented. Indeed, in this case, the decision by the participants does not seem to sufficiently ground the claim that nongovernmental stakeholders as a whole would consent to the policy proposal. Or suppose that the minority, even if small, is very strongly opposed to the majority decision. In our example, if the Watershed Council votes for fertilizer regulations that Farmer Brown vehemently insists will put farmers out of business, it seems wrong to claim that the Watershed Council as a whole has consented; the intensity of Farmer Brown's opposition is an indication that other farmers will also oppose the council's decision. The last condition on genuineness of consent therefore is that consent must be sufficiently broad and lack significantly intense opposition.[29]

In sum, criteria P1, P2, and P3 articulate standards that collaborative watershed management institutions must meet in order to ensure that their policymaking activities are procedurally legitimate. We believe that by meeting these standards, collaboratives enhance public acceptance of policy decisions, that is, they increase the likelihood of (hypothetical) consent among nongovernmental stakeholders.[30] But even as a matter of effectiveness rather than legitimacy, it is plausible that collaboratives that failed to meet the criteria would fail to produce policy because people would decline to participate in them.[31] But beyond the obvious goal of watershed policymaking, that is, improvements in the watershed, procedural legitimacy has an additional positive impact in the social domain: collaborative institutions that meet the criteria help strengthen what we called in chapter 1 civic culture. As the general public comes to understand that policymaking institutions are open to broad participation and are designed to embody respect for participants' autonomy, it will likely respond with deeper trust for the institutions and the officials in charge of them, contributing to a general improvement in social capital.[32]

Substantive Legitimacy

Let us now turn from the procedure by which policy is made to the actual content, or substance, of the resulting policy proposals. This section considers relevant features of the content of policy and offers a set of criteria as tests for substantive legitimacy.[33]

Whether a policy is substantively legitimate depends on policy outcomes—the effects the policy has (or is likely to have) on the world.[34] A policy is substantively legitimate to the extent that those outcomes can be justified. The question therefore is: What justifies a policy's outcomes? Our criteria start with the notion that the policy must have positive outcomes—but that these outcomes are not to be thought of strictly in terms of changes in the physical condition of the watershed. We also consider social and economic factors, involving how those physical changes are to be obtained, and how the costs involved are to be distributed. Thus, our criteria of substantive legitimacy (S1–S3) invoke the values of welfare and justice:

S1: The outcome of policy must be an improvement in the welfare of at least some nongovernmental stakeholders.

S2: Policy outcomes, and the means to attain them, must respect individual stakeholders' rights.

S3: The outcome of policy must be a fair distribution of welfare among all nongovernmental stakeholders.

Criterion S1: Improvement in Stakeholders' Welfare

The most obvious way to justify a policy's outcome is to invoke the value of welfare: in general, a policy is substantively legitimate if it makes people better off. We use the term *welfare* in a very broad way to refer to the general conditions of life. In the watershed example, the conditions of life include health, recreational opportunities, the situation of wildlife, and economic well-being.[35] To the extent that polluted water is unhealthy, improving water quality not only reduces health risks but also produces secondary benefits, such as increasing recreational boating and swimming, and increasing the number of fish and other wild species that will benefit people who enjoy fishing and observing wildlife. However, to the extent that improving water quality requires regulating fertilizer application, welfare will be decreased for others: rising costs for farmers affect their economic well-being, and higher agricultural costs make food more expensive for everyone. In other words, the goal of increasing welfare typically requires trade-offs: rules that improve water quality might be very good for people who fish and swim but very bad for farmers and their customers. This example is, of course, highly simplified, but it allows us to focus directly on the moral problem posed by the fact that the welfare of different groups of people can diverge as the result of a policy.[36]

Now precisely whose welfare is of concern? Nongovernmental stakeholders were previously defined as individuals who have an interest in or will be affected by a policy's outcomes. A restatement of this definition shows that a person is a stakeholder if his or her welfare improves or deteriorates depending on how the watershed is managed. It follows that because substantive legitimacy is based on a policy's outcomes, assessments of substantive legitimacy must consider the welfare of all nongovernmental stakeholders—that is, how a policy affects the interests of all those it does affect.

If we could imagine a policy that would improve the welfare of some stakeholders without harming any others, we would have an obvious example of a policy that was substantively legitimate under criterion S1.[37] Conversely, a policy that harms everyone it affected would, equally obviously, be illegitimate in the substantive sense. In reality, policies have different effects on different interests; typically, gains to the interests of one group involve losses to the interests of another. The more profound question of substantive legitimacy thus involves an evaluation of the balance a policy strikes between competing interests. The value that determines if such a balance is morally acceptable is justice.

Justice comprises two related concerns (Rawls 1999). On the one hand, it concerns rights: justice demands that people's rights be respected. On the other hand, justice concerns distribution: it demands welfare be shared in a fair manner. However, what are a person's rights, and what makes a welfare distribution fair? We shall address these questions as we consider criteria S2 and S3. As we shall see, answering these questions brings us back to the issue of stakeholder participation in policymaking.

Criterion S2: Respecting Stakeholders' Rights

The Watershed Council in the example might improve water quality dramatically if it could compel individuals to stop any activity that might lead to water pollution. Of course, such a policy would be unacceptable, indeed illegitimate: to the extent that an activity is within a person's rights, it is not subject to coercive interference. Individual rights function as limits on what society can compel an individual to do, even in the interest of increasing welfare (Dworkin 1977). However, precisely what lies within a person's rights is often contentious. For example, let us say that the farmers in the watershed believe that they are within their rights to use agricultural practices that increase their food production and lower their costs. If the farmers are correct, then the Watershed Council has a very narrow scope for proposing policy solutions to the water quality problems it faces.

But are the farmers correct? How is that question to be settled? This is, in effect, to ask, What are the farmers' rights? In order to flesh out criterion S2, we shall consider this question generally and at some length. In an obvious sense, a person's rights are a matter of the law; the law spells out what people can and cannot demand that the government protect. Obviously, however, there can be a divergence between what the law counts as people's rights and a wider moral sense of people's rights (Dworkin 1977). This divergence can indeed lead to changes in the law, as when the civil rights movement successfully demanded that the limited legal rights granted to African Americans and others be expanded to include what was seen as the full moral rights of human beings. Let us therefore begin with a fairly abstract moral conception of rights: the idea that people are entitled to be treated, by both the government and each other, in ways that acknowledge and respect their human dignity.

This abstract conception of rights has an important implication for watershed policymaking: in general, when determining whether a policy improves welfare, the interests of each individual nongovernmental stakeholder are accorded equal weight in calculating the effects of a policy on the welfare of the stakeholders as a whole.[38] In our example, if effects on farmers were ignored or given less weight than the interests of other stakeholders in determining whether a water quality rule increases welfare, we take it as obvious that the farmers' rights would be violated. Indeed, the environmental justice movement concerns cases where the interests of a specific group of stakeholders, typically members of an ethnic minority, are discounted in decisions on environmental matters (Cole and Foster 2001).

A person's rights thus involve the requirement that that person's interests be taken fully into account (Feinberg 1984). What it means to take account of interests will be considered more concretely in the next section. First, note an important complication in this general understanding of rights. There are obviously cases where something one person does to advance personal interests harms the interests of another. Preventing the harmful activity would set back the interests of the first person—but we would not conclude from this fact that his or her rights had been violated. For, of course, no one has the right to harm another unless there is an adequate justification.

In our discussion of watershed policymaking, what defines rights in practical terms is precisely the set of justifications that permits activities even if they work against the interests of others. A simple, nonwatershed case makes things clear: the right of self-defense justifies a person's harming an unprovoked attacker. In the watershed example, a similar case would be a regulation prohibiting the dumping of used motor oil into storm sewers. Although this sets back the interests of drivers by making it more expensive to operate cars, they have no right to do something that causes harm to the users of the water supply.

But what about the case of farmers applying fertilizer to their crops? Even assuming that the interests of people who fish are harmed by this activity, few would agree that the farmers' activity should simply be prohibited, without any consideration of the effect of such a rule on the farmers' interests. For it seems reasonable to hold that the farmers' activity is justified—that it is within their rights. An obvious justification is that applying fertilizer produces higher yields, which makes food more plentiful, which increases welfare.

When we consider the variety of activities that have potentially harmful effects on a watershed, it quickly becomes clear that a variety of putative justifications can be offered for them. For example, they might fall within the provisions of existing law or, of particular importance, follow from the ownership of private property. Whether such justifications hold up is vitally important. If an activity is rightful, then any policy that regulates it must take account of the interests of the people involved in it— but if it is not rightful, policy is free of that requirement.[39] Determining whether particular activities are justified requires an extremely detailed understanding of the full situation in which they take place. Persuasive determinations cannot be made in the abstract. Thus, rather than exploring in detail what sorts of activities might or might not be justified, we shall briefly touch on the question of the institutions in which these questions are settled.

Determining who is in the right is generally a matter for the courts, which apply standards expressed in common and public law. For example, the common law rules of nuisance deal with activities that impose unjustifiable burdens on others (Radin 1993). Note that public law, at least ideally, results from a legislative determination of what activities are acceptable in society. As noted above, there may be discrepancies between the law and moral values; movements for social change are geared in part to revise legislation in response to changing social norms. Much environmental law has this character: it reflects a broad social consensus that activities that were once tolerated are no longer justified, such as activities that threaten the quality of natural resources like air and water (Kubasek and Silverman 1997). Legislatures serve as fora for articulating this broad consensus; it typically falls to agencies, acting on a legislative mandate, to apply general guidelines to particular situations, hence to specify in detail which activities are rightful.

Legislatures, agencies, and courts thus elaborate and enforce the broad framework of rights that criterion S2 insists policy must respect. However, we hold that within this institutional context, there is a role for nongovernmental stakeholders in the determination of which activities are justified even if they produce harms. Considerations of procedural legitimacy suggest that the people whose interests are most directly at stake ought to have at least a share in the responsibility for determining exactly what are or are not rightful activities. Their deliberations should contribute to the process of aligning a society's law with its moral values (Sagoff 1999).

Thus, suppose that the Watershed Council determines that although farmers are justified in applying fertilizer, they are not justified in allowing their cattle to water directly in streams.[40] That is, the council determines that farmers have the right to use fertilizer, but have no right to let cattle trample stream banks. This determination ought to have some standing within the broad legal framework just discussed. Because the former activity is rightful, whatever policy was established would have to take account of the farmers' interests regarding fertilizer application. However, because the latter activity is not rightful, policy could simply prohibit farmers from giving cattle access to streams. Thus, though it is ultimately justified on procedural grounds, stakeholder participation can also contribute to substantive legitimacy. By helping determine the boundaries of rightful activity, hence the constraints within which policy must operate, stakeholders help specify legitimate policy goals.

Criterion S3: Fair Distribution of Welfare

The ongoing example illustrates a crucial fact about watersheds: they are tightly connected systems in which activities one group undertakes to improve its own welfare can ultimately damage the welfare of others. Let us focus on the simplified case that applying fertilizer makes the farmers' welfare go up but lowers the welfare of the people who fish, and limiting fertilizer use would raise the welfare of the people who fish but would lower the welfare of farmers. The effect of watershed policy can be understood as involving the redistribution of welfare among stakeholders—raising the crucial question, by what standard are changes in the distribution of welfare morally acceptable? That standard is fairness.

What then is a fair distribution of welfare? Note that in the example, it is unfair both for the farmers to gain welfare at the expense of the welfare of the people who fish and for the people who fish to gain at the expense of the farmers.[41] In the terms used by moral philosophers, in each case one group is using the other as a "means" for increasing its own welfare (Kant 1981). On this view of morality, to use other people as no more than a means to benefit oneself is inconsistent with the kind of treatment due to human beings as a matter of their fundamental moral rights. Basic respect for a person's rights, that is, consideration of the effect of a policy on his or her welfare, is therefore deeply linked to the idea that it is morally impermissible to treat human beings as if they were merely instruments for producing welfare gains for others. To treat a person this way is exploitation.

Thus, the key to fairness in the distribution of welfare is that, in general, no group of nongovernmental stakeholders can be used as a means to increase welfare for another group of stakeholders. At the very minimum, fairness requires meeting criterion S2: with the crucial exception of preventing people from acting beyond their rights, the effects of a given policy on each group of stakeholders must be counted. However, fairness goes beyond this basic requirement; it specifies more concretely how those effects should count, as we shall see in a moment. First, we emphasize that fairness does not demand that policies must never harm any interest of any nongovernmental stakeholder.[42] Such a demand makes policymaking impossible. Rather, fairness holds that policy cannot be justified by a simple benefit-cost analysis. Benefit-cost analysis might be taken to justify a policy if the benefits to some were greater than the costs to others, so that the policy's net effect is to increase welfare overall.[43] However, such a justification treats the cost bearers as a means to increase the welfare of the beneficiaries. This is precisely what fairness rules out.

What fairness requires is that if one group of stakeholders enjoys a welfare gain at the expense of a second group of stakeholders suffering an (unjustifiable) welfare loss, the second group must be compensated (Sagoff 1988). Compensation restores fairness to the distribution of welfare by ensuring that, on balance, no one is made worse off by the damage to a particular interest imposed to provide benefits to others.[44] Compensation ensures that stakeholders whose interests are harmed are not treated as nothing more than the means to advance others' interests. Compensation is thus deeply connected to the notion of respect for rights: policymakers must take note of the effects of a given policy on all stakeholders in order to determine who may need to be compensated and to what extent.[45]

What does fairness demand in the watershed example? We assume that the farmers gain welfare by imposing welfare costs on the people who fish; a prohibition on fertilizer use would increase the welfare of the people who fish by imposing welfare costs on farmers. To make this situation fair, the welfare gainer should compensate the welfare loser. Thus, a policy designed to improve the situation of the people who fish must compensate the farmers for their loss in income, perhaps, by dedicating part of the fee for fishing licenses to a farm subsidy. Alternatively, the farmers might compensate the anglers by paying into a fund that restocks the river with fish.[46]

In general, then, criterion S3 reflects a broad goal for watershed policy: policy must fairly balance the exchange of welfare that results from the physical interconnections found in watersheds so that one group's gains are not accomplished at the expense of uncompensated losses to others. This demand for fairness has two implications for stakeholder participation in watershed policymaking.

First, in line with the discussion of criterion S2, compensation is not due to anyone whose activities are not rightful: they are not entitled to the welfare they gain through wrongdoing. In the example, say the authorities shut down an illegal toxic waste dump. Although the welfare of all stakeholders increases at the "cost" of the dump operator's decreased welfare, no one would suggest that the operator should be compensated for his loss. His actions were harming the public, and fairness demands compensation only for those who act within their rights.[47] However, what counts as rightful activity is not defined as what is legal. Rather, the complex process of articulating legal standards—involving legislatures, agencies, and courts—can be interpreted as society's effort to have its laws reflect its moral standards. Stakeholder deliberations ought to have an important role in this effort.

In the example, we supposed that the Watershed Council determined that farmers are within their rights to apply fertilizer but have no right to allow cattle to enter streams. The practical effect of this determination is that if the council decided to regulate fertilizer use, it would have to compensate the farmers for their loss in welfare, because that loss would come despite the fact that the farmers were doing nothing wrong. But if the council decided to prohibit farmers from allowing cattle in streams, no compensation would be required, because that activity has been determined to be beyond the farmers' rights. The council's rulings ought to have some standing within the broader legal framework in which it operates: it should be respected by judges or given legal force by legislatures (Sagoff 1999).

Second, if compensation is a means of "operationalizing" fairness, because compensating people for their welfare loss is a way of treating them fairly, then an obvious test of fairness is the extent to which stakeholders extend or withhold their consent to a compensation plan. Here considerations of substantive legitimacy (whether a policy proposal is aiming at the proper target, that is, a fair distribution of welfare) overlap considerations of procedural legitimacy. For it is reasonable to suppose that unless adequate compensation was offered to offset their losses, people would not consent to a policy that harmed their own interests while furthering the interests of others. Note that the requirement of consent allows the sidestepping of the vexing problem that different groups' interests are very different in character and cannot be compared in a way that allows for an easy decision about how the losers should be compensated. In our example, while the farmers might think about regulation of fertilizer use in strictly financial terms, the people who fish might attach a sentimental (or aesthetic, or spiritual) value to their activity, independent of what it costs them to have that experience. From the outside, therefore, it is not at all obvious how to weigh the financial value of crops against the sentimental value of fishing, and hence how to strike the proper balance between these two interests. However, requiring that both sides consent to a trade-off allows each to determine for itself whether it has received compensation adequate to its own sense of any losses it will suffer.

More concretely, it is plausible to think that if the Watershed Council provides for collaboration among representatives of all nongovernmental stakeholder groups in accordance with the criteria of procedural legitimacy, it will be well placed to formulate a policy that meets criterion S3. As representatives of one group offered one proposal, representatives of another could respond that the scheme would impose undue costs on them and suggest a revision. Through bargaining, the representatives might strike a balance, according to which their respective groups are treated fairly.[48] Thus, nongovernmental stakeholder participation in policymaking can be justified not only as something that is right in itself, but also as something that helps fashion proposals with fair outcomes. A policymaking process that is legitimate on procedural grounds is well structured to produce policy proposals that are legitimate on grounds of their substance.

Finally, then, we hold that considerations of substantive legitimacy are linked to considerations of procedural legitimacy. Specifically, the ability of collaborative institutions for watershed management to attain the substantive goal of producing watershed outcomes that improve the welfare of stakeholders in a just way is linked to the collaboratives' implementation of the norms of procedural legitimacy. This is true for welfare outcomes, and we believe it is also true for an important further social benefit. As noted, procedurally legitimate collaborations contribute to a community's civic culture (Putnam, Leonardi, and Nanetti 1993). As individuals collaborate within a legitimate procedure, with an eye toward providing for a just distribution of welfare within their watershed, they are called on to increase their knowledge of the watershed and their understanding of other stakeholders' interests and concerns. By carrying out their responsibilities as representatives of nonparticipating stakeholders and by interacting with the other participants, they strengthen the networks of communication within their communities—

networks that are used for social functions other than watershed planning. To the extent that their collaborations are effective at producing policy proposals, and even more to the extent that their watershed proposals are implemented, their general sense of political efficacy will grow. Indeed these aspects of social capital themselves contribute to successful watershed collaborations; a community with very low social capital would have trouble sustaining an involved participatory procedure.[49] However, collaborations designed to meet the standards of procedural legitimacy can initiate a "virtuous cycle," whereby the elements of social capital needed for the deliberations are cultivated, leading to improved deliberations, leading to enhanced social capital, and so on.[50] In sum, just as legitimate policymaking procedures foster the stewardship of a watershed, they also foster the stewardship of social capital.

Conclusion: Legitimacy and the Survival of Watershed Collaboratives

Collaborative watershed management institutions are relatively new on the scene. Often they are chartered to address a particular problem and then disbanded. The question thus arises, Will this sort of institution survive within the tangled web of already existing governmental agencies? Ultimately, of course, this is an empirical question, and it is simply too early to answer it. But it is a question that intersects with the issue of legitimacy in two important ways.

First, there is already evidence that at least the perception of legitimacy among the participants in watershed collaborations is a condition of institutional survival. As chapters 7 and 8 show, participants will continue to contribute to the work of their collaboratives at least in part on the basis of their belief that these institutions meet the standards of procedural legitimacy. Further, on the basis of their beliefs that their collaboratives are procedurally legitimate, participants seem to believe that their policies have positive watershed outcomes. That is, at least the perception of procedural legitimacy leads to at least the perception of substantive legitimacy. And the perception of substantive legitimacy—the belief that the collaborative is accomplishing a worthwhile goal—is a crucial factor that motivates participants to continue investing their efforts in it. Thus, the perception of legitimacy contributes to survival. Conversely, the perception that a collaborative is not legitimate could lead to its demise. People who feel they are treated unfairly will cease to participate, as will people who believe that their efforts are not repaid by success.

The dependence of participation on perception poses a tremendous risk for collaboratives, in particular with respect to perceptions of substantive legitimacy. It seems reasonable to think that people are good judges about procedural legitimacy: they can tell if collaboratives are representative or if their consent to policy proposals is being solicited. But there are profound uncertainties about watershed outcomes due to the complexity and unpredictability of the ecological and physical systems, and the truth may not emerge for a long time. In the interim, participants may well give up: the fact that its procedures are acceptable may not compensate for the uncertainty about whether a collaborative is actually improving watershed conditions.[51]

Beyond this account of how perceptions of legitimacy influence whether collaborative institutions will survive, there is the question of whether they ought to survive. To the extent that they conform to our criteria of legitimacy, we say yes, since these criteria express our conception of how watershed policy ought to be made. More specifically, the commitments expressed in our procedural criteria reflect our belief that as an element within a broader democratic political culture, watershed management ought to be conducted in a democratic fashion. And, as observed in the discussion of substantive legitimacy, watershed collaborations can serve a crucial role in identifying proper goals for watershed policy. This observation points out how the survival of collaborations as ongoing institutions can serve substantive legitimacy. Ongoing participation by stakeholders in watershed collaborations can provide a source for good evidence of whether the actual outcomes of a policy increase welfare in a way that respects rights and is fair. In other words, the survival of watershed collaborations can help make watershed management responsive to its actual outcomes, in the sense that ongoing collaborations are in a better position to adjust their policies to the specific circumstances in which they are applied.[52]

Nonetheless, we certainly acknowledge what the succeeding chapters in this book show. Successful collaboration requires a substantial commitment of time and resources: it is a costly undertaking, and its payoff in terms of outcomes is unclear. Our discussion of legitimacy thus raises this broad and perhaps unsettling question: Are we willing to shoulder the burden of all our normative commitments, procedural as well as substantive? Although legitimacy is an ideal moral standard, this unsettling question is meaningful only with respect to concrete cases. We close with the hope that this chapter might focus attention on the normative stakes in specific watershed management situations.

Notes

1. This book has a rich conception of effectiveness. We distinguish between a procedure's effectiveness at producing policy and the policy's effectiveness at producing the desired result (see note 34). And while that result certainly involves improvements in water quality, it can also involve improvements in social factors in the given watershed, such as greater trust between participants or better economic conditions. For now, we will simply conflate these diverse aspects of effectiveness.

2. Consider the references to these values in the Declaration of Independence and the opening words of the U.S. Constitution.

3. Although these values mention only living human beings, we acknowledge that for many, concern for the environment extends to future human generations, or to nonhuman animals, or to ecological systems. It is not hard to imagine how (at least) the values of welfare and justice can be reconceived to take these broader moral subjects into account. However, for reasons of space and simplicity, this chapter will address only the moral requirements associated with human beings living today.

4. The question of evaluation runs two ways: not only do our criteria bear on the legitimacy of collaborative watershed management, empirical evidence about collaboration likewise bears on the reasonableness of the criteria. In chapter 9, we will return to comment on whether the experience of collaboration presented in other chapters supports these criteria as reasonable normative goals.

5. It might seem that if the wider regime (e.g., the federal or state government) is legitimate, legally authorized actions by its agencies would be legitimate as a matter of course; thus, the most important criterion for the legitimacy of a particular policy would be its legality. However, because our focus is on moral evaluation, we do not construe the legitimacy of watershed policymaking as simply a formal question settled by its legal consistency with a legitimate political system. As a result, we do not list legality as a separate criterion of legitimacy; rather, we assume that any policy whose legitimacy is to be evaluated is in fact legal. Furthermore, we have in mind the dissatisfactions noted in chapter 2 with top-down systems of watershed management; these may have met legal mandates, but their legitimacy was seen as compromised by their (fully legal) limitations on public input.

6. To appreciate the importance of the distinction between procedural and substantive legitimacy, consider that, as chapter 2 showed, public participation has hardly been the norm over the history of resource management in the United States. Rather, it typically has been seen as the domain of scientific experts and government officials, whose knowledge and legal jurisdiction legitimated their authority. Historically, legitimacy has been primarily a substantive matter: what counted was whether policy enhanced the public's welfare by providing clean water, ample timber, attractive recreational opportunities, and so on. Procedural issues were of lesser concern to policymakers, for whom the mere legality of a decision-making process established its procedural legitimacy. However, recent years have seen an emphasis on direct public involvement in many policy domains (Crowfoot and Wondolleck 1990, Webler and Renn 1995, Yosie and Herbst 1998). (There has also been a strong interest in public participation among political theorists, who have discussed it under the rubric of "deliberative democracy"; Barber 1984, Bohman and Rehg 1997; Elster 1998; Gutmann and Thompson 1996). The varied explanations for this phenomenon all endorse the premise that legitimacy is not exhausted by considerations of substance. Although welfare (the foundation of substantive legitimacy) is certainly crucial, it is not the sole moral value relevant to political life. Legitimacy also involves the value of autonomy, and autonomy justifies robust public participation. Procedural legitimacy thus complements substantive legitimacy, and an understanding of each is necessary for a full analysis of the moral aspect of watershed policymaking.

7. For simplicity we will take *policy* to mean anything from a set of broad goals for a watershed to a specific plan for coming into compliance with a particular statute.

8. This distinction is meant to help limit the notorious ambiguity in the term *stakeholder*, which encompasses policymakers, agency implementers, experts both within and outside government who participate in policymaking and policy implementation, private sector businesspeople who are economically affected by policies, members of the general public who are economically or otherwise affected by policies, environmental interest groups that purport to represent nonhuman values, and others. This diversity of roles is perhaps one reason that the National Research Council adopted the term *interested and affected party* in lieu of *stakeholder* (Stern, Fineberg, and NRC Committee on Risk Characterization 1996). We use the governmental-nongovernmental distinction to help explain the justifications for including nongovernmental stakeholders in policymaking; we acknowledge that we are abstracting from the very wide range of characteristics that distinguish stakeholders in actual cases.

9. For simplicity we ignore the variety of overlapping jurisdictions (local, state, regional, tribal, national, and international) that may apply in particular watershed cases.

10. Other chapters in this book show how including officials from a range of agencies can contribute to the effectiveness of watershed policymaking procedures (see especially chapters 7 and 8).

11. We acknowledge that members of the public often provide local knowledge (Lindblom and Cohen 1979, Ostrom 1990) and that some policymaking processes stipulate public involvement.

12. It is standard to say that such systems are illegitimate because they compromise their citizens' individual rights to political participation, or indeed other civil rights. But rights can be understood in terms of autonomy: people assert rights in order to protect their autonomy. For simplicity, in this section we shall speak about autonomy directly, and not use the language of individual rights.

13. We appeal to both of two senses of hypothetical consent: the empirical claim that if a policymaking procedure meets our criteria, then stakeholders would in fact consent to the resulting policy proposal if asked, and the normative claim that if a policymaking procedure meets our criteria, then stakeholders have a sufficient reason to consent, and so ought to consent if asked (MacLean 1982). The former claim, at least, is subject to empirical testing. Both senses of hypothetical consent rest on the belief that the stakeholders are rational—that they evaluate policy proposals on the basis of reasons (Webler 1995). Rationality here is closely linked to the notion of self-interest: a compelling reason for people to agree to a policy is that it will benefit them. But self-interest can be narrower or wider, and we do not preclude the possibility that some stakeholders will support policies in virtue of the benefits they offer to others—including beings who have no voice in policymaking, such as nonhuman animals or members of future generations.

14. Thus, they represent normative constraints on the "process" element of the framework presented in chapter 1.

15. In practice, groups like this Watershed Council are typically strictly advisory, with final decision-making authority vested by law in an agency, elected officials, or the legislature. However, to make our case about procedural legitimacy clearer, we will treat the public participants as if they have a vote—if not on the policy that goes into effect, then at least on the recommendation to the ultimate decision maker.

Note, however, that as we develop this example, it will remain highly idealized. In particular, we will assume that people are generally self-interested, in that they participate to protect their own interests. But we will assume that they do not engage in highly strategic behavior. We acknowledge that this model of collaboration is abstracted from the complex details of the political contexts that mark actual watershed policy problems. We do this because our focus is not the empirical question of how collaboratives function, but rather the normative question of what makes them legitimate.

16. In what follows, we shall draw on a number of considerations from the political theory of representation, the details of which are not relevant here (Birch 1972, Pitkin 1967). For a discussion of the question of representation in environmental policymaking, see O'Neill (2002); for a more general discussion of representation and deliberative institutions, see Gargarella (1998).

17. Often citizens who are active in a policy area are appointed to policymaking groups. We will treat this as a form of volunteerism.

18. Thus, presumptively, local residents should have more representation than people whose stake in the watershed is more attenuated, such as visitors to the region who come occasionally to enjoy recreational opportunities.

19. See chapter 5.

20. As chapter 5 makes clear, this requirement is especially challenging with respect to groups that are reluctant to become involved in political processes, typically due to historical patterns of exclusion. The costs involved in soliciting their participation are quite high and do not guarantee success. We discuss the conflict between the demands of legitimacy and high transaction costs in chapter 9.

21. See Webler's (1995) use of Habermas's theory of communicative rationality to articulate norms governing public participation in policymaking.

22. We assume stakeholders have broad trust of decision makers here; otherwise, it is doubtful that they would consent to their decisions in any case. See chapter 4 for a fuller discussion of trust issues.

23. This also raises the issue of trust. Unless there is trust of decision makers, a policy decision that favors one side will likely not garner the consent of all stakeholders. See chapter 4.

24. Webler (1995) provides detailed criteria that articulate a range of ways coercion can enter into deliberations. But see Przeworski (1998) for a discussion of the possibility of ideological domination in deliberations.

25. Such an argument underlies judicial rules that forbid withholding exculpatory evidence and refusing to turn over evidence requested during discovery.

26. As Webler (1995) observes, experts can be taken to be responsible to stakeholders; their role can be construed as helping stakeholders distill useable knowledge from otherwise recondite technical information.

27. Indeed, many watershed collaboratives do use a consensus decision rule. See chapters 7 and 8.

28. This problem has long bedeviled democratic theory. For an early solution, see Rousseau (1987). See also Wollheim (1962).

29. It is important to distinguish between sincere disagreement over the merits of a policy from obstructions raised by participants who are simply unwilling to compromise. We assume that narrow opposition raises an important moral issue only if all participants share a commitment to decide on a mutually acceptable policy through their deliberations (Cohen 1997). This commitment points to what might be called the responsibilities of participation: participants must demonstrate their respect for each other by hearing each other out and responding constructively. No doubt strategic behavior, stemming from the desire to further one's own interests whatever the effect on others' interests, is all too common in actual stakeholder processes. But because it thus reflects a refusal to respect the autonomy of other stakeholders it does not present a conceptual challenge to our understanding of procedural legitimacy. We thank Dan Poor for bringing this point to our attention.

30. This claim calls for further empirical research.

31. The theoretical and empirical work presented in chapters 6–8 bears on this point.

32. See chapters 4, 7, and 8 for additional discussion.

33. Ideally, procedural and substantive legitimacy go hand in hand: policy is made in legitimate ways, and it seeks to obtain legitimate ends. However, the actual relation between the two forms of legitimacy may be more intricate: typically trade-offs between them are required. There is no absolute rule that gives one type of legitimacy priority over the other. Rather, their relative importance depends strongly on the detailed circumstances of the given policy problem, including such factors (among others) as the urgency of the problem and the trust stakeholders have in government officials, experts and in each other. See the discussion in chapter 1 about context; in this chapter, we must abstract from the complex details of a watershed collaborative's context, in particular from the political factors that might influence a collaborative's work. We do, however, revisit trust issues in much more detail in chapter 4.

34. We understand "policy outcomes" in the light of the following distinction. A policymaking institution might be effective at producing policy recommendations; this can be called "output" effectiveness. But it is a further question as to whether the recommended policy makes those changes happen; actually bringing those changes about can be called "outcome" effectiveness. What makes a policy effective in this outcome sense, however, is a complex matter. Factors that contribute to outcome effectiveness include technical competence (i.e., the skills of the scientists and others who help design the instruments the policy uses to attain its goals), economic efficiency (i.e., whether these instruments provide the greatest impact at the least cost), and administrative implementability (i.e., whether the agencies charged with implementing the policy have the resources, skills, and bureaucratic will to do so). For simplicity, we will conflate the "output" of the policymaking procedure (the effects proposed for the watershed) with the policy's outcome (the actual changes that occur).

35. For simplicity, we are referring only to benefits to living human beings. For many theorists, and certainly for many activists, the welfare of future human beings, nonhuman species, or of ecological systems is of paramount importance in determining whether a policy's outcome is justified. These possibilities raise complex and controversial questions, but we do not have room to incorporate an adequate discussion of them into this chapter.

36. Indeed, different aspects of a given individual's welfare can likewise diverge: the same person can both enjoy fishing and want low food prices. We are simply passing over the enormously complex questions about how the elements in an individual's welfare should be weighted to determine his or her overall welfare and how the welfare of different individuals should be compared to determine the welfare of society as a whole. For a survey of theories of welfare see Hargreaves Heap et al. (1992).

37. This example recalls the Pareto criterion used by economists, whereby one situation is better than another if it improves the welfare of at least one person

but does not diminish the welfare of anyone else (Sugden 1981). But note that criterion S1 represents a "moralized" version of the Pareto criterion, since, in combination with S2 and S3, it allows the reduction of welfare of parties whose existing level of welfare results from wrongful activities.

38. In Bentham's famous phrase, "Each to count for one and none for more than one." Note that we are not here dealing with a right (grounded on autonomy) to participate in decision making.

39. It may nonetheless be politically prudent to take account of the interests of people whose activities are found not to be rightful.

40. Note that we have chosen these two activities for this example somewhat arbitrarily, to illustrate our claim that stakeholders ought to have a role in determining what counts as rightful activity. We are not offering a position on which specific activities ought or ought not be considered rightful—we take that determination to be a matter for local deliberation.

41. Both situations would fail the Pareto criterion. Economists would say that one group is externalizing costs involved in raising its own welfare by making the other group bear them; the discussion that follows bears on the issue of internalizing these external costs.

42. For this reason, we hold that the strict Pareto criterion is ultimately too limiting: virtually every policy change will produce winners and losers (Hausman and McPherson 1993).

43. This is called a "potential Pareto improvement," since at least potentially the "winners" could compensate the "losers." The idea that one situation is better than another if it involves a potential Pareto improvement, but where compensation is not actually paid, is known as the Kaldor-Hicks criterion (Hausman and McPherson 1993).

44. We acknowledge the profound challenge raised by the extreme difficulty (if not outright impossibility) of comparing different parties' interests, hence of calculating the proper amount of compensation (Hausman and McPherson 1993). As we suggest below, stakeholder participation offers a potential solution to this problem.

45. There is a parallel here to the requirement of fair compensation in cases where the government seizes private property through eminent domain.

46. These admittedly simplistic examples are meant solely to illustrate the idea of compensation. But note that market-like schemes for tradable permits to increase nutrient loading have as their moral basis the notion that the voluntary exchanges that market mechanisms facilitate are fair in the sense we have explained.

47. In line with the parallel cited in note 45, where government seizes private property to prevent a harm (an exercise of what is called the "police power"), no compensation is necessary (Freund 1904).

48. Our endorsement of bargaining is based on the assumption that the safeguards discussed with respect to procedural legitimacy are in place, so that, in

particular, the representatives of less powerful groups are protected from being pressured into accepting a bargain that is disadvantageous.

49. See chapter 4 for a theoretical discussion of this point.

50. See chapter 7.

51. We return to this problem in chapter 9.

52. Cf. Perez's (2002) discussion of dispute resolution in environmentally sensitive international construction contracts.

II
Collaborative Engagement Processes in Watersheds

4

A Trust-Based Guide to Stakeholder Participation

Will Focht and Zev Trachtenberg

In chapter 3, we argued that considerations of legitimacy demand that stakeholders participate in the processes that formulate watershed policy. However, this general moral imperative covers a wide range of situations that present distinct challenges to—and opportunities for—public participation. In this chapter, we consider how specific details of the context in which policy is to be made (specifically, stakeholders' trust of policy actors) influences the kind of participatory process that is likely to be most effective in generating policies acceptable to stakeholders.

The fact that context is crucial in determining the appropriate strategy for participation has been recognized at the federal level. For instance, the U.S. Environmental Protection Agency urges agency officials to "identify and select the public consultation or involvement process appropriate to the decision being made."[1] Likewise, the National Research Council (Stern, Fineberg, and NRC Committee, 7) advocates stakeholder involvement in processes for evaluating and managing environmental risks, arguing that "those responsible for a risk characterization should begin by developing a provisional *diagnosis of the decision situation* so that they can better match the analytic-deliberative process leading to the characterization to the needs of the decision."

Despite their recognition of the importance of context in the design of successful participatory strategies, neither the EPA nor the NRC offers concrete recommendations on how to act on this recognition; both organizations stop short of providing specific guidance on when to use which strategy, leaving this up to the discretion of decision makers. In this chapter, we address this gap by developing and then testing a framework that offers context-specific guidance for designing participatory strategies that satisfy stakeholders' expectations and preferences.

We suggest that the most important aspect of the watershed management decision context is trust. Consistent with the conclusions of Hupcey (2002) and Castelfranchi and Falcone (2000),[2] trust relates to stakeholders'[3] willingness to defer to the competence and discretion of others to manage risk on their behalf. Two dimensions of trust are most relevant: stakeholders' judgments of the trustworthiness of other stakeholders (which we label social trust) and stakeholders' judgments of the trustworthiness of policy officials (which we label official trust). The overlap of these two dimensions yields four decision contexts for which four distinct stakeholder participation strategies are recommended. We first describe the theoretical framework. Then we present empirical support for the framework by testing predictions generated with data obtained from interviews of 150 stakeholders in the Illinois River watershed in eastern Oklahoma. We close with a discussion of how the analytic-deliberative framework proposed by the National Research Council (Stern, Fineberg, and the NRC Committee 1996) is ideally suited to stakeholder participation in watershed management contexts involving both low social and official trust.

Theoretical Framework

Trust, Participation and Policy Effectiveness

Over the past four decades, the decline of social capital (norms of reciprocity, thriving social networks) and negative perceptions of government performance have contributed to a decline in the general levels of trust within society (Carnevale 1995; Chanley, Rudolph, and Rahn 2000; Coleman 1990; Craig 1993; Nye, Zelikow, and King 1997; Orren 1997; Rosenstone and Hansen 1993; Uslaner 2000), prompting concerns about the effectiveness of policymaking institutions (Lipset and Schneider 1983) and the legitimacy of government generally (Brown 1994).[4] This concern is especially acute regarding bureaucratic structures that have downplayed stakeholders' desires to participate in policymaking. Indeed, the renewed emphasis on stakeholder participation that is a theme of this book is in part a response to the erosion of public trust in bureaucracies. The stakeholder participation framework offered here is meant to address this concern about effectiveness by prescribing participation strategies that improve the chances for policy formulation and adoption, that is, output effectiveness.[5]

Policy output effectiveness, we argue, is enhanced when stakeholder participation strategies embodied in policy processes appropriately match stakeholders' participation preferences. In turn, stakeholders' participation preferences are strongly influenced by their judgments of the trustworthiness of each other and of policy officials. These judgments underlie stakeholders' willingness to cooperate with officials and each other in formulating policy that will be successfully adopted by policymakers. Moreover, selection of appropriate participation strategies can itself enhance trust. Thus, the possibility exists for a recursive, mutually reinforcing, relationship among trust, participation, and effectiveness.

Dynamic and Recursive Relationship among Trust, Participation, and Effectiveness   Trust judgments are dynamic (though this has been rarely studied by trust researchers).[6] Particularly when stakes are high, stakeholders continually monitor the policy environment for new information that may produce changes in their judgments of trustworthiness—of both policy officials and each other. Stakeholders may move between trust, which prompts deference toward others, and distrust, which prompts vigilance.[7] For example, stakeholders who distrust policy officials may initially insist on participating to protect their interests. During the participation process, however, they might learn that the officials can be trusted, thus reducing their incentive to participate—a move toward deference. Alternatively, stakeholders initially may be willing to defer to the competence and discretion of policy officials and later, but after learning that the officials are not acting in their interests, they may demand to be more involved—a move toward vigilance.

With respect to social trust, stakeholders who trust other stakeholders may be initially willing to collaborate in finding a solution. If they then learn that other stakeholders are working hard to maximize their own private interests at the expense of the collective interest, they might adopt a more defensive role—a move toward vigilance. Alternatively, distrusting stakeholders may learn that their perceived opponents share important values with them, which motivates a greater willingness to collaborate and cooperate—a move toward deference.

In sum, stakeholder participation strategies should change as trust judgments change in order to maintain the proper mix of deference and vigilance. Failure to adapt participation strategies to changing trust contexts can jeopardize policy effectiveness just as surely as adopting the wrong strategy in the first place.[8]

The dynamic and recursive relationship between trust and participation strategy presents both opportunities for and obstacles to increasing policy output effectiveness. If the appropriate strategy is selected, trust is increased and vigilance is decreased. Thus, if stakeholders have confidence in those responsible for policymaking, political demands are decreased and policy output effectiveness is enhanced. But if an inappropriate strategy is selected, trust is eroded and the demand for participation is increased.[9] Erosion of deference can render policymaking more inefficient and ineffective.[10] Thus, trust matters because institutions that enjoy higher trust, built through good policies, function better (Uslaner 2002).

Our argument that the relationship between trust and participation is recursive should not be interpreted as an endorsement of a goal of eventually eliminating the need for stakeholder participation in policy formulation. On the one hand, it seems entirely plausible to assume that as one problem becomes more tractable, another intractable one will arise in its place. On the other, as we argued in chapter 3, stakeholder participation is intrinsically important to policy legitimation. Moreover, trust is not simply an instrument used to define appropriate stakeholder participation strategies but rather an end that is valuable in itself. As Putnam (2000) makes clear, trust and social capital are essential to a well-ordered and flourishing society. Thus, trust is important not only to considerations of policy legitimacy but also to social cohesion and cooperation more broadly.

Relationships among Stakeholders' Trust, Stakeholders' Participation Preferences, and Policy Output Effectiveness   Stakeholders' participation preferences influence policy output effectiveness because they set the context for how policy should be formulated. This influence is mediated by the translation of stakeholder participation preferences by policymakers in their design and implementation of a stakeholder participation program.

Figure 4.1 illustrates our conceptualization of the influence of stake-holders' trust judgments on their participation preferences and on policy output effectiveness.[11] We recognize, of course, that output effectiveness is not directly affected by participation preferences but rather by the participation itself. The shaded box in figure 4.1 emphasizes that the product of the translation of participation preference to participation strategy is that which ultimately influences output effectiveness as well as its impact on stakeholders' subsequent trust of policymakers.[12]

Foundation of the Framework
A key motivation for developing the framework is our belief that past failures to gain stakeholder support for watershed management policies are due to the failure of policymakers to match stakeholder participation strategies to stakeholders' preferences for participation. Moreover, we believe that stakeholders' participation preferences are influenced by their judgments of the trustworthiness of other participants in the policy process. The more they trust other participants, the more stakeholders are willing to defer to their policy judgments; the more they distrust, the more vigilant stakeholders will be in protecting their interests and the more insistent they may be on participating in the policy process.[13] A means to increase policy output effectiveness therefore is to assess stakeholders' trust of the other participants[14] involved in a particular policy context[15] and then to select the stakeholder participation strategy that matches their preference.

We posit that two judgments of trust influence the willingness of stakeholders to defer—or, alternatively, to be vigilant—in the policy process: social trust and official trust:

Social trust.   Trust is a key enabler of cooperation (McKnight, Cummings, and Chervany 1995). Stakeholders' judgments of the trustworthiness of other stakeholders are influenced primarily by their own, and their perception of others', willingness to cooperate in the policy process. Cooperation can be stimulated by identifying shared goals and values—if not about desired policy outcomes, then about a shared desire to enhance policy effectiveness (to see that "something gets done"). If stakeholders do not trust other stakeholders, they are more likely to adopt a defensive strategy to protect their own interests in regard to those of other stakeholders.

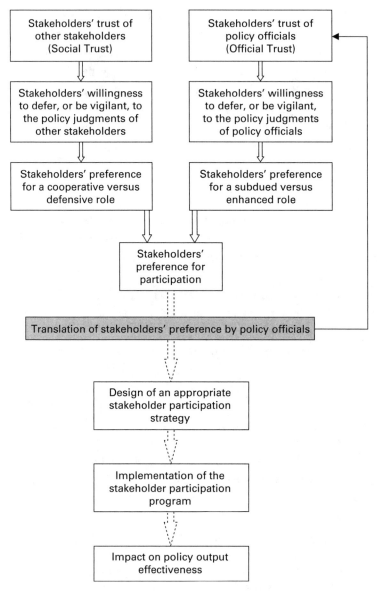

Figure 4.1
Influence of stakeholders' trust judgments on policy output effectiveness

Official trust.   Stakeholders' judgments of the trustworthiness of policy officials are influenced primarily by their perception of how well officials honor their responsibility to act as stewards of stakeholders' interests. If they trust officials, stakeholders will adopt a more subdued role in the policy process. If they distrust officials, however, stakeholders will adopt a more enhanced and intense role to safeguard their interests in relation to policy officials.

Influence of Trust on Vigilance   Stakeholders are more likely to be vigilant and insist on participation if they believe that other policy participants may harm their interests (Baier 1986, Hupcey 2002, Sztompka 2001). The judgment that harm may occur due to another's actions may be based on two beliefs: suspicion about another's intentions and sensitivity to opportunism (Markóczy 2002). Both beliefs motivate an increased willingness to be vigilant, and both can be related to distrust.[16]

This definition of trust thus equates judgments of trustworthiness to judgments of risk acceptability (Coleman 1990, Earle and Cvetkovich 1995, Luhmann 1979, Ruscio 1996). Risk is often operationalized as the interaction of two parameters: the severity or magnitude of an adverse consequence and its associated probability of occurrence (National Research Council, Committee on the Institutional Means for Assessment of Risks to Public Health 1983). Thus, risk increases when either the severity of the adverse consequence or its probability of occurrence increases. Analogously, trust can also be defined as the product of the interaction between the perceived stake that is at risk should trust be betrayed (equivalent to the severity of an adverse consequence) and the perceived likelihood that the trustee will fail to act to protect the stakeholders' stake (equivalent to the probability of occurrence of the adverse consequence).[17]

Attribution of trustworthiness involves complex judgments about risk to the trustor's well-being—about his or her vulnerability to harm. It combines judgments about the stake that is at risk and the likelihood that the stake will be successfully safeguarded by the trustee. The greater the stake (potential harm) to the stakeholder, the more trustworthy the trustee must be before the risk is voluntarily assumed. The probability of stake protection is itself a combined judgment of the ability of the trustee to manage the risk (a competency judgment) and the belief that the trustee will indeed honor an obligation to do so (a judgment of the trustee's motives and intentions).[18]

In sum, stakeholders are inclined to distrust those whom they judge will cause them harm, due to either incompetence or ill will. In this case, they will maintain (or increase) their vigilance. But if stakeholders judge other participants as competent and willing to protect their interests, they are more inclined to relax their vigilance and defer to the other participants' judgments.

Influence of Vigilance on Participation Preference   Stakeholders' willingness to defer to others' policy judgments influences their desire to participate in the policy process. If trust is high and stakeholders are more willing to defer, then their desire to participate will be lower. Distrust is expected to increase stakeholders' vigilance against threats to their interests; thus, they will be more willing to participate.[19] This relationship is based on the belief that stakeholders rationally want to minimize transaction costs of participation by free riding whenever feasible.[20] Where trust is high, the transaction costs of participation may outweigh the benefits—especially considering the opportunity costs of alternative activities that compete for stakeholders' attentions—and therefore, stakeholders are more likely to defer to others. (Chapter 7 explicitly considers the role that the transaction costs of cooperation play in stakeholder collaborations.)

Influence of Participation on Policy Output Effectiveness   Our framework prescribes how participation should be designed to enhance policy output effectiveness in the light of whether stakeholders trust or distrust other participants. Thus, the framework recognizes that the participation–effectiveness relationship is contingent on the trust context and makes appropriate prescriptions. If the participation design fails to match stakeholders' preferences, then trust is eroded and output effectiveness is threatened. For example, if policy institutions in high-trust contexts demand intensive participation by stakeholders, they are likely to meet with inadequate attendance since stakeholders see no reason to spend time on what they do not regard as a problem requiring their attention. But if the translation from preferences to participation design is appropriate, then trust is increased and output effectiveness is enhanced. For example, if policy institutions in contexts marked by distrust allow for power sharing and robust deliberation, they can build official trust (by demonstrating policy officials' respect for stakeholders) and social trust (by providing an institutional setting in which stakeholders can recognize common values), thus increasing policy output effectiveness and moving the context toward one marked by deference.

From Trust to Policy Output Effectiveness: Questions Raised   The conceptual linkage from stakeholders' trust of other policy participants to policy vigilance to participation preference to participation design to policy output effectiveness prompts four questions:

• How much trust is required before stakeholders are willing to defer to the discretion and expertise of others to manage risk on their behalf in a watershed policy arena?
• Is stakeholders' trust of other policy actors related to their participation preferences?
• If stakeholders do not defer initially, will appropriate participation strategies succeed at raising their trust and thus encourage deference in the future?
• Even if trust (hence deference) is not increased, do appropriate participation strategies in fact promote policy output effectiveness?

We will address only the first two questions in this chapter, after we lay out the structure of our framework. Chapters 7 and 8 consider the fourth question in detail and the third question only indirectly. Careful consideration of the third question requires a longitudinal research design, which was not incorporated into any of the studies presented in this book.

Structure of the Framework: Stakeholder Trust Dimensions
The purpose of this framework is to characterize the contexts in which particular watershed policy decisions are made. We hold that context should be understood in terms of the trust stakeholders have for two groups of policy participants: other stakeholders and policy officials. Thus, social trust and official trust are two dimensions of stakeholder trust. We identify two positions along each dimension (trust and

Table 4.1
Hypothesized stakeholder participation roles related to level of trust

Trust dimension	Level of trust	Stakeholder participation role
Social	Trust	*Cooperative role* Stakeholders are willing to cooperate in the policy process
	Distrust	*Defensive role* Stakeholders wish to participate defensively to protect their interests
Official	Trust	*Subdued role* Stakeholders are willing to allow policy officials to lead the policy process
	Distrust	*Enhanced role* Stakeholders wish to participate energetically in the policy process

distrust), and accordingly identify four corresponding roles, or types of participation, that we hypothesize stakeholders will prefer in the respective contexts.[21] These roles are summarized in table 4.1.

Social Trust—Cooperative versus Defensive Role in Stakeholder Participation   Social trust refers to stakeholders' tendency to accept the judgments of other stakeholders in the policy process. In contexts of social trust, stakeholders are inclined to cooperate with each other in a spirit of positive collaboration toward a shared goal (Gambetta 2000, Hardin 1997, Yamagishi 1988).[22] Indeed cooperative efforts should proceed quickly and smoothly, since they will not be hindered by stakeholders' suspicions of each other's motives. This may result from stakeholders' agreement that achieving a policy outcome is best, since they will accept the judgments of people with whom they already agree. But consensus on a specific policy goal is not necessary for high social trust, since stakeholders might all recognize the importance of finding a solution to the policy problem, and they might judge each other to be competent and of goodwill despite their disagreements. This judgment is facilitated by the existence of sufficient social capital in the stakeholder community (Putnam 2000) and the civic mindedness that it sustains.

Where social distrust exists, stakeholders are less inclined to cooperate with each other. Nonetheless, their suspicions of each other's motives or abilities induce them to participate in policymaking to defend their own interests. This defensive form of participation might result from profound disagreement over policy goals or the lack of shared commitment to the idea that they ought to collaborate to solve a shared problem— that is, a lack of social capital. In either case, the paradoxical situation where stakeholders do not wish to cooperate, but nonetheless insist on participating in the policy process, poses a strong challenge for the development of effective policy. The proper participation strategy in this situation should aim at building consensus on the importance of policy effectiveness, if not on policy ends. Collaboration may help cultivate social capital by producing familiarity, identification of shared values, respect for demonstrated competence, tolerance for different perspectives, and a civic orientation—all of which build social trust.

Official Trust—Subdued versus Enhanced Role in Stakeholder Participation Official trust refers to stakeholders' willingness to defer to policy officials' policy judgments. According to Barber (1983), trustworthiness implies both a judgment of technical competence and fiduciary responsibility. In other words, policy officials are trusted if both their ability (competence) and motives (discretion) are judged as trustworthy.

Where official trust exists, stakeholders have confidence that officials have their best interests at heart and the ability to make policy decisions that will successfully protect those interests. Thus, they see no reason to participate intensively in the policymaking process. Accordingly, they are willing to assume a subdued role in policymaking, whereby they tend to defer to officials' policy judgments.

In contexts of official distrust, however, stakeholders assume a much more enhanced role, motivated by the belief that officials are incompetent or irresponsible, or both.[23] In this case, independent policy experts are required (if competence is at issue) or officials participate only with the same status as other stakeholders (if they are seen as pursuing their own interests instead of those of stakeholders), or both. To the extent that officials accept the enhanced role for stakeholders by sharing power with them, it is plausible that stakeholders' trust of officials will increase sufficiently to allow stakeholders to take on the subdued role.

Table 4.2
Stakeholder participation strategy prescriptions

			Social Trust	
			Trust	Distrust
			Cooperative role	Defensive role
Official Trust	Trust	Subdued role	Confirmation strategy	Facilitation strategy
	Distrust	Enhanced role	Consultation strategy	Negotiation strategy

Stakeholder Participation Prescriptions

The combination of the two stakeholder trust dimensions defines four contexts (see table 4.2). For each trust context, a stakeholder participation strategy is prescribed that will improve policy output effectiveness.

Confirmation Strategy: Officials Lead, Stakeholders Confirm   In this context, produced from the combination of social trust and official trust, stakeholders judge that policy officials are both competent and well meaning, and they share with other stakeholders the desire to produce a policy output, if not a common policy goal. As a result, the framework suggests that stakeholders will be willing to accept a subdued and cooperative role in the policy process. In this case, a *confirmation strategy* is recommended in which policy officials assume a lead role in policy formulation, then seek confirmation from stakeholders that they share the need for policy, if not policy goals. Trust along both dimensions is maintained by the continuing effectiveness of policy—in particular, its ability to provide what stakeholders want.

For example, suppose a municipality owns a wastewater treatment facility from which raw sewage overflows during heavy storms. The river into which the waste is discharged has a limited capacity to assimilate the waste, and the adverse health and environmental impacts are well understood. Downstream stakeholders are universally opposed to these continuing discharges. However, the municipality argues that it would be too expensive to upgrade the treatment plant. Municipal officials hold that the increased amount of water in the river that results from high rainfall is enough to dilute contaminants safely from the sewer overflows. Though downstream stakeholders disagree with this claim, they agree that further analysis could be definitive. Trusted state policy officials, relying on data provided by both municipal and downstream stakeholders, as well as data obtained from their own study, find that dilution is not always adequate to reduce contaminants to safe levels, especially during the winter. The officials recommend, after a cost-effectiveness study, that the municipality can replace manhole covers with holes in them quickly and easily with solid covers that can be sealed to prevent excess storm water from entering the sewage system, thus preventing the overflows. This policy recommendation is circulated to stakeholders for their comment. The plan triggers no significant opposition and is adopted by the municipality.

Consultation Strategy: Officials Consult with Stakeholders   In this context, produced from the combination of social trust and official distrust, stakeholders doubt the competence or good faith of policy officials, but they are willing to cooperate with each other in the policy process. Since stakeholders cannot rely on officials to develop effective policies alone, they prefer to participate in a more deliberate way. However, given the high level of social trust, their participation need not involve resource-intensive deliberation among themselves; rather, the officials need only consult with stakeholders first before formulating policy to determine their preferences and ensure that adequate analyses have been conducted. In this case, effectiveness is most improved when policy officials demonstrate in advance that their policy will safeguard stakeholders' interests. Official trust is increased as officials demonstrate that they are willing to adopt policies that stakeholders find acceptable.

For example, suppose that stakeholders in an area are socially and economically dependent on tourism and the relatively undisturbed state of the surrounding watershed. In fact, many residents moved there because they cherish its pristine nature. They agree that threats to tourism caused by damage to the watershed should be minimized. A timber company has proposed purchasing large tracts of land in the watershed to harvest trees for lumber, which stakeholders perceive as threatening. The timber company has responded to stakeholder concerns by offering to cut timber in a responsible manner and then to replant trees after harvest. Because policy officials have historically sided with economic development interests in the past, stakeholders believe that the pristine nature of the watershed and the tourism that it attracts will be sacrificed for timber harvesting. Aware of this history, policy officials consult with key stakeholder representatives from all perspectives to ask for their preferences and the analyses they would like to see performed to make an informed decision. The officials undertake appropriate studies and present the results to the stakeholders. After reviewing these data, stakeholders agree that limited and careful harvesting with replanting can take place on a restricted portion of the watershed without any significant damage to the environment or to tourism. The officials adopt the limited harvesting policy and require that periodic inspections be conducted and reports submitted for public inspection to ensure that unacceptable damage does not occur. This assurance helps build stakeholders' trust of officials.

Facilitation Strategy: Officials Facilitate Stakeholders' Negotiation   In this context, produced from the combination of social distrust and official trust, stakeholders have full confidence in policy officials, but are unwilling to set aside their differences with each other in order to cooperate. Since stakeholders do not trust their peers to make decisions on their behalf, they are inclined to insist that they be allowed to represent themselves in the policy process to defend their interests from damage by other stakeholders. Since policy officials are trusted, they can facilitate these negotiations. Effectiveness results from stakeholders' willingness to allow officials to mediate stakeholder differences; this willingness rests on their belief that officials are competent, impartial, and fiduciarily responsible. To the extent that officials are successful at brokering a solution to the policy problem, stakeholders may come to appreciate their mutual willingness to negotiate, thus improving social trust.

Suppose that a watershed contains a large number of poultry feeding operations and that the waste from the animals is applied to local land as a fertilizer.[24] Officials agree that phosphorus runoff from the land is a major contributor to eutrophication of the lake that receives the water. They also agree that human-generated organic waste from local residents' septic tanks and from the large numbers of visitors to the river also contributes to the problem. Fearing loss of business, operators who rent canoes and rafts to tourists argue that chicken producers should institute controls to prevent runoff from their operations. However, the producers blame residents for their septic tanks and recreationists for their trash dumping, beer drinking, and biological waste discharges, and instead argue for increased enforcement and trash collection policies. Attempts to forge a collaborative approach between the two groups fail because each side believes strongly that the facts uniquely support its own case.

Both sides appeal to state policy officials to do something to protect the river. The officials convene a series of meetings with both sides, individually and together, to learn about their concerns and design a study to quantify nutrient sources and impacts. Both sides agree that a properly designed study of causes and effects will authoritatively determine responsibility for the problem. Moreover, both sides agree that any solution must balance economic costs and benefits.

The officials commission a comprehensive study of eutrophication, which shows that poultry farmers are most to blame for eutrophication of the lake but that septic tanks are most to blame for eutrophication of the river during the warm season; recreationists are shown to be a minor contributor. Policy officials develop a plan that includes grants, educational programs, and a phased implementation strategy for poultry farmers to manage better the application of chicken litter as fertilizer. The officials also impose stricter regulations on septic systems. The officials present this plan to the stakeholder groups, who agree to the plan after receiving satisfactory answers to their concerns about costs and effectiveness. The ability of the stakeholders to reach agreement builds social trust and enhances social capital.

Negotiation Strategy: Officials and Stakeholders Negotiate Together   In this context, produced from the combination of social distrust and official distrust, stakeholders are disaffected from officials as well as from each other. In this most challenging context in which to produce effective policies, stakeholders are unwilling to cooperate among themselves to find a solution and are reluctant to accept officials as policy brokers. In this case, effectiveness is bolstered when stakeholders and policy officials jointly participate as parties to a policy negotiation. A neutral third party, acceptable to both stakeholders and policy officials, should facilitate. Moreover, independent experts may be required to conduct analyses. The willingness of policy officials to share power in deliberating over policy gives them an opportunity to build official trust through demonstration of their expertise and their commitment to protect stakeholders' interests. Social trust can be increased by sharing values, building social capital, and working toward consent. In other words, the pairing of analysis (building knowledge and competence) and deliberation (building trust and social capital) recommended by the National Research Council (Stern, Fineberg, and the NRC Commission, 1996) is most appropriate to enhancing policy effectiveness in this context.

Suppose that competing land uses in a watershed have produced chronic controversy. Residential and recreational developers argue that their activities produce vast economic benefits and produce important public amenities. Long-standing agricultural interests feel threatened by these developments and view them as impositions on traditional lifestyles and infringements on personal liberties, particularly property rights. Disagreement on the types and magnitudes of threats to water quality, economic growth, personal freedoms, and cultural traditions dominates the discourse among stakeholders. Policy officials are viewed by agricultural interests as biased in favor of economic interests, by economic interests as incompetent, and by environmental interests as both.

After years of failed attempts to produce an effective watershed management plan, officials decide that they need an outside facilitator. They obtain a federal grant; a team of independent technical experts conducts a comprehensive study of watershed impacts on water quality, and independent professional facilitators obtain an assessment of stakeholder concerns and management preferences. The findings of these studies are presented first to policy officials and stakeholders in separate meetings. Each group's reactions are presented to the other, leading to a common realization that development within riparian zones, inappropriate behavior by recreationists, and illegal trash dumping must be halted. These issues had not been considered before by policy officials, and they reveal a solid basis for common ground. The facilitators use this joint recognition of common interest as the occasion to convene a joint meeting of officials and stakeholders.

Eventually a consensus emerges on a policy for restoring riparian zones, cleaning up illegal dumps, regulating littering and socially undesirable behavior by recreationists, and consolidating utility permitting to ensure that properly designed septic tanks are installed before water use permits are issued. In addition, the group agrees that it should meet once a year to review progress and consider future actions. All agree that an incremental policy approach is best and that policies should be revised whenever new information becomes available that indicates that policies are not effective. Over time, social and official trust is built among the participants, and meetings become less acrimonious and frequent.

Framework Summary
Table 4.3 presents a summary of the four trust contexts and their associated stakeholder participation prescriptions.

Empirical Test

Thus far, we have presented a theoretical framework that links trust with policy output effectiveness. We proposed a scheme for analyzing the context in which watershed policy is to be made in terms of the trust that stakeholders have for policy officials and for each other, and using this analysis to choose the strategy for stakeholder participation that has the best prospect for producing an acceptable policy.[25] We now turn to an empirical test of our framework: an investigation of the extent to which stakeholders' trust in officials and themselves predicts the participation strategy they would prefer for the resolution of a watershed policy conflict. Our data are drawn from detailed research on the Illinois River Basin in eastern Oklahoma.

Introduction to the Illinois River Watershed
The Illinois is Oklahoma's most prized scenic and pristine river. It and its two major tributaries (Flint Creek and Barren, or Baron, Fork Creek) flow freely from their headwaters in northwestern Arkansas to a dam that forms Tenkiller Ferry Reservoir, south of the town of Tahlequah. Together the three streams comprise a corridor 191 kilometers long and drain a watershed of 2,331 square kilometers in three counties in Oklahoma (combined population, 80,000) (Meo et al. 2002). The Illinois

Table 4.3
Context-specific stakeholder participation recommendations

Social trust (preferred role)	Official trust (preferred role)	Stakeholder participation recommendation	Participation strategy description
Trust (cooperative)	Trust (subdued)	Confirmation	Policy officials formulate policy in conformance with their understanding of stakeholder preferences and then submit the policy proposal and its rationale to stakeholders to *confirm* stakeholder acceptance before adoption
Trust (cooperative)	Distrust (enhanced)	Consultation	Policy officials *consult* with stakeholders to identify their policy preferences before they formulate and adopt policy
Distrust (defensive)	Trust (subdued)	Facilitation	Policy officials *facilitate* a policy dialogue among stakeholders to formulate a policy, which officials then adopt
Distrust (defensive)	Distrust (enhanced)	Negotiation	Policy officials assist and participate in a stakeholder *negotiation*, which is facilitated by an independent mediator and informed by independent analysts, to formulate a policy, which officials then adopt

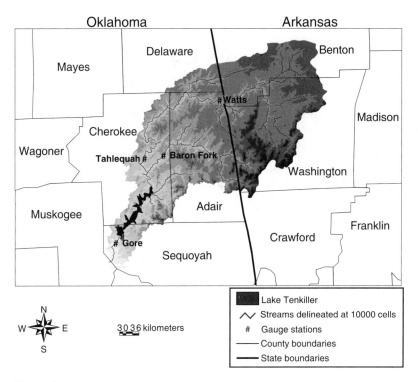

Figure 4.2
Illinois River watershed

River provides multiple social benefits to the citizens of the state and region. It provides drinking water for Tahlequah and Watts and irrigates farms and nurseries. It also provides habitat to an abundance of wildlife, including several threatened and endangered species of plants and animals. In addition, the river corridor is a popular tourist and recreation attraction and in 1977 was the first river designated as a wild and scenic river by the state. Tourism is the major industry in the area. Annually, more than 180,000 people float the Illinois River by canoe, raft, or kayak. An estimated 350,000 enjoy swimming, fishing, camping, hiking, birding, and hunting opportunities, drawing users from Oklahoma, Arkansas, Missouri, Kansas, and Texas (Bality et al. 1998). Figure 4.2 provides a map of the watershed.

Though the economy is based primarily on tourism, a substantial portion of economic activity derives from agriculture—especially from poultry farming and cattle ranching—and from plant nurseries, forestry, and gravel and limestone mining. The city of Tahlequah, which hosts Northeastern Oklahoma State University and the tribal government of the Cherokee Nation, also helps anchor the regional economy (Bality et al. 1998).

Despite these benefits, threats to the watershed are apparent. The area has seen increasing agricultural development, particularly with large-scale poultry feeding operations. Recent studies have indicated that the water quality in the Illinois has deteriorated, particularly from nutrient loading. Although both point and nonpoint sources contribute nutrients, nonpoint agricultural sources are responsible for most of the phosphorous loading. Recreational users and agricultural users blame each other for the decline in water quality. Riverfront property owners also blame recreationists for trespassing on their land, littering stream banks, and rowdy behavior. Many in Oklahoma blame effluent discharges from the wastewater treatment plant near the Arkansas city of Fayetteville. Oklahoma's dispute with Arkansas eventually led to a U.S. Supreme Court decision in 1992 and is still continuing with a judicial dispute concerning the Oklahoma's recent definition of more stringent phosphorus concentration limits.[26]

This pattern of stakeholder groups trading blame for the river's problems has meant that management of the Illinois River watershed has been the center of political controversy for more than twenty-five years. Since 1970, management has been held by Oklahoma Scenic River Commission (OSRC), which has attempted to balance stakeholder claims. The OSRC has been frustrated, however, in its efforts to implement a comprehensive management plan. The need for a plan was recognized as early as 1979, when a study showed that the Illinois River was not ready for designation under the federal Wild and Scenic Rivers Act. In the early 1990s, the OSRC undertook five years of difficult work and released a draft plan in late 1998 that proposes water quality protection goals and implementation strategies. Despite this work, the OSRC too had come under intense criticism by more recently elected members of the commission.[27]

The watershed policy management challenge that exists in the Illinois River watershed is the persistent inability of stakeholders to reach agreement about how to protect this shared resource. In recognition of this problem, the U.S. Environmental Protection Agency, in cooperation with the National Science Foundation, awarded a water and watersheds research grant to a team of collaborators at the University of Oklahoma, Oklahoma State University, and the University of Oklahoma Health Sciences Center to conduct a five-year study of impacts in the watershed and test a protocol for policymaking' that will lead to impact management policy that is simultaneously technically effective, economically efficient, administratively implementable, and sociopolitically acceptable. In the course of conducting research associated with this grant, we collected data that bear on the topic of this chapter.

Interview Methodology
The data were obtained from open-ended interviews conducted with 150 respondents in 1999. To maximize the representativeness of the sample of stakeholders and policymakers contacted for participation, the watershed population was divided along two dimensions: geographic and demographic. These dimensions were selected because it is reasonably predicted that opinions regarding impacts and their management vary by location and occupation (due, for example, to different stakes, values, relationships with the river, and experiences). Individual participants were selected by either reputation (known opinion leaders, agency representatives, policy elites, organizational leaders, attendees at Oklahoma Scenic River Commission meetings, and others) or snowballing (reference by previous interviewees based on their having different perspectives). The interviews were conducted at the homes of or other locations chosen by the participants and lasted an average of two and a half hours. The participants received no remuneration for their participation.

Tables 4A.1 and 4A.2 (in the chapter appendix) present categorical and demographic profiles, respectively, of the participants.

Results and Discussion
Interviewers asked stakeholders to give their judgments of the trustworthiness of policy officials and other stakeholders and to indicate their preferences for participation in policymaking. The stakeholder trust data and participation preference ranking data were analyzed to determine how well our framework predicted stakeholders' preferences for participation, given the level of their trust of policy officials and each other.

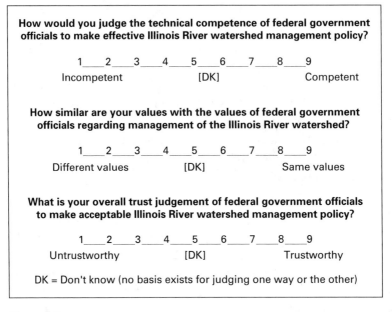

Figure 4.3
Example trust judgment scales

Trust Judgments   Stakeholders' judgments of their trust of policy officials and other stakeholders were obtained using nine-point scales, which
were recoded as 1 (very high distrust) to 9 (very high trust).[28] The three
scales relating to the trustworthiness of federal government officials
shown in figure 4.3 were repeated for state government officials, expert
officials and other stakeholders.[29]

Table 4.4 presents a summary of stakeholders' trust judgments. Several observations may be made about these data. First, as anticipated,
experts are judged as most highly technically competent, followed
by federal officials and state officials; stakeholders are judged least
competent.[30]

Second, stakeholders judge federal officials as sharing fewer values
with them, followed by state officials and, finally, fellow stakeholders.
This finding was also anticipated. However, it was surprising to find
that stakeholders believe that experts share their values more than other
policy actors do. Following Braithwaithe (1998), we anticipated that
value congruence with experts would be less salient than technical com-

Table 4.4
Stakeholders' trust judgments

Trust dimension	Trust component	Mean	Median	Mode
Social trust	Technical competence	5.58	6	7
	Shared values	6.22	6	8
	Overall social trust	6.26	7	7
Official trust	Federal official competence	6.33	7	8
	Federal official values	5.30	5	5
	Overall federal official trust	5.66	6	7
	State official competence	6.73	7	7
	State official values	6.03	6	7
	Overall state official trust	6.18	7	7
	Expert official competence	7.51	8	8
	Expert official values	6.92	7	8
	Overall expert official trust	7.11	8	8
	Overall official trust	6.32	7	7

petence.[31] However, Sztompka (1999) offers an explanation. He identifies three types of expectations involved in trust judgments: instrumental (competence, predictability, efficiency, and reasonableness), axiological (civility, truthfulness, and justice), and fiduciary (dispassion, generosity, and responsibility to others). Given that the instrumental trust dimension concerns competence and not value congruence, we conclude that stakeholders' value-similarity judgments are based on axiological and fiduciary trust attributes.[32]

Third, stakeholders trust each other more than they trust federal and state officials, presumably because they believe they do not share values as much with government officials who do not live in the watershed communities. However, they trust experts more than they trust each other due to both technical competence and shared values.

Fourth, we found stakeholders' overall trust judgments of federal officials, state officials, and each other correlated more closely with their shared value judgments than to their technical competence judgments (see table 4.5). Only stakeholders' overall trust of experts correlated more closely with technical competence than to shared values. Stakeholders trust public officials and fellow stakeholders based more on their value similarity than for their technical competence. Only experts, who

Table 4.5
Comparison of Pearson's bivariate correlations between overall trust-shared values and between overall trust-technical competency pairs (N = 150)

Trust dimension	Shared value judgment	Technical competence judgment
Overall social trust	0.735*	0.433*
Overall trust of federal officials	0.730*	0.522*
Overall trust of state officials	0.796*	0.562*
Overall trust of experts	0.633*	0.743*

*$p < 0.01$.

presumably are dispassionate in their analyses, are trusted more for their technical competence.

Development of a Composite Official Trust Scale   The similarity among trust judgments of federal government officials, state government officials, and experts suggested that we may be justified in combining these judgments into a composite "official" trust scale.[33] We first investigated the bivariate correlation between stakeholders' trust judgments of federal and state officials. The correlation between these trust judgments is 0.477 ($p < 0.01$). Moreover, when we measured the correlation of federal and state official trust judgments against a composite *government trust* judgment (constructed by averaging federal and state government trust judgments), we found the correlations to be 0.822 and 0.835, respectively.

We next investigated the correlation between the composite government trust and expert trust judgments to determine whether we could justifiably combine them into a composite official trust judgment scale. Theoretically, this combination is justified because stakeholders told us that they tended to judge the trustworthiness of experts the same whether they worked inside or outside government (supported by the finding that they tend to judge expert trustworthiness based more on competence than on shared values). The correlation between trust judgments of expert officials and government officials is 0.416 ($p < 0.01$).

Encouraged by these correlations, we averaged federal, state, and expert overall trust judgments to derive a composite official trust judgment. The correlations of these three trust judgments with the new composite policy official trust judgment are relatively strong ($r = 0.849$, 0.790, and 0.666, respectively). However, the decision to combine all three trust judgments into a composite official trust scale must be confirmed using a reliability analysis. Cronbach's alpha coefficient of scale reliability is 0.656. We thus conclude that we are justified in developing a composite official trust judgment with which to test the stakeholder participation framework.

Participation Preferences We now turn to stakeholders' preferences for their participation in the Illinois River watershed policy process. Participants indicated their preference for four alternative stakeholder participation strategies by judging each one as highly preferred, moderately preferred, or not preferred. The strategies were defined as follows:

Confirmation strategy. Government drafts a river basin management policy based on what it understands is the preference of its citizens. Government then seeks confirmation from citizens that the policy does in fact reflect their preference before it is adopted.

Consultation strategy. Government determines the river basin management policy that citizens prefer, then adopts the policy that reflects the citizens' preference.

Facilitation strategy. Trained *government* mediators facilitate public meetings that allow citizens ample opportunity to discuss and debate various river basin management policies. Any agreement on a policy reached at these meetings is adopted by the government.

Negotiation strategy. Trained *independent* mediators facilitate public meetings that allow citizens ample opportunity to discuss and debate various river basin management policies. Government officials participate in the meetings on an equal basis with other participants. Any agreement on a policy reached at these meetings is adopted by the government.

Table 4.6 presents a summary of stakeholders' participation preferences.

The results of stakeholders' preference ratings of the participation strategies show that the negotiation strategy is most preferred and confirmation is least preferred. Negotiation requires vigilance along both context dimensions (enhanced involvement and a defensive stance in relation to other stakeholders), whereas confirmation requires deference along both context dimensions (subdued involvement and a cooperative stance in

Table 4.6
Stakeholder participation preferences

Recommended participation strategy	Highly preferred	Moderately preferred	Not preferred	Median rank score	Preference order
Confirmation	21%	34%	45%	1	4 (lowest)
Consultation	33	37	30	2	3
Facilitation	44	35	21	2	2
Negotiation	64	21	15	4	1 (highest)

relation to other stakeholders). Thus, stakeholders prefer strategies that are based on an unwillingness to defer to the competence and good faith of both officials and fellow stakeholders to manage risks on their behalf. Moreover, table 4.6 shows that facilitation is preferred over consultation, suggesting that defense against assaults by fellow stakeholders is more important to their participation preference than their unwillingness to defer to policy officials. We return to this finding in the next section.

Propositions

Three propositions for empirical investigation will test the participation framework:

Proposition 1:   If stakeholders highly trust each other, they will rank cooperative strategies in the highly preferred category. Otherwise, they will prefer defensive strategies.

Proposition 2:   If stakeholders judge policy officials as highly trustworthy, they will rank deferential strategies in the highly preferred category. Otherwise, they will prefer vigilant strategies.

Proposition 3:   The framework will predict which of four participation strategies will be highly preferred based on the combination of social trust and official trust judgments by stakeholders as defined in the previous two propositions.

Because the model forces trust judgments to be dichotomous (trust or distrust),[34] it is necessary to determine the optimal location of the break point between trust and distrust along the two trust dimensions. In other words, if the framework is valid in this case study, then a specific point on each nine-point trust scale should be identified such that the intersection of the two dimensions at those points (the origin) should function well to predict stakeholder preferences.

The Demarcation between Trust and Distrust A popular aphorism states that trust is hard to win but easy to lose. Though this intuition is widely held, it has been rarely tested. Slovic, Layman, and Flynn (1991) noted that even a hundred trustworthy acts will not restore trust lost from a single untrustworthy act. Rothbart and Park (1986) found an analogous asymmetry: favorable traits such as trustworthiness were judged hard to acquire and easy to lose, whereas unfavorable traits such as dishonesty were judged as easy to acquire and hard to lose. Similarly, the National Research Council (1989, 120) noted that a short-term reversal of untrustworthy behavior is insufficient, as reflected by their statement, "One year of being honest with the public is not enough." Shapiro (1987) argued that trust is only slowly gained through a series of incremental acts that conform to social expectations. Hardin (1997), Meyerson, Weick, and Kramer (1996), Janoff-Bulman (1992), Dasgupta (1988), Baier (1986), Barber (1983), Luhmann (1979), and McGregor (1967) have all noted the fragility of trust. Kasperson, Golding, and Tuler (1992), reinforcing the fragility of trust, observed that "trust is probably never completely or permanently attained, but rather requires continuous maintenance and reinforcement."

Hardin (1997) explains the trust-distrust asymmetry by conceptualizing trust as grounds for cooperation. Distrust, he argues, comes more easily because it relies on very little evidence. Trust, in contrast, requires an understanding of the other's intentions deduced from repeated demonstrations of trustworthiness in continuing the cooperation. Similarly, Breton and Wintrobe (1982) observe that trust is conditioned on the trustee's continuing behavior, whereas distrust and refusal to cooperate further can be made permanent by a single violation of trust ("every betrayal begins with trust").[35]

The asymmetry of trust can also be explained by its conceptual equivalence to risk acceptability. Consistent with prospect theory (Kahneman and Tversky 1979), losses are feared more than gains are desired. People tend to be risk averse, which equates to being trust averse.

In one of the few studies that have examined the asymmetry of trust, Slovic et al. (1993) demonstrated that trust-destroying events have a much greater impact on trust judgments than trust-building events.[36]

Despite these studies and theories that posit or demonstrate the asymmetry of trust, none quantified the extent of the asymmetry. Perhaps the lack of reports that quantify asymmetry is not so much a shortcoming as the result of the implicit acknowledgment that the line between trust and distrust varies with context. Gambetta (2000, 222) states that "the optimal threshold [of trust in forging cooperative relations] will not be the same in all circumstances" and that the threshold can be expected to vary in response to both subjective risk predispositions and objective risk circumstances.[37] Bouckaert et al. (2002, 6) state, "Trust is never absolute but always conditional and contextual." Good (2000) and Johnson-George and Swap (1982) also find that trust is situation specific. Kramer (1994, 226) alludes to the contextual nature of the trust-distrust distinction in his observation that the issue "is not simply whether to trust or distrust, but rather how much trust and distrust are appropriate in a given situation." In the case of watershed management, the subjective contextual attribute of stakeholders' preexisting attitudes toward risk and objective contextual attributes such as sizes and types of stakes at risk, likelihood of risk imposition, level of personal risk controllability, sense of urgency, and level of compensating benefits can all be expected to influence the distinction between trust and distrust.

Since we did not ask respondents in this study to make this distinction, we were left to estimate where along the distrust-trust scale this distinction could be made. Ullmann-Margalit (2002) presents a convincing argument that full trust requires meeting three conditions: positive intention (the trustee intends to act to promote the trustor's interests), right reason (the trustee will act on the trustor's behalf even if the trustor's interests conflict with the trustee's own interests), and competency (the trustee is able to protect the trustee's interests). This would indeed raise the bar quite high for full trust to be accorded. She also argues that distrust is the most rational presumption in dealing initially with strangers.[38] Williams (1988) conjectures that full trust may require thick relations (a rich and lengthy history of relationships). Given the dearth of thick relationships among stakeholders across the Illinois River watershed, the long history of controversy and frustrated expectations in dealing with threats to water quality, and the high stakes in a policy outcome—as well as frequent expressions of distrust offered during stakeholder interviews—we believe that the trust asymmetry in this case is quite pronounced. In other words, we believe that very high levels of trust are required before stakeholders in the Illinois River watershed are willing to defer to each other or to officials. Given that the trust scale's values vary from 1 (completely untrustworthy) to 9 (completely trustworthy), we assumed that location of the dichotomy between trust and distrust is between 7 and 8 (thus, 1–7 was classified as distrust leading to increased vigilance and 8–9 was classified as trust leading to a willingness to defer).[39]

Framework Performance   Testing the framework also requires creating a dichotomy of the stakeholder participation preference ratings. Stakeholders were asked to judge each of the four participation strategies as highly, moderately, or not preferred. During interviews, stakeholders were instructed to give the "not preferred" rating only to those strategies that they would likely oppose, whereas the "moderately preferred" rating should be given to strategies that were not their first choice but would nevertheless be acceptable. A successful participation strategy prediction (based on stakeholders' social and official trust judgments) is therefore defined as that judged by stakeholders as "preferred" (moderately or highly), and a failed prediction is one that was judged as "not preferred." This dichotomization is justified by the claim that stakeholders will likely not fight a process unless they find it unacceptable, even though it may not be their top choice.

Table 4.7 presents the results of how well stakeholders' trust judgments predicted their participation preferences using the trust–distrust dichotomy and the preferred–not preferred dichotomy. From these results, we can evaluate the three propositions identified above.

Test of Propositions

Proposition 1: Social Trust Predictions of Participation Preferences Table 4.7 demonstrates that twenty-eight of the thirty-seven stakeholders who trusted other stakeholders preferred cooperative strategies—a prediction success rate of 75.7 percent. This finding suggests that the framework, though correctly predicting three out of four preferences, is somewhat biased toward cooperation. Thus, for at least some stakeholders in the Illinois River watershed, trust must be even higher than 8 (out of 9) before they are willing to prefer a cooperative role over a defensive one.

Table 4.7
Accuracy of framework's prediction of preferred participation strategies

Predicted stakeholder role	Predicted participation strategy	Frequency that predicted strategy was preferred	Percentage predicted correctly
Deferential (cooperative, subdued)	Confirmation	5/8	62.5
Mixed (cooperative, enhanced)	Consultation	23/29	79.3
Mixed (defensive, subdued)	Facilitation	10/11	90.9
Vigilant (defensive, enhanced)	Negotiation	88/102	86.3
All		126/150	84.0

The framework preformed even better in predicting vigilant strategy preferences. Ninety-eight of the 113 stakeholders who distrusted other stakeholders preferred defensive strategies, a prediction rate of 86.7 percent. This result confirms the prior finding that very high trust is required before cooperative strategies are preferred over defensive ones for the large majority of stakeholders in the Illinois River watershed.

Widespread social distrust among stakeholders in the Illinois River watershed has been exacerbated by persistent chronic controversy and threats from federal and state environmental regulatory agencies to expand or increase the stringency of their regulatory authorities. The imposition of regulatory costs has stimulated many stakeholders to seek escape from liability by either downplaying water quality deterioration or blaming others.

Proposition 2: Official Trust Predictions of Participation Preferences
Referring again to table 4.7, note that 15 of the 19 stakeholders who trusted policy officials preferred subdued participation strategies, a prediction rate of 78.9 percent. However, as with proposition 1, the framework performed even better in predicting vigilant strategies. Among those who distrusted policy officials, 111 of 131 stakeholders preferred enhanced participation strategies, a prediction rate of 84.7 percent. The framework again appears to work well in predicting participation preferences based on stakeholders' trust judgments.

Morgan, England, and Humphreys (1991) previously reported that the political culture of Oklahoma combines both individualist and traditionalist forms and thus exhibits a populist leaning with a strong preference for minimalist government. Government distrust thus is embedded in the social fabric of Oklahoma. Against this fabric, however, are the threatened regulatory burdens. This further motivates stakeholders to seek enhanced participation to protect their interests from government intervention.

Proposition 3: Combined Social Trust and Official Trust Predictions of Participation Preferences   The final proposition tests how well the model performed in combining both trust dimensions to predict stakeholders' participation preferences. As can be seen in table 4.7, the model predicted the participation strategies well, achieving an overall 84 percent accuracy in prediction. The lowest prediction success was recorded for confirmation strategies at 62.5 percent, but this relatively low rate may be explained by the low number of stakeholders (8 out of 150) who manifested both high social and official trust.

Framework Test Conclusions

How Did the Framework Perform?   This analysis demonstrates substantial empirical support for our claim that social and official trust influences stakeholders' preferences for participation in watershed management policy processes. Although the data were drawn only from the Illinois River watershed, this framework is sufficiently robust to show that stakeholders' trust judgments may explain their participation preferences in other locations as well. Nonetheless, our results do have specific salience for policymakers in the Illinois River watershed, illustrating the practical significance of this framework.[40]

What Stakeholder Participation Strategy Should IRB Policymakers Employ?   Illinois River watershed stakeholders manifest a strong preference for participation strategies in which their role is defensive (to protect their interests against assault by other stakeholders) and enhanced (to share decision-making power with officials). When these characteristics are viewed together, IRB stakeholders prefer to participate vigilantly. The most preferred strategy is negotiation, which requires third-party-facilitated consensus building and fact finding before decisions are made. The least preferred strategy is confirmation, which allows government officials to lead policy formulation with public input limited to postdecision approval.

Given these results, prudence dictates that policymakers accord Illinois River watershed stakeholders more involvement in watershed decision making if they wish to promote policy output effectiveness. Bradbury, Branch, and Focht (1999) find that Misztal's (1996) argument for communication ("trust is both the fruit of good communication and its necessary precondition") especially applies in environmental risk policy arenas. Sztompka (1997, 1) provides an interesting justification for increased stakeholder involvement to build trust: "Democracy breeds trust by institutionalizing distrust." Therefore, policymakers can build trust by increasing transparency, accountability, responsiveness, empowered participation, and so on. The relationship between trust and participation is paradoxical: in contexts of distrust, increasing participation can build trust, which can then decrease demands for participation. Alternatively, in such contexts, decreasing participation will only exacerbate demands for participation.

Specific suggestions follow. Since experts are accorded substantial deference, they can be trusted to conduct competent scientific impact studies. Voluntary and educational programs designed to improve stakeholders' understanding of water quality impacts and their causes are also recommended (and are not controversial). While studies and educational programs are underway, we further recommend that policymakers consider participating in policy dialogues with stakeholders. These dialogues, which should be facilitated by an outside neutral party, should consider information developed from prior and continuing studies, negotiate the design of further studies, and deliberate possible impact management solutions. These measures will build trust among policy participants and gain stakeholder support for the watershed management policy that is eventually produced.

Conclusions and Implications   In chapter 1, we pointed out that trust has traditionally been related to increased political participation in the traditional realms of voting and contacting. This chapter shows that trust can be associated with decreased participation when transaction costs are high, as in the case of watershed management. However, we are not offering a normative prescription that transaction costs should be increased as a means to discourage participation. On the contrary, Levi (1998) reminds us that democratic theorists from Hobbes to modern republicans have embraced distrust and vigilance as the basis of a flourishing democracy.

In chapter 9, we point out that the findings derived from our study of collaborative partnerships in chapter 8 indicate that trust is negatively correlated in young partnerships but positively correlated in old partnerships. We believe that the most coherent explanation of these seemingly disparate findings is that high stakes and low trust motivate the initial willingness to participate, but building trust is required to motivate continued participation. Since watershed management policy usually involves high stakes, this explanation can be paraphrased as "low trust will get you there but only high trust keeps you there."[41] Given that trust is asymmetric (hard to earn), it takes repeated interactions over time to build trust (by building competence, discovering shared values, and demonstrating willingness to move away from ideological commitments and toward mutually beneficial outcomes—see chapter 6). Moreover, if participation produces positive outcomes, perceived stakes decrease, and the willingness to continue participation decreases. The dynamic relationship among trust, vigilance, and participation seems, in retrospect, quite rational.

Chapter 1 reports that increased trust reduces the need for elaborate rules and procedural safeguards. This relationship is borne out by this study. Rules and safeguards are the province of vigilant participation, not deference motivated by trust.[42]

Chapter 1 also suggests that civic community variables such as social capital, cooperative attitudes, and human capital are highly related to trust. This is also supported by this study. The recursive relationship among trust and vigilance and participation suggests that the use of the proper participation strategy can build trust and thereby move the decision context toward more deference and less participation. As Gamson (1968) has observed, trust is important to increasing the efficiency and effectiveness of government; that is, policy outputs and compliance to secure policy outcomes can be obtained without resort to coercion. Failure to use a strategy appropriate to the trust context may decrease trust and amplify demands for participation.[43]

Finally, we believe that this study provides an important warning to policymakers: it is critically important to assess stakeholders' trust of each other and of policy officials before designing and implementing a participation program. This is especially true in watershed management policy processes since the risk to stakes, complexity, and uncertainty are typically high (circumstances especially relevant to trust according to Luhmann, 1979). If stakeholders' trust of policy actors is low, then policy output success will likely hinge on intensive stakeholder participation.[44] We will examine a particularly promising strategy for intensive participation next.

Watershed Management Using Analysis and Deliberation

This chapter opened with the lament that although the EPA and NRC have acknowledged the importance of context in designing stakeholder participation programs, they do not offer specific guidance on how to match context with participation. We have developed and tested a framework that provides such guidance. In the Illinois River watershed case, we found that stakeholders' distrust of policy officials and other stakeholders corresponds to their preference for negotiation participation strategies. While this provides some specificity, an enormous array of negotiation strategies exists. In this section, we defend our suggestion that the analysis and deliberation framework prescribed by the NRC in 1996 is an ideal candidate for structuring stakeholder collaborations in watershed management within a context characterized by widespread distrust.

In the first section of this chapter, we suggested that the self-reinforcing relationship among trust, participation, and effectiveness allows the possibility that the proper participation strategy can make highly problematic policy contexts more tractable over time. As Funtowicz and Ravetz (1992) argue regarding risk management policymaking, contexts characterized by relatively low decision complexity—those involving low stakes and high certainty—can be handled by "normal" science, that is, the routine application of standardized methods (Kuhn 1970). However, contexts of high complexity—those involving high stakes or low certainty—call for "postnormal" science, which incorporates stakeholder participation into the policy process.[45] In part, participation is required to ensure that in the anxious circumstances of high stakes or low certainty, stakeholders are confident that policy reflects their values and safeguards their interests. Thus, complex contexts place great stress on stakeholders' trust of officials and each other—and few watershed management policy contexts are characterized by low complexity.

Dietz and Stern (1998) define the characteristics of policy contexts in which participatory processes involving deliberation should be used:

Multidimensionality—contexts that possess complexity with regard to salient issues and possible outcomes

Scientific uncertainty—contexts in which important causal relationships remain unspecified or underspecified or their quantification lacks confidence

Controversy—contexts that involve value conflicts concerning, for example, issue frames, relative importance of decision criteria, and desired outcomes

Distrust—contexts in which decision-making institutions fail to meet their fiduciary obligation to protect watersheds, which may lead to judgments that the institutions are incompetent or corrupt (or both)

Urgency—contexts in which decisions cannot await long-term reductions in uncertainty and permanent resolutions of value conflicts

Following Dietz and Stern, we suggest that policymaking in the watershed management context in which the negotiation strategy is appropriate (due to social and official distrust) requires deliberative processes. As we argue, deliberation should be used not only to negotiate policy outputs but also to frame policy analysis designed to inform the deliberation. The challenge, of course, is to determine how these two activities should be integrated.

Frameworks of Environmental Risk-Based Decision Making

The Dominant Framework: Linearized Risk Analysis   The National Research Council (1983) has defined a process of decision making that embraces a linear process that attempts to separate facts from values. In the first stage, risk assessment, scientists are asked to conduct scientific

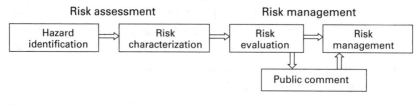

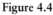

Figure 4.4
Dominant framework of risk-based decision making

analysis of risk using the best data and risk models available. This assessment is fed into the second stage, risk management, in which a politicized process of negotiating among competing values is conducted to select a risk-reduction strategy. While the 1983 framework acknowledges that stakeholders have a legitimate role in risk management, their involvement in risk assessment is considered less important in virtue of the expert scientific nature of the enterprise. The linearized approach to risk-based decision making is summarized in figure 4.4.

The linear risk analysis process begins with hazard identification—a technical investigation of the existence of a threat to human health or the environment caused by environmental exposure of biological receptors to an adverse condition. This is followed by risk characterization, a quantification of risk based on the probability of an adverse consequence multiplied by the severity of that consequence. In risk evaluation, the decision on whether the quantitative risk estimate produced in the risk assessment stage is acceptable depends on an a priori definition of acceptable risk. If the assessed risk exceeds the relevant acceptable risk level, it is judged as unacceptable, and risk management to reduce the risk is implemented.

The 1983 framework thus adopts the position that hazard identification and risk characterization should be scientific enterprises conducted by experts freed from the complications of political, economic, and social concerns. This approach still dominates risk-based decision making in most government environmental agencies. Nongovernmental stakeholders are permitted to participate only at the risk management stage.

The Competing Framework of Recursive Analysis and Deliberation   In 1996, another committee commissioned by the NRC to reexamine the

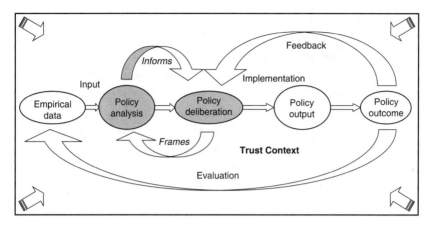

Figure 4.5
Framework of integrated policy analysis and policy deliberation

risk analysis framework derived a remarkably different approach (Stern, Fineberg, and the NRC, 1996). In their view, risk-based decision making should be prescribed as an integrated and iterative process of technical analysis and political deliberation.[46] The arbitrary separations of fact and value, expertise and dialogue, and assessment and management are abandoned in favor of a holistic integration that encourages the interplay of analysis and deliberation in both risk assessment[47] and risk management. No longer is risk seen as only probability and consequence, thus assigning its subjective and contextual attributes as accidental attributes (which Thompson and Dean 1996 argue is analogous to thinking of color as an accidental attribute of the eye). No longer are hazard identification and risk characterization viewed as the exclusive domain of science and scientists. Since risk is socially constructed and risk assessment is embedded in psychosocial contexts, "whoever controls the definition of risk controls the rational solution to the problem at hand" (Slovic 1999, 689). Therefore, risk assessment should be situated in a recursive relationship with value deliberation. We believe that this approach, referred to as analysis and deliberation (A&D), may increase the trustworthiness of policy actors and better resolve controversies than the former paradigm.[48] Figure 4.5 depicts an expanded version of the A&D framework by incorporating it into the traditional public policy process heuristic.[49]

Consistent with Slovic's (1999) elegant defense of stakeholder parti-cipation in risk assessment, figure 4.5 emphasizes the role that policy deliberants should play in framing policy analysis. Figure 4.5 is also con-sistent with the dynamic frameworks for watershed management pre-sented in chapters 1 and 9 of this book, which serve as organizing heuristics. Although figure 4.5 does not specifically identify civic commu-nity (which includes trust) as separated from the trust context, it does illustrate that both trust context and collaborative processes influence—and are influenced by—policy outcomes. Moreover, both figure 4.5 and the dynamic frameworks show that trust context influences policy output effectiveness.

In A&D, analysis informs policy deliberation so that the best informa-tion is brought to bear on the problem to be solved ("getting the science right"). In this respect, A&D does not differ remarkably from the older framework. The novelty of A&D is its prescription of participant delib-eration to frame the analyses ("getting the right science"). Thus, risk as-sessment no longer should be restricted to policy officials and experts. Nongovernmental stakeholders should also participate in framing the issues that are salient to the decision problem, such as what information should be considered, what further studies should be performed to re-duce uncertainty, how impact management alternatives should be eval-uated, what assumptions and defaults should be used in the impact assessment models, and so on. New information provided to the deliber-ants may stimulate other rounds of analyses.

To conceptualize the idealized A&D process, it may be most useful to begin at the deliberation stage. Based on information gained from analy-ses and outcomes of previous policies, adverse impacts make it onto the policy agenda.[50] Policy deliberation may result in a demand for (further) analysis of the impacts, alternatives for impact management, or both. The deliberants then frame the analyses that are needed to inform their deliberation and task expert analysts to conduct appropriate analyses. In response, the analysts obtain data necessary to incorporate into the analyses, select appropriate analytical models, conduct the analyses, and communicate their findings to the deliberants in ways that the deliber-ants find useful. This new information may trigger additional demands for analyses. At some point, based on the adequacy of the information provided and the urgency of the decision, deliberants move to produce a policy that, it is hoped, will be adopted and subsequently implemented. The outcome of policy implementation serves as a feedback mechanism to allow deliberants to judge the legitimacy of the policy and generates data for further analyses in more formal program evaluations. Referring again to the negotiation scenario described earlier in this chapter, stakeholders learn from a formal program evaluation commissioned by policymakers after a few years of policy implementation that illegal dumps have been successfully halted, septic tanks are being properly installed and maintained, and recreationist behavior is much improved. However, riparian area restoration is lagging behind goals set during policy deliberations. Based on trust built during the original policy deliberations and collaborative oversight of program implementation, stakeholders work with policymakers to encourage further riparian zone restoration using increased incentives for conservation easements and penalties for unauthorized riparian area destruction.

Figure 4.5 also illustrates that context-dependent exogenous variables (the four arrows operating within the contextual environment) exert influence on the A&D policy process and its outcomes. In this chapter, we make no claims about the importance of relevant elements of context beyond stakeholders' trust of policy actors. However, the studies reported in chapters 6, 7, and 8 demonstrate that context more generally affects collaborative partnership success.

Legitimacy Evaluation of These Frameworks   Because the 1983 NRC framework places the identification of hazards and the assessment of risks outside the reach of deliberation, it fails to consider procedural legitimacy criteria and the substantive legitimacy criterion of autonomy discussed in chapter 3. The consequence of a top-down, elite-driven process is that impacts important to stakeholders and the polity may be ignored or that the mechanisms for assessing the magnitudes of impacts are constructed in a way that delegitimizes nonscientific constructions. Thus, no attempt to ensure that nonscientific values are incorporated into the definitions and assessment of risk is included. Moreover, the 1983 framework is linear, which implies that new information gained later in the process may not be used in policy refinement. Finally, the

1983 paradigm violates democratic norms of decision making, which raises questions about procedural justice. As MacLean (1987) points out, failure to consent to the decision process may lead to failure to consent to the decision outcome.

The A&D framework avoids these difficulties because it is recursive and deliberation driven. It is an effective integrator of what have too often been seen as separate activities. When environmental policy elites deliberate about methods, assumptions, data, and meaning of findings developed from their analyses, these deliberations necessarily involve value-based choices. Moreover, policy deliberations have always relied on information provided by analysts. The missing piece has been the linkage of deliberation to analysis in such a way that deliberation among stakeholders and policy officials is not simply informed by analysis but also frames analysis. Thus, the linear process of top-down, elite-driven policy analysis is replaced with the recursive integration of analysis and deliberation that can more assuredly lead to policy that is more legitimate.

The A&D framework's emphasis on participation clearly addresses procedural factors, since it insists that all persons affected by a policy have an appropriate influence on its formulation. Participation is obviously meant to garner broad consent to the chosen policy. Its emphasis on scientifically valid analyses clearly addresses substantive factors, since it insists that policy formulation be guided by an accurate assessment of current and postintervention impacts. Note, however, that the concern with scientific results also motivates an emphasis on participation, since participation is meant to ensure that the right scientific questions are asked so that the impact assessments actually reveal outcomes considered positive by relevant nongovernmental stakeholders.

Perhaps more relevant to the question of legitimacy, the A&D framework engages the value of autonomy we discussed in chapter 3. In particular, the public good that is the goal of the A&D policymaking process is conceived in terms of values held by the public. Therefore, the conception of the public good cannot identify what is good for the public simply in terms of welfare. If it was simply a matter of subjective welfare (i.e., preferences), then participation by stakeholders in deliberation would be redundant since desires could be better aggregated by social scientific methods such as polling. But if it was simply a matter of objective welfare (i.e., scientifically determinable facts about human welfare), then there would be no normative reason to insist on participation by stakeholders.[51] Thus, the good must be defined in terms of beliefs about what is good, which can be expressed only in terms of values. Deliberation is precisely the means by which individuals' values are rationally revised and ultimately aggregated into public values (Sagoff 1999). This conception of the good thus motivates the A&D framework's insistence that deliberation frame analysis. More relevant to this chapter, A&D, appropriately used in the context of widespread distrust, can also restore trust.

A&D in Watershed Management Planning

It is unlikely that watershed management policy legitimation can be achieved if the policy is uninformed by relevant facts about watershed impacts—their causes and their mechanisms of propagation; therefore, expert analysis of impacts and the likely outcomes of policy interventions is essential. However, as we have seen, expert analysis is not sufficient if stakeholders prefer vigilant participation in the policy process due to their unwillingness to defer to (i.e., trust) other policy actors. In the Illinois River case, distrusting stakeholders preferred negotiation processes in which policymakers and stakeholders deliberate to reach agreement on acceptable policy outputs.

We have argued that the A&D framework, with its reliance on deliberation to both frame analysis and negotiate policy outputs, is well suited to contexts in which distrust of policy actors abounds and vigilant participation preferred. Unfortunately, documented attempts to apply the A&D framework to any environmental policy situation are rare (Tuler and Webler 1999, concerning U.S. nuclear weapons complex) and are even rarer in watershed management cases (Webler and Tuler 1999).[52] Nevertheless, we hope that the A&D framework will find additional application in future watershed management processes whose context is dominated by distrust.

Chapter 5 examines stakeholder participation in a watershed in Texas that used an analysis and deliberation procedure.

Appendix

Table 4A.1
Participant categorical profile

Occupational category	Geographic region							Outside Water-shed	Totals
	Upper Illinois River	Middle Illinois River	Lower Illinois River	Barren Fork	Upper Tenkiller Lake	Flint Creek	Caney Creek		
Agriculturalist	3	3	2	3	0	1	0	0	12
Animal feeding operator	2	0	1	2	0	2	0	1	8
Forester	0	0	2	0	0	0	0	0	2
Nursery worker	0	1	2	0	2	0	0	0	5
Recreation businessperson	1	6	0	1	1	2	0	0	11
Nonrecreation businessperson	0	4	4	4	7	2	2	0	23
Resident	4	9	5	2	5	4	6	0	35
Environmentalist	0	0	2	2	1	0	1	2	8
Recreationist	0	0	1	0	0	2	2	6	11
Local official	0	0	1	0	0	0	0	1	2
State official	0	0	2	0	0	0	2	9	13
Federal official	0	0	2	0	0	0	1	9	12
Tribal official	0	0	0	0	1	0	0	1	2
Policy elite	0	0	1	0	0	0	0	5	6
Totals	10	23	25	14	17	13	14	34	150

Table 4A.2
Participant demographic profile ($N = 150$)

Age	Gender	Race	Education	Household income	Length of residence
Less than 20 = 1	Female = 23	African American = 2	Less than high school = 7	Less than $10K = 8	Nonresident = 38
20–29 = 6	Male = 126	Hispanic American = 0	High school = 19	$10K–20K = 10	Less than 1 year = 3
30–39 = 27		Native American = 18	Trade school = 8	$20K–30K = 12	1–3 years = 6
40–49 = 47		Caucasian = 123	Some college = 32	$30K–40K = 22	4–10 years = 27
50–59 = 30		Other = 6	Bachelor's = 27	$40K–50K = 21	11–20 years = 22
60–69 = 17			Some graduate school = 15	$50K–60K = 28	21–30 years = 15
70–79 = 17			Master's = 19	$60K–70K = 8	31–40 years = 10
Over 79 = 4			Doctor/profession = 21	$70K–80K = 10	41–50 years = 11
				$80K–90K = 7	Over 50 years = 7
				$90K–100K = 7	
				$100K–125K = 6	
				$125K–150K = 3	
				Over $150K = 3	
Mean = 50			Median = Bachelor's	Median = $50K–60K	Mean = 16 years

Notes

We thank the U.S. Environmental Protection Agency for its funding of this research under the EPA/NSF Partnership for Environmental Research, Water and Watersheds Program, EPA Grant GAD R825791. The title of the project is, "Ecological Risks, Stakeholder Values, and River Basins: Testing Management Alternatives for the Illinois River." We also thank the reviewers for their insightful comments.

1. Draft Public Involvement Policy (65 Federal Register 82341-2, December 28, 2000).

2. Hupcey found the structural features of trust to include dependency on others to meet a need, willingness to accept risk, and expectation of fiduciarily responsible behavior by the trustee. Castelfranchi and Falcone believe that the trustor must have a "theory of the mind" of the trustee, which includes estimations of risk and a decision on whether to rely on the other based on the trustor's predisposition for risk acceptability. Their view is completely consistent with our own.

3. We define *stakeholders* here as nongovernmental stakeholders (see chapter 1)—members of the public who have an interest in, or will be affected by, policy outcomes. Governmental officials acting in their role as representatives of the public are not stakeholders. However, government officials who are or could be affected by policy outcomes can also be stakeholders. Thus, we are referring here to roles that policy actors play, not to policy actor identities per se.

4. We differ from Lewis and Weigert (1985a) in their definition of trust as a purely sociological phenomenon. We would label their holistic conception of trust as social capital (as Putnam does) and instead adopt their psychological or atomistic definition as trust. We do not dispute, however, their (1985b) and Barber's (1983) arguments that trust is socially constructed. Nevertheless, we believe that trust is psychologically applied by individuals to objects of trust. Piotr Sztompka (1999, 25) defines trust as "a bet about the future contingent actions of others."

5. We recognize that policy effectiveness can include both output and outcome effectiveness (see chapter 3). We focus only on output effectiveness in this chapter because we are concerned with stakeholder participation in policy formulation and adoption. However, it follows, we believe, that outcome effectiveness is enhanced if stakeholders cooperate with officials and each other in policy implementation and implementing agencies accomplish policy goals in ways that respect the stakeholders' values and interests.

6. Exceptions include Zucker (1986); Rempel, Holmes, and Zanna (1985); and Lewis and Weigert (1985a, 1985b).

7. Sztompka (1999) is one of many researchers who define distrust as an opposite of trust. We are aware, however, that some argue that trust and distrust are not bipolar concepts but rather distinctly separate. For example, Earle and Cvetkovich (1995) argue that distrust defined as the loss of trust (the traditional

trust characterization, which situates trust as individualist, pluralistic, and adversarial) fails to recognize that trust is socially constructed, cooperative, and unitary (their "cosmopolitan" trust). We, however, wish to focus on trust as leading to deference and its absence as leading to vigilance, the latter of which we define as distrust.

8. Two caveats concerning the relationship between trust and stakeholder participation preferences deserve attention here. First, our framework is concerned with predicting whether stakeholders will initially want to participate in a watershed management decision process, not whether they will want to remain in it. If, after joining the process, they learn that their involvement is token, their interests ignored, their influence minimized, and their information needs unsatisfied, then distrust may grow to the point that they defect from the process. It may be more accurate, therefore, to consider the relationship between trust and participation as a second-order phenomenon in which participation demands are greatest under conditions of moderate trust but fall off when trust is either very low or very high. Second, we are referring to persons and institutions as objects of trust rather than the participation process itself. However, we recognize that if the participation process fails to match stakeholders' expectations, then they may again decide to defect.

9. Again, we acknowledge that if distrust becomes so great that citizens become alienated, they may decline to participate because they believe that participation would be fruitless.

10. Robert Putnam (2000) makes a similar point about the role of social capital (the network of civic engagement and the norm of reciprocity it generates) as an essential foundation for democracy.

11. We do not wish to overstate the influences within the figure, however; the arrows are intended merely to suggest that the preceding component influences, but does not necessarily cause, the succeeding component.

12. A comparison of figure 4.1 against the dynamic frameworks for watershed management in chapters 1 and 9 shows that our conceptualization is compatible with, but not as complete as, these frameworks. Since our emphasis in this chapter is on the influence of trust on participation preferences, we do not include the complex influence of nontrust contextual parameters on other components of the frameworks or address the recursive influences of policy outcomes on participation processes and context.

13. We do not make a normative claim that distrust, and therefore vigilance, is to be avoided. From Ullmann-Margarit (2002), we learn that Hardin (2001, 517) insists that "large and modern democracies work better if we can be sure that there are professional distrusters or cynics or skeptics, people who act as watchdogs, raise alarms, or provide contrary information." Similarly, Kramer (1999, 590) states, "Vigilance and weariness about institutions, some have argued, constitute essential components of healthy and resilient organizations and societies. From this perspective, distrust and suspicion may, in a very fundamental sense, constitute potent and important forms of social capital." Ely (1980) and Warren (1999) express similar sentiments.

14. We wish to stress that we are referring to stakeholders' trust of other policy participants (policymakers and other stakeholders), not to their trust of the policy process as such.

15. The specific trust context in which a policy decision is being made may be more important than general trust of policymaking institutions and actors. Driscoll (1978) and Scott (1980) found that specific (situational) components of trust predicted outcomes, whereas global (attitudinal) components did not.

16. Markóczy (2002) draws a distinction between distrust and vigilance, the former being generalized and the latter being a willingness to protect oneself against opportunism. As a result, she develops a two-dimensional typology of individuals based on their willingness to trust and their willingness to be vigilant: prudent trusters (trustful and vigilant), naive trusters (trustful and less vigilant), ordinary distrusters (distrustful and vigilant), and passive distrusters (distrustful and less vigilant). She admits that passive distrusters are "almost nonexistent in practice." This leaves only "ordinary" distrusters who are distrustful and vigilant. We believe that her distruster distinction is less important in our study since we take the view that distrusting stakeholders are more vigilant and trusting stakeholders are more deferential (as opposed to less vigilant). This subtle but important distinction shows up in our later finding that stakeholders' willingness to defer does not mean that they do not wish to be involved. Thus, we do not find stakeholders in our case study who are naive trusters.

17. We intend that "stake" capture the concept of self-interest. A stakeholder is motivated to participate when his or her stakes are at risk, that is, his or her self-interest could be threatened by policy and decision outcomes.

18. The operationalization of trust as a combination of technical competence and fiduciary obligation was first suggested by Barber (1983). Another property of trustworthiness judgments is people's predispositions (attitudes) toward risk. Most people are risk averse, that is, they are predisposed to avoid unnecessary risk. Staying with the risk-trust equivalence hypothesis, this means that most people are also trust averse. This has been demonstrated by Slovic (1993) and others, who have shown that trust is asymmetrical: it is much harder to earn than to lose. This asymmetry of trust is consistent with Kahneman and Tversky's (1979) prospect theory.

19. One reviewer questioned whether distrust can become so great that alienation and cynicism motivate the distruster to decide that political participation is worthless. Generalized distrust can indeed lead to such detachment. However, we were interested only in specific trust and distrust related to watershed management decision. Moreover, the decision to participate is based on several variables other than trust, including perceived personal political efficacy, political ideology, transaction costs, and resources. Thus, we continue to believe that increasing distrust increases the willingness to participate but acknowledge that participation is motivated by other variables as well.

20. This proposition excludes motives to participate based on social capital developed from civic engagement (Brehm and Rahn 1997).

21. We distinguish between the forms of vigilance and deference appropriate to social and official trust.

22. Gambetta (2000) acknowledges that cooperation can be an outcome of trust but that competition is also essential to a healthy democracy. He also notes that cooperation can be induced without trust, for example, by coercion and contract.

23. Hardin (1997) suggests that inequalities of power block the possibility of trust. This may make stakeholders much more likely to distrust government (at least nonlocal levels) and thus motivate their insistence on enhanced participation.

24. This example and the next are loosely based on our research on the Illinois River in eastern Oklahoma, explained in greater detail later in this chapter.

25. Policy acceptability is a complex judgment that includes consideration of both substantive and procedural legitimacy criteria (see chapter 3). Policy effectiveness is subsumed within these criteria.

26. Arkansas v. Oklahoma, 503 U.S. 91 (1992).

27. The criticism emanated from agricultural interests on the OSRC who believed that the plan favored tourist interests. Criticism waned as agricultural concerns were addressed in subsequent commission decisions.

28. We instructed the participants to record their trust judgments in the light of their earlier open-ended discussion of their preferences for participation in Illinois River policymaking. We did not provide them a specific definition of trust for at least two reasons: we wanted to avoid steering them to render trust judgments in tautological conformance to our framework, and, in any case, stakeholders do not share the same definition of trust—therefore, a more robust test of the framework would not impose a definition that may not be operational for the participant. Despite the flexibility afforded to participants in judging trust, however, we found substantial empirical support for the framework, as we explain later. Trust was treated somewhat differently in the other studies discussed in this book (see, for example, the trust attributes examined in chapters 6 and 8).

29. Additional scales were used to obtain stakeholders' judgments about social controversy, factual certainty, factual salience, and value salience. Results of analysis of these data are not included in this chapter.

30. The National Science Board (2000) also found that medical and scientific institutions were most trusted among the institutions rated. In fact, the trust of scientific institutions has remained constant for the past thirty years. However, their study does not distinguish between technical competence and shared values.

31. Braithwaite argues that people react to complexity in one of two ways. Those with a "security" orientation collect knowledge and engage in rational calculations of outcome risks. Those with a "harmony" orientation are more concerned with shared values and process legitimacy. We had anticipated that experts would be judged from a security, rather than harmony, orientation.

32. Ullmann-Margalit (2002) offers another reason. She argues that intention is weighted more than competence in trust judgments. Following Sidney Morgenbesser, she argues that competence is more closely associated with confidence or reliance than it is on trust. If this is true among our stakeholder sample, then trust would be expected to be more closely associated with shared values than competence regardless of the object of trust, including technical experts.

33. We did not combine social trust with official trust for theoretical and statistical reasons. Theoretically, stakeholders told us that they do distinguish between officials and fellow stakeholders insofar as trustworthiness is concerned. Statistically, this is borne out by the very low correlation between official and social trust judgments ($r = 0.027$, $p = 0.743$). Moreover, although we did not specifically test whether stakeholders define social and official trust as we do, our constructions are supported by the correlations reported here.

34. We do not deny that trust and distrust are judged in degrees; however, our framework requires a binary operationalization in which trust contributes to a willingness to defer and distrust contributes to a desire for vigilance. As we explain, we argued theoretically for an extreme asymmetry between trust and distrust and verified this division empirically (see note 37).

35. Hardin (1993, 1997) suggests that distrust hinders learning by discouraging cooperation that could provide evidence of trustworthiness. This observation lends additional support for the argument that stakeholder collaboration, particularly when alternative venues are not feasible, provides a powerful opportunity to build trust. See chapter 9 for further discussion.

36. Slovic (1993) offers four reasons for trust's fragility: (1) trust-destroying events are more visible (and attract more media attention), (2) trust-destroying events carry more weight in influencing trust judgments, (3) trust-destroying events are seen as more credible, and (4) distrust tends to reinforce and perpetuate distrust due to people's aversion to trust-destroying agents (that inhibit contact with persons or experiences that could rebuild trust) and to framing effects (coloring of event interpretation). In addition, Cvetkovich et al. (2002) find that the trust asymmetry exists only in contexts in which distrust is already present. Thus, when trust is high, trust-destroying events have less erosive effects than they would when trust is low. Similarly, Earle (2000) finds that arguments supporting trust asymmetry ignore the role of existing attitudes and beliefs in trust judgments.

37. Similarly, Ajzen and Fishbein (1980) argue that behaviors are better predicted by proximal variables, which vary with context.

38. Ullmann-Margalit (2002), arguing from a Hobbesian view of social interaction, states that the presumption in favor of distrust is justified. No one wants to expose himself or herself to exploitation. In our opinion, this is the reason that misplaced trust ("mistrust") triggers more regret and thus is more feared than opportunity lost from failing to trust.

39. We tested the optimal location of the trust-distrust demarcation by independently determining the score on the nine-point trust scales for social trust

and official trust against respondents' preference for social deference and official deference, respectively. We found that social deference is accorded most often when social trust is rated as either 8 or 9. Similarly, official deference is also accorded most often when official trust is rated as either 8 or 9. We therefore cannot claim that this method for determining the break point between trust and distrust was independently obtained from the model. Instead, we must rely on the literature that suggests that the trust-distrust relationship is asymmetrical in favor of distrust and the magnitude of the asymmetry varies with context. Based on our interviews and the long history of controversy and failed expectations, we believe that we are justified in selecting a rather extreme asymmetry. If the break point between trust and distrust is moved down one unit (trust = 7–9 and distrust = 1–6), the model's performance is reduced from 84 percent to 77 percent.

40. A random sample telephone survey was conducted in 2001 to test a variant of the framework discussed here. The variant examined the ability of stakeholders' trust judgments of experts to predict their preferences for evidentiary processes (those in which stakeholders provide evidence to decision makers, which we hypothesized would be appropriate if stakeholders express high expert trust) versus constitutive processes (those in which stakeholders themselves serve as decision makers, which is more appropriate in low-expert-trust contexts). The variant model did not perform well in this test. We conclude that the Illinois River watershed controversy inextricably involves both facts and values, and stakeholders do not easily distinguish between facts and values in choosing between evidentiary and constitutive processes. Regardless of their trust of experts, stakeholders prefer processes that require substantive participation. Another conclusion is that stakeholders do not easily distinguish government experts from government policymakers. This lends further support for our combination of expert and policymaker trust judgments into a composite "official" trust measure. Insofar as generalizability is concerned, one of us (Focht) is currently engaged in two projects to test further the framework discussed in this chapter. The first involves the Eucha-Spavinaw watershed in northeastern Oklahoma and northwestern Arkansas in a study funded by the U.S. Department of Agriculture. The second involves bioremediation of subsurface radioactive and heavy metal contamination at three sites in Hanford, Washington, Los Alamos, New Mexico, and Oak Ridge, Tennessee, in a study funded by the U.S. Department of Energy. The results of these studies will be reported later.

41. Similarly, Levi (1998, 9) concludes that "distrust raises the transaction costs of cooperation ... trust can play a role in reducing these transaction costs and provide a means for moving out of an equilibrium of non-cooperation."

42. Bella, Mosher, and Calvo (1988, 29) included in their definition of *distrust* that order is attained only through coercion and a proliferation of rules and rule enforcers.

43. Also important is the caution offered by many trust researchers (Bateson 1986, Dasgupta 1988, Gambetta 2000, Hirsch 1977, Hirschman 1984) that trust is depleted through disuse. Trust, to be sustained, must be continually renewed.

Hardin (1997, 10) eloquently made this point in his distinction between trust and social capital: "It is argued by some that trust is similarly a resource, indeed that it is a matter of 'social capital.... Trust is not a kind of resource and is therefore not a candidate for social capital. Rather, if there is social capital, it is the capital of rich relationships that enable trust and therefore cooperation. Trust is not, as altruism may be, a motivation that must be used sparingly because of limited amounts. Rather, it is a cognitive judgment that depends on perceived facts. It may or may not be in short supply, but using it—that is to say, acting on it—does not reduce the supply.... Trust can build on trust."

44. Earle and Cvetkovich (1995) appropriately point out that distrust is risk averse and trust is risk accepting. We take their point. Given the complexities, stakes, and uncertainties of watershed management decision making, it is best if decision makers build trust (through appropriate participation) to motivate stakeholders to accept the inevitable risks of watershed management. Failure to do so may encourage further risk aversion, thus jeopardizing both policy output and outcome effectiveness.

45. Luhmann (1979) stresses that trust is used to reduce cognitive complexity and uncertainty by substituting for knowledge. In other words, if adequate knowledge is already available to allow stakeholders to predict future actions of others, then trust would not be required. Thus, knowledge cannot be used to build trust. However, involving stakeholders in decisions about what knowledge is needed (through framing analyses, discussed later in this section) can build trust by demonstrating fiduciary interest and respect for democratic norms (as well as meeting Sztompka's, 1999, axiological requirements for trust; see the earlier discussion regarding expert trust findings).

46. This prescription was earlier defended by Frank Laird (1993), who persuasively argued that participatory analysis in technological decision making is consistent with the norms of democratic governance.

47. *Risk assessment* is the term used to combine hazard identification and risk characterization, which yields quantitative risk estimates.

48. Despite this (r)evolutionary change in thinking, there is little accumulated evidence to date that environmental agencies have abandoned the earlier paradigm. This may be due to the emphasis on natural sciences and engineering in the professional training of government policy elites.

49. The reader should not attribute too much to the classic policy process model. Though no model comprehensively mimics reality, we believe that the analysis-deliberation model possesses heuristic value in its depiction of the analysis-deliberation cycle embedded within a larger policy framework with its own recursive relationships.

50. David Truman (1951) discussed the important role that interest groups' demands play in agenda setting. We are reminded of his disturbance theory in our discussion of the role that stakeholders can play in deliberation as they frame policy analyses.

51. There might still be pragmatic reasons, but only if the participation was rigged to produce the result that is determined to be scientifically good.

52. Variants of this approach such as adaptive management (Bormann et al. 1994) are gaining popularity, however. These variants generally focus on an iterative process for developing and adapting the technical implementation of some remedial or management strategy, with little or no integration of the policy or social components. These approaches are, in effect, technical optimization tools. Improving trust among stakeholders and policymakers requires a more integrated approach.

5

Citizen Participation and Representation in Collaborative Engagement Processes

Charles D. Samuelson, Arnold Vedlitz, Guy D. Whitten, Marty Matlock, Letitia T. Alston, Tarla Rai Peterson, and Susan J. Gilbertz

This chapter explores citizen participation and representation in collaborative projects using a case study involving two watershed restoration councils in San Antonio, Texas. Our research team formed these councils to develop long-term watershed restoration plans. We describe a theoretical framework for representation of participants in these councils as well as our attempt to use this framework in recruiting stakeholders to participate in watershed restoration councils. The findings, based on surveys of citizens at large as well as participants in the watershed restoration councils, suggest that representation may be the most difficult legitimacy criterion to accomplish in the collaborative engagement process.

This chapter, building on the discussions of chapter 3, focuses on the question of political legitimacy. In particular, we address the relationships among public perception, representation, and legitimacy (criteria P1 and P2 in chapter 3). This chapter provides an empirical investigation of the normative principles proposed by chapter 3 in a multiyear study conducted in San Antonio.

The study, funded in 1998 by the U.S. EPA STAR Water and Watersheds Initiative, was designed to develop improved methods for stakeholder-driven watershed restoration planning. Working with the San Antonio River Authority, a nonregulatory agency in San Antonio, we implemented a three-year program to (1) design and implement a large-scale, representative survey of residents in the San Antonio metropolitan community; (2) test hypotheses that predict citizen willingness to participate in a collaborative engagement process dealing with watershed management; (3) recruit citizens into long-term collaborative stakeholder forums; and (4) evaluate stakeholder representation patterns and the stated goals for citizen participation. Interpretation of the results of these quantitative measures of participation requires an explicit statement of our theoretical framework for legitimacy, as well as a discussion of the context in which the collaborative engagement within the councils occurred.

Theoretical Framework

Democratic nations expect citizens to participate in important matters governing social, political, and economic life. In maintaining the relationships that hold a democratic nation together, citizen representation and participation play significant roles in generating support and compliance, providing important information, and shaping direction on complicated choices for the nation. Electing representatives through public voting and contact with those representatives are seen as the primary channels linking citizen preferences to policy outcomes and legitimizing the overall process of policymaking (Almond and Verba 1963, Coulter 1988, Verba and Nie 1972).

The participatory role of individual citizens and organized interest groups in the regulatory rule-making process received its first real legal boost with the passage of the Administrative Procedure Act of 1946. Sections of the act specifically encouraged greater public access to agency information and rule making through public hearings and open meetings processes. The act increased agency solicitation of individual and group input into the rule-making process through both written statements and in-person attendance at meetings and hearings. This access was expanded in the 1966 Freedom of Information Act (FOIA), the FOIA Amendments of 1974, and the 1976 Government in the Sunshine Act (Heffron and McFeeley 1983).

In political decision-making and regulatory processes, governments at all levels in the United States have been working to involve citizens in ways other than voting, contacting representatives, and the relatively formal, limited public hearing processes encouraged in the Administrative Procedure Act (see chapter 2). The new trend involves diverse sets of individuals in longer-term relationships facilitating interactions, initiating integrated efforts, establishing goals, and reaching solutions to complex problems. These longer-term, relationship-building, solution-oriented stakeholder processes could potentially foster new avenues for citizen representation and participation on matters of important concern. In the process of civil government, these pathways enrich the overall quality of governance by endowing the government with a particular kind of legitimacy and providing significant channels of communication through which agreement on specific policies can be generated.

However, gaining participation in these community activities is increasingly difficult. Robert Putnam (1995, 1996) ascribed this civic disengagement to the prominence of television in modern life. Regardless of the cause, Putnam and others agree that if this trend in disengagement is not reversed, our democratic processes are at risk. This chapter investigates who is more willing to participate, why they participate, and what basic values about democracy and society they represent. In any assessment of civic attitudes, place matters; therefore, we provide a brief description of the San Antonio area for context.

The Watershed Context: A Description of the San Antonio Area

The San Antonio metroplex, with approximately 1 million people, was one of the fastest-growing metropolitan areas during the 1990s (San Antonio Economic Development Foundation, 1999). The metroplex and surrounding areas experienced a 25.2 percent increase in population from 1990 to 1998 and are expected to grow at an average annual rate of 1.9 percent through the year 2010. Bexar County, which primarily comprises the San Antonio metroplex, was 53.9 percent Hispanic, 37.5 percent Anglo, and 6.6 percent black in 1995.

This complex urban system is located in the upper reaches of the San Antonio River basin. Three watersheds drain the entire San Antonio metroplex: Leon Creek, the Upper San Antonio River, and Salado Creek (see figure 5.1). Water quality in the basin is declining due to nonpoint source pollution from urban runoff from the city of San Antonio and its surrounding urbanizing and agricultural areas (Texas Natural Resource Conservation Commission 1996).

The Telephone Survey

This project began with a large-scale survey of the San Antonio community. From March 13, 1999, to May 5, 1999, we conducted a telephone

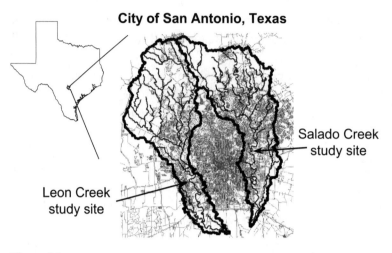

City of San Antonio, Texas

Salado Creek
study site

Leon Creek
study site

Figure 5.1
Watersheds that cross the San Antonio, Texas, area

survey of adults in Bexar County, Texas. The two principal goals of the survey were to measure public opinion in the county on a variety of issues relevant to watershed condition and management and to identify possible participants for our stakeholder process. The next step in this project was to recruit citizens into long-term stakeholder forums (watershed restoration councils). Survey respondents who reported interest in participation in discussions were one source of recruits. Toward the end of the phone survey, respondents were asked, "Would you be willing to represent your community by participating in discussions on the topic of clean water in San Antonio?" Those who said yes were later contacted and invited to participate in the stakeholder forums. Participants for these forums were also recruited using a snowball technique that started with lists of community organizations.

In summary, the study includes two distinct groups: (1) a representative survey sample of San Antonio residents comparing respondents willing to participate in subsequent stakeholder processes versus those not willing to participate, and (2) a recruited group of citizens who actively participated in the stakeholder forums. A few of the participants in the stakeholder forums were interviewed in the original citizen survey, but the vast majority was recruited through the snowball technique. We examine each of these groups in detail regarding the correlates of their willingness to participate in stakeholder forums and then directly compare them later in the chapter.

Representative Survey Sample

We first examined the survey sample of citizens. Of the 1,017 adults interviewed in the phone survey, 245 reported that they would be willing to participate in discussions. To evaluate what factors influenced Bexar County residents' willingness to participate in discussions on the topic of clean water, we used existing theories to develop a set of hypotheses about what would make an individual more or less willing to participate. We then evaluated these hypotheses in a multivariate model of respondents' answers to a survey question asking them whether they would be willing to participate. If respondents said yes, they were coded as willing to participate. Those who refused to answer this question or had dropped out of the survey by the time this question would have been asked were excluded from these analyses. Thus, all calculations are comparisons between those who answered yes and those who answered no.

Hypotheses about Participation

Using these respondents, we first test several hypotheses about democratic participation that emerge from the literature on individual political participation. This literature suggests at least three distinct sets of variables that may be appropriate in this environmental policy context: general outlook attitudes, specific environmental attitudes, and demographic characteristics. We discuss each set separately and then test them together in a multivariate context.[1]

Willingness to Participate: General Outlook Attitudes   The literature discusses three general outlook concepts deemed very important in predicting a citizen's willingness to participate in the political process: personal efficacy, trust in government and other people, and financial optimism. It is almost an accepted truth in the participation literature that a sense of personal efficacy is strongly related to political participation (Clarke 1996; Smidt 1971; Verba and Nie 1972; Verba, Nie, and Kim 1971; Verba, Schlozman, and Brady 1995). Personal efficacy, or a sense that one has some power to influence events outside one's personal sphere, has been evaluated for all levels of government—national, state,

Table 5.1
Hypotheses regarding efficacy and willingness to participate

Hypothesis 1: The greater the personal efficacy in the local government context, the greater the willingness to participate in watershed stakeholder decision processes.

Hypothesis 2: The greater the personal efficacy in the national government context, the greater the willingness to participate in watershed stakeholder decision processes.

and local. For the purposes of this study, we focus on national and local contexts. The hypotheses regarding efficacy and willingness to participate are outlined in table 5.1.

In the literature, trust, like efficacy, has a fairly consistent relationship to the two more traditional forms of participation, voting and contacting. Researchers as varied as Putnam (with Leonardi and Nanetti, 1993), Farrand (1983), Anderson and Yaffee (1998), and Gandy (1991) report consistently higher levels of voting and contacting associated with higher levels of trust.

However, as explained in chapter 4, the type of involved, long-term, direct participation we investigate in stakeholder decision processes may relate to trust very differently. We argue that due to the significant investment required in long-term stakeholder processes, those who trust other participants will not need to make the substantial investment required to protect their interests, while those who are more distrustful of other participants will participate to protect their interests. This is really a transaction costs argument—if I, a potential stakeholder participant, trust other actors to represent my interests, then it is not worth the transaction costs for me to participate. If, however, I do not trust other participants to represent and protect my interests, then I will not think the transaction costs of my participation are too high. This chapter's analysis of trust focuses on traditional measures examining levels of trust that respondents place in other people and government generally. Table 5.2 lists the hypotheses examined in this chapter regarding trust and willingness to participate, formulated following the instructions and arguments of chapter 4.[2]

While efficacy is relatively consistently found associated with political participation, the literature on financial optimism shows, like trust, more ambiguous possibilities. For example, Putnam (2000) finds no relation

Table 5.2
Hypotheses regarding trust and willingness to participate

Hypothesis 1: The lower the level of interpersonal trust held by a respondent, the greater the willingness to participate in watershed stakeholder decision processes.

Hypothesis 2: The lower the level of trust in government held by a respondent, the greater the willingness to participate in watershed stakeholder decision processes.

Table 5.3
Hypotheses regarding financial optimism and willingness to participate

Hypothesis 1: The greater the sense of personal financial optimism, the greater the willingness to participate in watershed stakeholder decision processes.

Hypothesis 2: The greater the sense of national financial optimism, the greater the willingness to participate in watershed stakeholder decision processes.

between financial optimism and American civic engagement. But Farrand (1983) and Day, Beiner, and Masciulli (1988) report that financial optimism strongly relates to political participation. Verba, Schlozman, and Brady (1995) argue that, at least among high-SES citizens, financial optimism is associated with less civic engagement in some of its forms. There appears, then, to be no consistent picture emerging from the literature about the direction of the relationship between financial optimism and political participation. For the purposes of directional clarity and comparative examination across all the hypotheses, we assume a positive relationship between financial optimism and political participation. We examine two aspects of financial optimism here. The first relates to personal finances and the second relates to the national economy. The hypotheses tested regarding financial optimism and willingness to participate are given in table 5.3.

Willingness to Participate: Specific Environmental Attitudes People who are more interested in politics are more likely to participate in political activities like voting, contacting, and campaign activities. Studies of particular policies also indicate that people with an interest in a policy area are more likely to be knowledgeable about that area, to talk about that area to others, and to participate in activities related to that issue area (Verba, Schlozman, and Brady 1995). The question arises about directionality of this interest and its effects on participation.

In order to evaluate these distinctions, the study examined three specific categories of environmental attitudes. The first is general attitudes relating to national and international concerns like population growth, resource availability, and role of animals. Interviewers asked twelve environmental questions that gave respondents a chance to select a pro- or anti-environmental protection position on each. We created an index of environmental beliefs from this battery of questions ranging from -2 for the most antienvironmental set of beliefs to $+2$ for the most proenvironmental set of beliefs (see note to table 5.5).

The second environmental attitude area looks at local attitudes about San Antonio's most important problem (those respondents who mentioned in an open-ended question format "water" or "environment" versus those who did not). The question asked is whether those who mentioned water or a related environmental problem will participate more than their less concerned citizens. The literature suggests this greater salience should be reflected in a greater willingness to participate.

The third question examines ratings of local water quality. Respondents rated the quality of San Antonio's water on a scale of very good to very bad. Again, the literature gives no indication of which responses are more or less likely to be associated with willingness to participate. Although the literature on salience does suggest that greater perceived importance should result in higher levels of participation, because of the uncertainty in directionality for two of these policy-specific attitudes, we will present null hypotheses for them. The hypotheses outlining the relationship between issue salience and willingness to participate are given in table 5.4.

Demographic Characteristics and Willingness to Participate   In addition to these specific categories of variables, we include a number of demographic indicators frequently used to differentiate populations on attitudinal dimensions—sex, age, race, and education, for example. A large number of political participation studies find that increases in socioeconomic status indicators like income, education, and occupation are positively associated with higher levels of participation (Verba and Nie 1972). These variables are included in the overall model tested.

Table 5.4
Hypotheses on the relationship between issue salience and willingness to participate

---

Hypothesis 1: There will be no difference in levels of willingness to participate in watershed stakeholder processes between pro- and antienvironmental protection policy attitude holders.

Hypothesis 2: There will be no difference in levels of willingness to participate in watershed stakeholder processes between those who give high and low ratings of local water quality.

Hypothesis 3: Those for whom water and environmental issues have higher salience as major local problems will be more willing to participate in watershed stakeholder decision processes than those who do not express this concern.

To test the hypotheses, we estimated a single multivariate model. The results of this model are presented in table 5.5. The dependent variable for this analysis was dichotomous, representing each respondent's yes or no answer to the question of whether that person would be willing to participate. With such a dependent variable, a binary probit model is the most appropriate for simultaneously evaluating all the hypotheses (Aldrich and Nelson 1984).

Summary of Telephone Survey Results

This section identifies respondent characteristics that predict willingness to participate in discussions on clean water in San Antonio. Only a handful of the variables expected to influence respondents' willingness to participate were statistically significant in this model. An examination of demographic characteristics of survey respondents indicated that women were less likely to express willingness than men. Among ethnic groups, we were mildly surprised to find evidence that Hispanics were more likely to express a willingness to participate than were other ethnic groups. People working more than forty hours per week were slightly less willing to participate.

In terms of general outlook attitudes, only financial optimism toward personal finances was positively related to participation: more optimistic individuals reported greater willingness to participate than less optimistic residents (providing support for hypothesis 1 in table 5.3). For specific environmental attitudes, the rating of San Antonio's water quality was a significant predictor of willingness to participate in discussions on clean

Table 5.5
Multivariate model of respondents' willingness to participate in discussions on clean water in San Antonio

Variable	Maximum estimated effect
Female	**−12.2%**
African American	*
Asian	*
Hispanic	**+12.1%**
Native American	*
High school dropout	*
High school graduate	*
Took some college	*
College graduate	*
Some postgraduate Schooling	*
Household income less than or equal to $25,000	*
Household income greater than or equal to $40,000	*
Age	*
Working	*
Retired	*
Working more than 40 hours per week	−3.9%
Number of years living in greater San Antonio Area	*
Named a water problem as San Antonio's greatest problem	*
Rating of San Antonio's water quality	−3.0%
Self efficacy—City government	*
Self efficacy—National government	*
Believes most people can be trusted	*
Frequency with which government can be trusted	*
National economy—Expectations	*
Personal finances—Expectations	*+4.5%*
Environmental beliefs index	**+5.5%**

Note: Entries in the second column indicate the estimated maximum effect of the variable in the first column on the probability that the respondent will be willing to participate, holding all other variables constant. There were 996 observations; 76.2 percent were classified correctly.

Entries in bold type in the second column indicate that the estimated effect of the variable in the first column of that row was significant at conventionally accepted levels for statistical hypothesis testing in the social sciences (a two-tailed p-value less than or equal to .05). Entries in italics in the second column indicate that the estimated effect of the first column variable of that row was close, but not quite significant, at conventionally accepted levels (a two-tailed p-value between .05 and .10). An asterisk in the second column indicates that the estimated

Table 5.5
(continued)

effect for the first column variable was not significant at conventionally accepted levels (a two-tailed p-value of .10 or greater).

The ethnic categories should be interpreted as the predicted effect of each category relative to Anglos. The educational categories should be interpreted as the predicted effect of each category relative to people who had a ninth-grade education or less. The household income categories should be interpreted as the predicted effect of each category relative to people whose reported household income was between $25,000 and $40,000.

Almost all of the variables on which analyses are reported are dichotomous, indicating that the respondent either had the characteristic or not. Exceptions to this are:

• Age, measured in years.
• Individuals' rating of San Antonio's water quality, varying from 4 ("very good") to 0 ("very bad").
• Self efficacy-city/national government, which were based on whether respondents strongly agreed (0) to strongly disagreed (4) with the following statement: "People like me don't have any say about what the city/national government does."
• Frequency with which government can be trusted, ranging from 1 ("almost all the time") to 4 ("almost never").
• National Economy/personal finances—Expectations, which ranged from +1 ("better") to −1 ("worse").
• The variable "believes most people can be trusted" was based on respondent's agreement (coded as 1) or disagreement (coded as 0) with this statement.
• Environmental Beliefs Index, constructed from responses to a set of twelve environmental statements from the New Environmental Paradigm (NEP) scale (Dunlap and Van Liere 1978). We created this summary index ranging from −2 (antienvironment) to +2 (proenvironment). This instrument has been used extensively in past research on environmental concern and is presumed to assess three dimensions: the desire to protect the balance of nature, the belief that there should be limits to growth and that humans should be regarded as part of rather than ruling over nature (Scott and Willits 1994). We used the original four-response version of this scale (see Dunlap and Van Liere 1978), with respondents being asked if they strongly agree, agree, disagree, or strongly disagree with each of the twelve statements (see table 5.8 for a listing of the twelve items in the NEP scale).

water in San Antonio, with respondents who thought that water quality was worse being more willing to participate. The environmental beliefs index was also significant: respondents who evidenced a more proenvironmental set of beliefs were more likely to participate than those who evidenced less supportive environmental positions. Trust and efficacy were not significant.

In a separate study, we examined how an individual's proximity to the watershed affected his or her evaluations of the watershed. We created a variable for the actual driving distance respondents lived from the two watershed creeks under study. We then correlated that distance measure with knowledge and perceptions of the creeks. Controlling for other independent variables such as those noted above, residential closeness to the creeks was positively associated with greater knowledge of the creeks and the belief that they are polluted (Brody, Highfield, and Alston 2004). Although this second study did not measure distance and participation directly, based on the findings noted in table 5.5, we infer that distance could be another significant factor in encouraging or discouraging participation in watershed-based stakeholder decision-making processes.

Recruiting Participants to Achieve Representation in Watershed Restoration Councils

After identifing factors that predict the expressed willingness of citizens to participate in collaborative engagement processes, the next step in the research project was to recruit participants for two collaborative stakeholder forums. A major objective was to ensure the procedural legitimacy of the watershed policymaking process by meeting the autonomy criterion (see chapter 3) in recruitment efforts. We used alternative recruitment techniques to accomplish this task.

We recruited people willing to make a year-long commitment to serving on the Watershed Restoration Council that would bring together research scientists, agency personnel, and citizen groups to share watershed information and develop management recommendations. Two councils were organized in San Antonio—one for the Leon Creek watershed and one for the Salado Creek watershed (Figure 5.1). We describe those recruitment methods and associated results.

The Collaborative Process in the Watershed Restoration Councils

The research team facilitated thirteen meetings over a period of fourteen months, from November 1999 to December 2000, in each of the two watersheds in the San Antonio area. Each meeting took the form of a four-hour workshop and was both audio and video recorded for review by researchers. The meetings were designed to enable stakeholders to work together to develop an acceptable, workable plan for watershed development and protection.

The team employed the collaborative learning (CL) process as the mechanism to facilitate analysis and deliberation (see chapter 4) in the watershed restoration council meetings (Daniels and Walker 2001). The CL process intervention is grounded in theoretical work on soft systems methodology (Checkland and Scholes 1990, Wilson and Morren 1990) and alternative dispute resolution (Fisher, Ury, and Patton 1991; Gray 1989). It uses information as the foundation of communication between conflicting parties, with a clear objective that participants are expected to achieve not consensus but, rather, improved understanding of the watershed processes being managed and the basis for each other's perspectives. Thus, this process is characterized by extensive facilitated conversations about attitudes, experiences, and values of the participants, as well as the more standard training and discussions on watershed environmental sciences. Participants were first trained in the CL process and in collaborative discussion and debate. Second, organizers created a common knowledge base on the major issues affecting water quality in the watershed using external experts, predominantly university faculty members. Information was conveyed and deliberated using panel question-and-answer sessions and informal small group discussions. Third, the recruits participated in active learning exercises to help them think systemically about the watershed ecosystem and enable them to identify key issues, concerns, and interrelationships among variables affecting water quality. During this phase, participants generated specific suggestions for improvement of the current situation (existing water quality in watershed), then shared and refined their ideas with other participants through a structured small group discussion process. Fourth, through collaborative debate with other stakeholders, a final set of improvement suggestions was organized, discussed, and refined. The structured set of CL activities moved participants away from positional strategies and toward the identification of mutual interests and joint gains from collaboration. Moreover, the presence of outside facilitators during CL sessions permitted use of effective principles from mediation theory and research (Gray 1989).

Stakeholder Recruitment Process

We adopted two perspectives essential to understanding the recruitment of citizen stakeholders as council members. First, we held the view that all who participate in a particular "cultural domain" are "experts" of that domain (Lindlof 1995). This perspective allowed us to be highly inclusive; virtually anyone whose life experiences included the Leon Creek watershed or the Salado Creek watershed was seen as a potential citizen stakeholder. With attention to the geographic character of the two watersheds, council members were recruited from the various segments of the watershed, including those living in the most affluent and the most disadvantaged neighborhoods.

Second, we used the snowball technique to recruit participants. We developed a set of initial community contacts that gave us access to potential council members. Each contact was approached for two reasons: to determine whether the individual would serve as a council member, and to generate additional referrals. (The technique is referred to as the snowball technique because contact with one individual leads to the identification of two or three additional participants, and so on.) Briefly, citizen stakeholders were recruited as follows:

1. A list of community groups and organizations was generated.
2. San Antonio city officials were asked to identify organizations and leaders with an interest in watershed management issues.
3. Community gatekeepers were contacted for further recommendations of potential participants.
4. Citizens were recruited directly by telephone and personal interviews.

Some recruitment was done over the telephone. In addition, many of the recruits were interviewed by members of the research team in one-on-one settings prior to the first council meeting. This is an important recruitment technique because people often need encouragement to follow through on their commitment to serve on such councils.

The goal of the recruitment activities was to achieve representativeness in public participation for an ethnically diverse population. We attempted to construct the councils as representative of the variety of demographic categories in these watersheds: race, age, sex, socioeconomic status, and education. It became apparent early on that we had primarily tapped into two groups of people: middle-class citizens, mostly Anglo, who were active in local government and community functions and a group of retirees committed to using their time to making their communities better places to live. Although this second group was much more racially diverse than the first group, they also tended to represent the middle class.

To widen the diversity, we adjusted our recruitment efforts to target missing groups. One approach was to use a pool of names generated in conjunction with the telephone survey described earlier. Survey respondents who indicated they would be willing to participate in discussions on clean water in San Antonio ($N = 245$) were asked for their contact information. To maximize the representativeness of the stakeholder groups in terms of Bexar County's basic demographic profile, these 245 respondents were ranked in terms of the importance with which contact with them should be pursued.

Overall, the recruitment methods yielded agreements to participate from twenty-six agency or government officials, forty community or civic organizational contacts, twenty-two personal referrals, and five phone survey respondents. In sum, following up to the phone survey was the least effective and efficient method of recruiting potential stakeholders to participate, and relying on participants in relevant existing organizations was the most effective.

Representation: Comparison of CL Stakeholder Groups with Telephone Survey Samples

The criterion of procedural legitimacy can be satisfied in two distinct ways (see criteria P1 and P2 in chapter 3). One approach suggested by chapter 3 is based on statistical representation—that is, to what extent the composition of the stakeholder groups represents the larger populations from which these participants were recruited. Survey data collected in this project allowed us to address this question quantitatively. This section presents survey results using two subsamples from the Bexar County population (Salado and Leon Creek watersheds), as well as the corresponding CL stakeholder groups from these watersheds, who were given a series of overlapping questions with identical content. Concerning demographic attributes, inspection of table 5.6 reveals a general picture of the similarities and differences between the stakeholder councils and the corresponding watershed subsamples of the Bexar County population.[3]

On balance, table 5.6 reveals that the composition of the two stakeholder groups was reasonably similar to the statistical profile of residents in the Salado and Leon Creek watersheds for the demographic attributes of age, income, and median hours worked. However, for the characteristics of sex, race, educational level, marital status, children in household, and employment status, there were some apparent differences. Women in both councils were underrepresented relative to men. African Americans were overrepresented to some degree in the Salado Council. However, the percentage of Anglos in the Leon Council was substantially higher than in the Leon watershed subsample proportion. One striking finding in table 5.6 was that Hispanic participants were substantially underrepresented in both council groups (particularly the Leon Creek Council) relative to the proportions in the corresponding watershed subsamples. Both college-level and graduate education was overrepresented in both stakeholder councils, relative to the watershed subsample populations.[4] In addition, individuals with children (under age eighteen) in the household were somewhat overrepresented in the Salado Council, but this pattern was reversed in the Leon Council. Finally, members of both councils were employed in higher proportions than in the relevant watershed subsample.

General political beliefs and ideology (see table 5.7) were assessed with the same set of four questions in the telephone survey and in the stakeholder council surveys. One item asked respondents to indicate which of the following two statements was closer to their own views: (1) "The less government, the better" or (2) "There are more things that government should be doing." (A third option offered was "Indifferent.") The next two questions were identical to the national government and city government self-efficacy items described in the first section of this chapter. The final question asked, "Generally, when you think about politics, which

Table 5.6
Demographic characteristics of Salado and Leon Creek stakeholder councils compared to corresponding characteristics of watershed subsamples and total Bexar County sample

Demographic characteristic	Bexar County 1990 Census	Total Bexar County sample (N = 1,017)	Salado Creek Watershed subsample (N = 194)	Salado Creek Stakeholder Council (N = 60)	Leon Creek Watershed subsample (N = 218)	Leon Creek Stakeholder Council (N = 35)
% female	51.4	52.6	55.7	41.7	54.1	42.9
% married	53.9	59.9	52.1	76.3	60.6	57.6
% children 18 or under (in household)	—	62.2	34.0	41.7	47.3	36.4
Median age	35–39	47	49	48	45	51
Median income ($)	25–29K	50–59K	50–59K	60–69K	50–59K	60–69K
% high school graduate	72.5	90.5	25.8	5.0	17.4	3.0
% some college/college graduate	41.1	68.1	52.6	45.0	62.4	42.4
% some graduate/Masters'/doctorate	5.9	15.4	12.4	46.7	15.1	54.5
% African American	4.7	6.9	11.9	20.7	3.7	0.0
% Anglo	49.7	58.7	62.4	67.2	59.2	78.1
% Hispanic	33.0	27.4	19.1	6.9	30.3	3.1
% employed	—	60.6	55.7	67.8	65.6	81.3
Median hours worked (weekly)	—	40	40	40	40	48

Table 5.7
General political beliefs and ideology of Salado and Leon Creek stakeholder councils compared to corresponding political beliefs and ideology of watershed subsamples and total Bexar County sample

General political beliefs and ideology	Total Bexar County sample	Salado Creek Watershed subsample	Salado Creek Stakeholder Council	Leon Creek Watershed subsample	Leon Creek Stakeholder Council
Less government, the better	41.6%	44.3%	31.6%	42.7%	31.3%
Government should do more	54.2	53.6	54.4	53.2	56.3
Indifferent	2.8	1.0	14.0	2.8	12.5
Self-efficacy/national government (% disagree)	56.7	54.1	71.7	59.7	69.7
Self-efficacy/city government (% disagree)	62.3	64.4	80.0	64.3	81.8
Democrat	26.1	30.6	39.2	26.3	16.2
Independent	43.1	38.3	42.9	38.3	58.1
Republican	30.7	31.0	17.9	35.5	25.9

of the following best describes you?" (strong Republican; weak Republican; independent, but lean Republican; pure independent; independent, but lean Democrat; weak Democrat; and strong Democrat).

Table 5.7 presents the results on these four items for the Salado Creek and Leon Creek stakeholder groups using a similar format to table 5.6. On the role of government question, there appear to be no differences between the two stakeholder groups and their respective watershed subsamples in terms of support for statement that "government should do more." However, we did observe less frequent endorsement of the "less government, the better" ideology in the stakeholder council groups relative to the corresponding watershed subsamples. Another consistent result across both the Salado and Leon watersheds was that the stakeholder councils reported a higher sense of self-efficacy in influencing national and city government policies. In terms of political affiliation, the patterns varied depending on the particular council group: the Salado Council is typical with respect to percentage of independents, although Democratic representation was somewhat higher and Republican representation lower relative to the Salado watershed subsample. For the Leon Creek Council, however, independents were overrepresented compared to the statistical profile in the Leon watershed subsample. Democrats and Republicans were underrepresented in the Leon Council.

Environmental attitudes were measured in the stakeholder surveys using the same twelve-item New Environmental Paradigm (NEP) scale described earlier in this chapter for the telephone survey. Table 5.8 lists the percentage agreeing for each group. The table shows that, in general, the Salado Council members were representative of the watershed in terms of their support for the NEP.

Table 5.8 also shows that the Leon Council was considerably stronger in its support for the NEP than was the corresponding Leon watershed subsample. In addition to the limits to growth items, the Leon Council rejected the notion of humans ruling over nature to a greater extent than the broader Leon watershed population.

Finally, table 5.9 presents the results from five survey questions dealing specifically with water quality in the Salado and Leon Creek watersheds of San Antonio. We wanted to assess how familiar respondents were with Salado and Leon creeks and how safe they considered various activities that required contact with the water. In general, Salado

Table 5.8
New Environmental Paradigm beliefs of Salado and Leon Creek stakeholder councils compared to corresponding beliefs of watershed subsamples and total Bexar County sample

New environmental paradigm scale item	Total Bexar County sample (% agree)	Salado Creek watershed subsample (% agree)	Salado Creek Stakeholder Council (% agree)	Leon Creek Watershed subsample (% agree)	Leon Creek Stakeholder Council (% agree)
We are approaching the limit of the number of people the earth can support.	46.4	45.3	62.7	40.8	60.6
The balance of nature is very delicate and easily upset.	76.2	76.8	81.7	73.4	68.8
Humans have the right to modify the natural environment to suit their needs.	42.1	30.9	35.6	46.8	35.5
Mankind was created to rule over the rest of nature.	41.7	36.6	35.0	46.3	31.0
When humans interfere with nature, it often produces disastrous consequences.	75.8	75.3	83.1	68.8	86.7
Plants and animals exist primarily for human use.	36.2	34.5	28.8	39.5	17.2
To maintain a healthy environment, we will have to develop a steady-state economy where industrial growth is controlled.	75.2	80.9	71.4	74.8	82.8
Humans must live in harmony with nature in order to survive.	90.9	87.1	95.0	89.5	90.9

The earth is like a spaceship with only limited room and resources.	69.1	68.6	83.1	69.7	84.4
Humans need not adapt to the natural environment because they can remake it to suit their needs.	24.2	20.6	16.7	23.4	9.4
There are limits on growth beyond which our industrialized society cannot expand.	59.2	57.2	77.6	55.1	77.4
Mankind is severely abusing the environment.	77.3	77.8	84.7	73.4	84.4

Table 5.9
Knowledge and beliefs about San Antonio water quality of Salado Creek and Leon Creek stakeholder councils compared to corresponding knowledge and beliefs of watershed subsamples and total Bexar County sample

Knowledge/beliefs about San Antonio water quality	Total Bexar County sample, Salado Creek	Salado Creek Watershed subsample	Salado Creek Stakeholder Council	Leon Creek Watershed subsample	Leon Creek Stakeholder Council
Familiar with creek (% yes)	73.0	86.1	85.0	60.1	91.4
Safety of water—drinking (% safe)	11.0	8.4	3.4	22.1	0.0
Safety of water—swimming (% safe)	16.3	10.2	1.7	34.4	5.9
Safety of eating fish (% safe)	20.0	16.8	6.9	29.0	8.8
Safety of water—livestock drinking (% safe)	46.3	45.5	27.6	62.5	29.4

Creek was quite familiar to both stakeholders and watershed subsample respondents alike. With respect to water quality assessments, the overall picture in table 5.9 is that Salado Council members were consistently less convinced of the safety of Salado Creek water for human consumption, swimming, eating fish, and livestock consumption than were residents in the broader Salado watershed sample.

Table 5.9 also presents the comparable results for Leon Creek. In general, Leon Creek was not as familiar to watershed subsample respondents as to Leon Council members. More striking, however, was the large disparity in the water safety beliefs between the Leon Council and the broader Leon watershed population. This pattern of results suggests that knowledge of water quality in Leon Creek may be less widely distributed among residents living in this watershed compared to Salado Creek. In sum, table 5.9 demonstrates that Leon Council members were both more familiar with the creek and rated the water as less safe for all uses compared to the corresponding Leon watershed subsample. These effects appear to be more pronounced than for the Salado Council (see table 5.9). The differences between the watershed subsamples and the council groups in perceived seriousness of water quality problems may be related to the demographic differences in education level and ethnic status (percent Hispanic) documented in table 5.6 (see note 6).

Summary of Recruiting Results in Achieving Representative Participation

This section addresses the following basic research question: "To what extent did the combined effect of the snowball, interview, and survey recruitment techniques achieve statistical representation of the relevant watershed populations in our watershed councils?" We explore this question along four dimensions: demographics, general political beliefs and ideology, environmental attitudes, and evaluations of water quality. The council groups were representative of their respective watershed populations on three of nine demographic characteristics: age, income, and number of hours worked. Despite dedicated efforts to achieve adequate representation of the watershed communities at large, the recruitment methods did not fare as well for two specific subgroups of citizens: women and Hispanics. However, our recruitment efforts were effective with the African American community in the Salado Creek watershed.

With respect to political beliefs and ideology, we succeeded in representing residents holding the belief that "government should do more"
but underrepresented residents with the belief that "the less government,
the better." Moreover, our methods did not reproduce distributions of
political affiliation mirroring the respective watershed populations. For
environmental attitudes, the council groups demonstrated higher environmental concern (support for NEP) than their corresponding watershed samples. Finally, the council groups were composed of residents
who reported both greater familiarity with the creeks and more negative
beliefs about water quality than the larger Salado and Leon watershed
populations.

Goals and Reasons for Citizen Participation in Watershed Councils
The quantitative survey results provide a refined profile of our CL participants. These data, however, do not tell why citizens participated in these
collaborative stakeholder forums. To address this issue, we collected additional data at the fourth (February 2000) of the series of stakeholder
meetings. The final section of the chapter presents a qualitative analysis
of CL participant responses.

Researchers asked participants at the fourth CL meeting to complete
the following statements: (1) "My participation in the Council will have
been worthwhile if: _____," and (2) "My participation in the Council
will *NOT* have been worthwhile if: _____." Providing context for this
request was the meeting agenda, which focused on having the groups discuss their mission as a council, with the unstated process goal of developing their collective identity as citizen groups. Forty-eight participants
provided responses across the two councils ($N = 28$ in Salado Creek;
$N = 20$ in Leon Creek). This sample of meeting attendees represented
47 percent of the total number of survey respondents in the Salado
Council ($N = 60$) and 57 percent of the total number of survey respondents in the Leon Council ($N = 35$). We report a brief qualitative summary of these data in this section because council members' responses
provide important insights into why citizens choose to engage in collaborative watershed management processes.

Fifty-nine responses to the first question were content analyzed and
divided into eight distinct categories.[5] Table 5.10 presents these eight response categories along with two representative examples of statements

Table 5.10
Citizen goals and reasons for participation in watershed councils

Protection or restoration of watershed (N = 11)	"Creek is brought back to lush, green, living, flowing creek that I grew up with." "Nature is preserved and enhanced. Wildlife is conserved."
Information, education (N = 9)	"Other participants have a better understanding of watershed and water quality management issues." "Useful information to help preserve the creek in its natural state will be gained from Council meetings."
Political action, implementation (N = 8)	"City Council and public approval of Council plan." "Council recommendations are implemented."
Community good (N = 7)	"Something progressive and meaningful comes out of it. We accomplish good for the city as a whole." "Quality of life for Bexar County residents in watershed has improved 10 years from now."
Water quality and quantity improvement (N = 7)	"We get a reliable/sustainable quantity of quality water." "We can clean up the creek."
Parks, greenbelt, recreation (N = 7)	"Three miles of hike/bike trails opened by June 2001 on the creek." "Process furthers city/county commitment to watershed linear parks and dedicated buffer zones along San Antonio's watersheds."
Flood control (N = 4)	"Necessary flood prevention of lower creek is accomplished." "Flooding and erosion is prevented. Master plan for drainage adequate to development is created."
Idiosyncratic motives (N = 6)	"Develop working relationships with stakeholders from different areas of watershed to protect the resource." "Incorporate procedure for contacting Native American descendants when sites/remains are uncovered."

coded in each category. The categories are arranged in table 5.10 from most to least frequent. The final category ("idiosyncratic motives") includes a number of diverse statements that did not fit clearly into the other seven categories.

The responses to the second statement ($N = 43$) about what would make participation not worthwhile were more tightly clustered: 77 percent of responses were captured by four categories. The modal response (42 percent, $N = 18$) was expressed as follows: "Nothing is done/No implementation/Council recommendations—plan gathers dust on shelves." The next most common response (19 percent, $N = 8$) was: "Council disbands/Can't reach agreement on plan." Less frequent were the following two categories: "No useful information is obtained for community education/Willingness to inform and be informed stops" (9 percent, $N = 4$) and "Channelization of creek with concrete occurs" (7 percent, $N = 3$). The remaining ten responses fell into a fifth category labeled "idiosyncratic." The majority of these idiosyncratic responses were simply the opposite of the reasons stated in response to the first question.

In summary, two general conclusions emerge from this content analysis. First, the stated goals and reasons for worthwhile participation are quite varied, being distributed fairly evenly across the eight categories. Moreover, over 40 percent of the responses (three categories) focus on rather abstract reasons not tied to the specific content of the council's recommendations: information/education, political action/implementation, and community good. The remaining majority of responses, however, do reflect objectives that depend on specific issues (protection or restoration of creek environment, water quality, parks and greenbelts, flood control) being addressed directly by the council's final action plan. Second, the outcomes of the council's work making citizen participation not worthwhile are not necessarily mirrored by those cited that make participation worthwhile. Citizens seem most concerned about two possible outcomes: no implementation of council recommendations by relevant political entities and the inability of the council to reach consensus on a set of policy recommendations. It is instructive to note that neither of these concerns depends on the substantive issues addressed by the council's action plan. One possible implication, at least for a majority of citizen participants (61 percent), is that the minimum criteria for worthwhile participation in the CL process are that the council agree on some set of specific recommendations, and that actual "on-the-ground" implementation in the community of at least some council recommendations occurs by the relevant political authorities.

Conclusions

The chapter began by posing three fundamental questions about stakeholder participation and representation in collaborative engagement processes: (1) Who participates in these collaborative processes? (2) Why do they participate? and (3) What basic values, beliefs, and attitudes about democracy, society, and the environment do they represent? In this concluding section, we begin by discussing the empirical results with respect to these questions. Next, we consider whether the stakeholder recruitment techniques used to structure the watershed councils satisfied the normative criteria—autonomy, welfare, justice—proposed in chapter 3 for evaluating procedural legitimacy. Finally, we explore implications of empirical results for practitioners and researchers working on collaborative engagement processes in watershed management.

Who Participates in Watershed Collaboratives and Why?

The survey and qualitative results suggest some initial answers to our three questions. First, with respect to the first question—Who participates?—three attitudinal variables in the large-sample telephone survey positively predicted willingness to participate: optimism about personal finances, negative evaluations of water quality, and proenvironmental attitudes. Survey responses of actual participants in the CL stakeholder groups also confirmed the importance of negative water quality evaluations and proenvironmental beliefs. They also suggested the important role of self-efficacy, specifically relating to city government. In terms of demographic characteristics, the larger survey of San Antonio residents indicates that Hispanic citizens would be more willing to participate in discussions on clean water in San Antonio. However, data on actual participation in collaborative stakeholder groups supported the opposite conclusion: Hispanic citizens were significantly underrepresented in both stakeholder forums.[6] In addition, women in both survey samples were found to be less willing to participate than men.

People participate in collaborative engagement processes for two similar types of reasons.[7] Not surprisingly, the majority state that they participate because they believe specific policy issues—such as environmental protection and restoration, flood control, or parks and green belt development—can be addressed directly by the collaborative process. Participation is worthwhile for this subgroup if the final recommendations that emerge from the collaborative process include their personal issues and deal with them satisfactorily. The second category of citizens participates because they believe that the collaborative process has the potential to enhance the public good by improving the quality of life for all residents in the watershed.

This group is less concerned with specific issues and more concerned that the collaborative process produces any tangible, positive results "on the ground" for their community. Personal efficacy appears to be the underlying theme for this subgroup. Participation is valued by these citizens as long as something worthwhile gets done in their watershed. This response pattern reveals that many citizens in the stakeholder groups were often frustrated by numerous planning processes soliciting citizen input and then not culminating in successful implementation by elected political authorities and government agencies.

Survey results from both watershed restoration councils present a fairly consistent picture of what basic values, beliefs, and attitudes are represented by those who actually participate in collaborative engagement processes. In terms of political beliefs and ideology, while participants represented both ideological positions on the role of government in society, there was greater participation among those who believe that "government can do more" compared to citizens who subscribe to the "less government, the better" ideology. We also found that personal efficacy (both city and national government) was generally higher in both watershed restoration councils than in the watershed subpopulations from which these stakeholders were recruited. With regard to environmental attitudes, clear evidence existed in both watershed restoration councils of greater support for the NEP (Dunlap and Van Liere 1978) relative to those residents surveyed in the respective watershed populations. Finally, citizens who rated water quality in the watershed as "unsafe" were overrepresented in the watershed restoration councils compared to citizens in the respective watershed subsamples.

One interpretation of this pattern of participation is that our councils may have overrepresented "problem perceivers." Prospect theory (Kahneman and Tversky 1979) from the behavioral decision literature may help explain this outcome. According to this theory, people value losses more than gains; thus, they may be more willing to accept the costs of participating in a council if they perceive problems to be solved (impending losses) rather than opportunities for gains. In these council groups, water quality perception and education level were positively related: citizens with higher levels of education also believe that water quality is poor in the watersheds. From a representation perspective, this is not necessarily a problem. In fact, one could argue that problem perceivers should be overrepresented because these individuals have stronger beliefs and attitudes toward the policy issue in question. An implication for practitioners is that they should expect these problem perceivers to represent a significant segment of their stakeholder audience when using recruitment methods similar to those used here.

Theoretical Implications: Evaluating Normative Criteria for Legitimacy
In chapter 3 we proposed a normative framework for evaluating procedural and substantive legitimacy of watershed management policy. The research design permitted a quantitative evaluation of whether the recruitment techniques succeeded in meeting the normative criterion of autonomy. Specifically, do the empirical results support the conclusion that the demographic composition of the watershed council stakeholder groups matched the corresponding statistical profiles of the watershed subpopulations from which these participants were selected? Overall, we conclude that the actual demographic profile of the stakeholder councils differed in important respects from the statistical characteristics of the Leon and Salado Creek watershed subpopulations. As noted earlier, women and Hispanic residents were clearly underrepresented in the watershed restoration councils.

Note that representatives from the San Antonio business and development community were visibly absent from the majority of the watershed restoration meetings. State and local agency and city government officials were active participants, as were citizens from a wide variety of interest groups and neighborhood associations. Despite dedicated efforts to recruit business and development representatives, relatively few small business owners participated actively in the watershed restoration councils, and large corporations in the watersheds declined to participate.

In our view, the underrepresentation of Hispanics is the most serious threat to the goal of ensuring autonomy because they represent the largest non-Anglo group in San Antonio, with substantial numbers living in proximity to the watersheds in question. Any policy with regard to the management of these watersheds will affect this population and vice versa. While the proportion of women in our watershed restoration groups was lower than the statistical incidence in the respective watershed populations, we still had roughly 40 to 45 percent women in these stakeholder groups. The openness of the process for recruiting watershed restoration council participants helps mitigate the potential for negative consequences of having underrepresented interests.[8]

Implications for Practitioners and Researchers

The findings of this project underscore how difficult it can be to fully satisfy the legitimacy criterion proposed in chapter 3. Researchers and practitioners must think carefully about what will constitute adequate representation in a particular geographical area and about how they will recruit from socioeconomic groups with which they have little familiarity. Although we expended considerable time and effort to achieve adequate representation of all-important stakeholders in these collaborative processes, there were gaps in representation, particularly regarding Hispanics.

The decision about which groups to include as stakeholders requires, at a minimum, familiarity with the social categories of people who make up the population potentially affected by policy and management decisions. While it may be relatively easy to acquire information about the population characteristics of the general geographic area in question, it may take more effort to acquire information on the population nearest the management area. This, however, is the population most likely to be directly affected by decisions and most likely to have strong feelings about the feature or area in question, both of which have obvious implications for the sustainability of management policies and practices.

Almost a quarter of the respondents (24.1 percent) from the initial survey indicated interest in participating in a citizen forum on watershed issues. This was also true of the Hispanic citizens who were contacted.

While only five of the survey respondents (2 percent) who expressed interest in participation actually became members of one of the watershed councils, other recruitment methods were relatively more successful, except for Hispanic residents of the watershed.

Our experience suggests that issues of community consultation should be of special concern to practitioners and researchers who seek to involve underrepresented populations, including Hispanics. This consultation should begin during the planning stage of the project and continue through the project's completion. Community consultation integrates several approaches, including public forums, immersion, and interaction with key informants and the use of consultants. Field researchers should become well informed about the local community, going beyond census data and obtaining information that will help the researchers better understand the way in which a community functions. In research projects where personal contact is involved, same-ethnicity data collectors enhance rapport, willingness to disclose, and the validity and reliability of the data provided. Other similarities in background between researchers and participants are equally valuable in motivating participants to complete the research process and provide accurate information.

A practical implication of the elaborate process needed to acquire representation is the time and staff needed to accomplish it. Research teams can budget adequately for the effort, but agencies rarely have the staff and other resources required. These observations are consistent with the findings of the EPA Science Advisory Board (2001).

Persistence is a more complicated question. The Leon Creek Restoration Council did not persist after the completion of the collaborative learning activities. The Salado Creek Restoration Council, however, resurrected an inactive nonprofit entity, the Salado Creek Foundation, as a vehicle for its continuation. (www.saladocreek.org). The Salado Creek Foundation is active in community policy advising, education, and cultural preservation of the riparian zone of the Salado Creek system. The variables that give longevity to collaborative organizations are certainly too complex to define in this project; however, we speculate that several fundamental differences in the two watersheds resulted in the different ends. The Salado Creek system is heavily urbanized and relatively well developed, and it has a history of conflict over management issues. The Leon Creek watershed, in contrast, is only recently urbanizing, resulting in rapid land use changes and degradation of water quality. The citizens in the Leon Creek watershed are a broad mix of urban fringe poor with little formal education and well-educated ranchette owners (1- to 2-acre lot size homes), resulting in very little common experience among the stakeholders (see table 5.6). A few motivated citizens who committed themselves to the task organized the Salado Creek Foundation. No such leadership emerged from the Leon Creek Watershed Restoration Council. The obvious complexity of this process suggests that designing watershed collaboratives for persistence may be very difficult indeed.

The experience of this process in San Antonio can provide useful information for those in similar circumstances in other parts of the country. Long-term citizen interactions to address watershed issues require significant investments in individual and organizational time, monetary resources, and the application of a great deal of interpersonal skill and team-building values.

Notes

1. The dependent variable we use to test these hypotheses is the respondent's self-report of willingness to participate in a collaborative stakeholder process. As can be seen from the question wording, respondents were not told in detail what exactly would be involved in the collaborative stakeholder process. Instead, they were asked whether they would be willing to participate in discussions "on the topic of clean water." There is no doubt that had survey interviewers taken the time to explain what exactly is entailed in a collaborative learning process, some respondents might have changed their answer to this survey question. This was, however, beyond the scope of our phone survey.

2. Not all researchers agree with this direction. Traditional research has found a strong positive relationship between trust and participation.

3. Note the disparities in sample size in the stakeholder groups relative to the telephone survey subsamples. All individuals in each group who attended at least one council meeting were asked to complete a survey. The combined response rate for the stakeholder groups was 90 percent. However, because the marked differences in sample size preclude reliable tests of statistical significance, we restrict our descriptive analysis to the largest differences (in percentages) between the stakeholder council groups and the corresponding watershed subsamples drawn from Bexar County.

4. These educational differences between the watershed subsamples and the stakeholder councils may provide an explanation for the large differences between these groups in perceived water quality evident in table 5.9. Thus, college or graduate education may be positively correlated with perceived severity of

water quality problems in the watershed, which may lead these individuals to participate in the councils.

5. $N = 59$ because some participants listed more than one goal or reason for their participation.

6. We return to this apparent paradox later in this final section.

7. We did not find much evidence that council members participated for purely defensive reasons—that is, to prevent the council from recommending actions that they would oppose.

8. Some researchers would argue that the absence of a significant business or development interest group in the council meetings is a more serious problem for solving water quality problems in the watershed than the underrepresentation of a specific ethnic group. The assumption here is that changing the behavior of a specific target group is extremely difficult if that target group is not at the table during the council deliberations.

III

Measuring and Explaining the Success of Watershed Partnerships

6

Theoretical Frameworks Explaining Partnership Success

Paul A. Sabatier, William D. Leach, Mark Lubell, and Neil W. Pelkey

In chapter 1, we presented a flow diagram linking context (e.g., ecological and socioeconomic conditions), process (rules governing collaborative institutions), civic community (e.g., human and social capital), policy outputs (management plans and restoration projects), and watershed outcomes (environmental and other impacts). That diagram has served as a useful framework guiding our understanding of the factors affecting the performance of collaborative watershed arrangements in the United States over the past ten to twenty years.

As a scientific theoretical framework, however, the flow diagram has two important limitations. First, it is not very general, since it was designed to explain the success of collaborative watershed partnerships in the United States. We have no idea if variables, such as civic community, that appear to be important in explaining watershed partnerships are important in explaining the performance of other policymaking institutions, such as city councils, irrigation districts, or school boards. Similarly, there may be factors important in explaining school performance, such as the professional norms of teachers, that are not included in the flow diagram because they do not contain critical analogues explaining the behavior of watershed partnerships.

Second, the flow diagram does not have a clear sense of process, of the mechanisms by which the unemployment rate in a community affects social capital, which in turn affects management plans. The principal reason is that the flow diagram contains no explicit model of the individual. Since we are dealing with human behavior, it seems obvious that most processes run through human beings. The assumptions made concerning an actor's goals, information processing capabilities, and decision rules can dramatically affect a wide variety of relationships. For example, assuming actors are self-interested income maximizers, trust and norms of reciprocity are much more difficult to develop than if one assumes that people frequently consider others' welfare in their decision calculus. Similarly, trust is more difficult to develop if one assumes that actors possess very strong perceptual filters screening out any information coming from opponents.

Thus, in this chapter we supplement the flow diagram by examining three relatively general theoretical frameworks that have been used to explain the success of a variety of policymaking institutional arrangements:[1]

• Institutional rational choice (IRC), as represented by Lubell et al.'s (2002) use of transaction cost economics (TCE) and Ostrom's (1999) institutional analysis and development (IAD) framework.
• The social capital approach grounded in the work of Putnam (Putnam, Leonardi, and Nanetti 1993) and Coleman (1988).
• The advocacy coalition framework (ACF) developed by Sabatier and Jenkins-Smith (1988, 1993, 1999). Here we focus on a more recent version that borrows extensively from the literature on alternative dispute resolution (Carpenter and Kennedy 1988; Susskind, McKearnan, and Thomas-Larmer 1999) to suggest ways in which stalemate may eventually lead to policy agreement.

In each case, we briefly outline the theoretical framework's basic structure and assumptions and then identify several hypotheses derived from the framework that help explain the formation and outcome of collaborative watershed processes.

We present several theoretical frameworks—rather than one—for a number of reasons. First, it is not clear that one of them is demonstrably superior to the others. Institutional rational choice is certainly the best known, but it is also among the most criticized (Green and Shapiro 1994). Second, Graham Allison's classic analysis of the Cuban missile crisis (1971) amply demonstrates the advantages of looking at the same set of phenomena through several theoretical lenses. Each tends to illuminate a different portion of the total portrait. Third, scholars adept at applying multiple perspectives will not assume a priori that a particular lens is automatically superior. They are psychologically and intellectually free to let the evidence reject a particular perspective, knowing they have alternatives at hand (Platt 1964, Stinchcombe 1968). Additionally, they are free to compare the relative merits of different perspectives. Scholars committed to a single perspective tend to view any confirming evidence as conclusive, without bothering to consider that an alternative perspective might explain twice as much of the variance in a given phenomenon.

Chapter 7 combines elements from IRC and ACF, while chapter 8 contains variables from all three frameworks in its analysis.

Institutional Rational Choice

Institutional rational choice (IRC) refers to a set of theoretical frameworks (such as IAD and TCE) that seek to explain the patterns of interactions and outcomes emerging from actors making decisions and behaving within a set of institutional constraints. IRC frameworks start with models of the individual specifying actors' goals, information processing capabilities, and decision rules. The frameworks then examine how institutional rules and other factors affect actors' behavior and cumulative outcomes (Ostrom 1998, 1999; Scharpf 1997).

IRC frameworks assume actors are self-interested, but relax the strict rational decision maker of neoclassical economics in favor of Simon's (1955) notion of bounded rationality. Individual decision makers seek to engage in behaviors that further their self-interest, but their ability to do so is bounded by limited cognitive and information processing abilities. In the context of watershed management, we would expect stakeholders to engage in a great deal of trial-and-error learning as they try different management approaches and react to emerging watershed problems. The evolution of cooperation depends on the benefits of long-term cooperation outweighing the short-term incentives for noncooperation.

At a general level, institutions are defined by the set of formal rules and informal norms that structure human behavior. Formal rules define sets of required, forbidden, and allowable behaviors; the agents responsible for monitoring compliance; and the punishments for violating the rules. Formal rules are generally written down in some fashion in legislation, judicial rulings, agency rule making, management plans, or some other type of authoritative statement. Informal norms are shared prescriptions typically enforced through individuals using reciprocal strategies, with punishment meted out through withdrawal of cooperation or social sanctions. As Ostrom (1999) notes, institutions are one of the main features of a watershed that structure the process of collaboration.

In this section, we examine two variants of IRC frameworks that are particularly promising for explaining the formation and success of watershed partnerships: the institutional analysis and development framework developed by Ostrom (1990, 1999) and the political contracting framework derived from transaction cost economics by Lubell et al. (2002) and Libecap (1989). As will become evident, these two IRC variants are linked in many ways, differing primarily in the level of detail achieved in specifying causal relationships and describing institutional structures. Hence, we derive a set of hypotheses about partnership formation and success, drawing on both IRC variants.

Institutional Analysis and Development Framework

The IAD framework was first articulated in Kiser and Ostrom (1982) and has since been developed through numerous empirical studies by researchers from a wide range of social science disciplines (Ostrom 1990, 1999; Ostrom, Gardner, and Walker 1994). The IAD has primarily been applied to the governance of common pool resources and is therefore directly applicable to the case of watershed management. Figure 6.1, adapted from Kiser and Ostrom (1982), and from Ostrom (1999, 42), summarizes the critical features of the IAD framework.

The central focus of the IAD is a conceptual unit called the action arena, consisting of two elements: (1) a set of actors behaving according to an explicit model of the individual and (2) a decision-action situation. The model of the individual specifies the assumptions being made concerning actors' preferences, information-processing capabilities, current information, personal resources, and decision rules. The decision-action situation comprises a set of resources and constraints defining which actors are allowed to participate in a policy game, the positions and moves available to them, the information available, the outcomes for various patterns of individual actions, and the associated payoffs for the actors for each outcome. Taken together, the decisions and behaviors of actors within the structural constraints of the action arena produce the observable patterns of interaction and outcomes in a particular policy setting.

a.

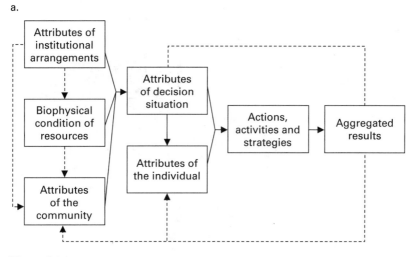

Figure 6.1
Institutional analysis. *Source:* Kiser and Ostrom 1982, Ostrom 1999. *a.* The working parts. *b.* Three levels.

The structure of a decision-action situation is determined by three sets of variables: the biophysical structure of the resource under consideration, the attributes of the community, and institutional rules-in-use. The biophysical structure of the resource refers to whether the resource is overexploited and the nature and complexity of the causal relationships between human behaviors and environmental outcomes. For example, nonpoint source pollution and point source pollution feature quite different temporal and spatial attributes that require appropriate management strategies. "Attributes of the community" encompasses the homogeneity of behavioral norms, cultural differences, people's discount rates (the extent to which they discount future benefits and costs), and the community's aggregate levels of human and social capital (Ostrom 1999). The characteristics of the actors involved in a particular watershed management institution are often heavily influenced by the nature of the community from which they come. Institutional rules refer to the existing sets of social choice or management rules structuring how new rules are made or how resources are used. Taken together, these broad categories of variables determine the details of a particular decision-action situation. Because broad classes of variables are easier to conceptualize and

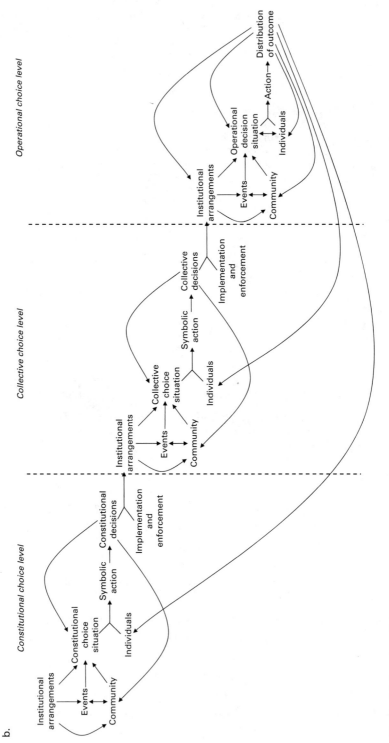

b.

Constitutional choice level

Institutional arrangements

Constitutional choice situation

Symbolic action

Constitutional decisions

Individuals

Events

Community

Implementation and enforcement

Collective choice level

Institutional arrangements

Collective choice situation

Symbolic action

Collective decisions

Individuals

Events

Community

Implementation and enforcement

Operational choice level

Institutional arrangements

Operational decision situation

Action

Distribution of outcome

Individuals

Events

Community

Figure 6.1 (continued)

measure, they often become the central focus for empirical analysis (Lubell et al. 2002).

Another important characteristic of the Ostrom IAD framework is that it includes multiple levels of rules, with decision outputs at higher levels producing rules at lower levels. Operational rules are the specific rules and norms directly governing the use of natural resources. "Collective choice" rules govern the process by which operational rules are changed and "constitutional rules" govern the changing of collective choice rules. Thus, an actor dissatisfied with the decision outputs at a given level has the option of appealing to higher-level authorities to change the rules at the lower level. This is generally quite difficult, however, as changing higher-level rules usually involves more people with more diverse interests and thus much higher transaction costs.

In the complex system of federalism in the United States, it is often difficult to define collective choice rules because a myriad of agencies, governments, and statutes govern the operational rules applying to a particular geographic area or watershed. However, we argue that collaborative processes are in fact an experiment in environmental governance occurring at the collective choice level, and the management actions produced by collaborative institutions are new sets of operational rules governing the use of resources in a specific watershed. Hence, the question of effectiveness hinges on whether watershed partnerships produce a set of operational rules that, when combined with a culture of cooperation, encourage stakeholders to put projects on the ground and engage in other behaviors that ultimately improve watershed health.

The Political Contracting Framework

The political contracting framework developed by Lubell et al. (2002) is based on the contracting for property rights ideas of Libecap (1989) and more generally the literature on neoinstitutional economics and transaction costs (Eggertsson 1990, North 1990, Williamson 1975). Applied to watershed management, the political contracting approach starts with the same assumption as IAD: watershed resources are subject to the tragedy of the commons and feature severe collective action problems. Solutions to watershed collective action problems emerge from a political contracting process in which the various stakeholders agree on a set of institutional rules to govern how the watershed resources are managed and used, then cooperate to implement those rules. The resulting political "agreement" can be analyzed very much like a contract in economics.

The key problem is that political contracting is plagued by three sources of transaction costs: searching for information required to estimate the benefits and costs of various alternatives, negotiating about which of the various alternatives will be incorporated into the final agreement, and monitoring compliance with the agreement and sanctioning violators. Transaction costs are a problem for both the formation and maintenance of collaborative institutions because both stages involve some type of political contracting. The formation of a collaborative institution entails agreeing on a set of institutional rules that will be used to structure decision making about specific watershed management plans. Ongoing maintenance requires successful contracting about management actions, which takes place within the structure of the collaborative institution. In Ostrom's terms, the collaborative institution defines the rules for collective choice, and the management plan defines operational rules.

The general argument of the political contracting framework is that the likelihood of partnership formation and success increases with stakeholder valuations of the benefits of partnerships, decreases with the magnitude of transaction costs involved in forming and running a partnership, and increases with the resources available to pay those costs. This conceptualization is analogous to Ostrom's (1990, see especially pp. 192–210) idea of an institutional choice situation, where people evaluate the net benefits (benefits minus transaction costs) of adopting a new set of collective choice or operational rules. It is this similarity that forms a crucial theoretical nexus between the IAD and political contracting frameworks. The benefits and transaction costs of collective action are determined by the same three broad categories of variables that affect the structure of the action arena: biophysical structure of resource, institutional rules, and attributes of community. Thus, it is possible to derive a set of hypotheses about the formation and success of watershed partnerships common to both frameworks, where the hypotheses are grouped under the main categories of variables. The basic logic of analysis is to determine the characteristics of the watershed decision-action situation that work to increase or decrease the benefits and transaction costs of collaboration, or provide resources for absorbing transaction costs. Table 6.1 presents hypotheses about partnership formation for the three categories of variables, mostly derived from Lubell et al. (2002) Ostrom (1990) and Schlager (1995).

The benefits of partnerships are higher in situations where pollution sources are heterogeneous and dispersed rather than homogeneous and concentrated—for example, nonpoint versus point sources of water pollution. Such dispersed problems create enormous transaction costs for centralized command-and-control regulation, which is thus likely to be both ineffective and inefficient. Anyone wishing to address such dispersed problems effectively is likely to push for a new institution, such as a watershed partnership, involving both local target groups and the proponents of environmental improvement in the development of a solution. However, it is unlikely anyone will be willing to bear the costs of a partnership if environmental threats are not severe or at least perceived as severe by the majority of stakeholders. Transaction costs are also significantly reduced when scientific knowledge about the problem is adequate, allowing people to reach consensus on estimates of the effects of various management options.

If existing institutions are willing to subsidize the initial costs of partnership formation by providing grant money, personnel, facilities, or other in-kind contributions, then partnership formation is more likely. Once they are up and running, most partnerships will continually seek new resources. However, if existing institutions are adequately addressing the problems in a watershed through either traditional regulatory approaches or existing regional governance structures (e.g., CALFED), then a partnership is most likely not needed. Partnerships are also unlikely to form if existing institutions deprive local stakeholders of the autonomy needed to engage in collaborative actions. For example, many agencies may refuse to grant their staff extra time to pursue collaborative activities outside the scope of their existing standard operating procedures.

Clearly, the large majority of hypotheses regarding partnership formation relate to community attributes. Partnerships are more likely to form in areas with sufficient human capital (e.g., income, education) and social capital (e.g., trust, networks) to absorb transaction costs. Partnerships are more likely to form in places where people value long-term benefits, which often occurs in areas of low population mobility where people

Table 6.1
IRC hypotheses about the factors affecting formation of watershed partnerships

---

Attributes of the resource

Partnerships are more likely to form where environmental problems are heterogenous in nature and geographically dispersed, such as nonpoint source pollution.

Partnerships are more likely to form where environmental problems are severe or perceived by most actors to be severe.

Partnerships are more likely to form where scientific knowledge about the problem is very good.

Attributes of institutions

Partnerships are more likely to form when an existing institution has enough resources to subsidize initial transaction costs.

Partnerships are more likely to form when existing institutions are not actively addressing watershed problems.

Partnerships are more likely to form where higher-level institutions grant local autonomy.

Attributes of community

Partnerships are more likely to form in communities with high existing stores of human and social capital.

Partnerships are more likely to form in communities where stakeholders have low discount rates, which equates to a willingness to trade short-term costs for long-term benefits.

Partnerships are less likely to form in situations of high cultural or belief heterogeneity.

Partnerships are more likely to form in communities where the costs and benefits of management actions are spread equitably over different segments of the community.

Partnerships are less likely to form in communities dominated by extractive industries.

Partnerships are more likely to form in communities dominated by service industries.

---

develop a sense of place and learn to value watershed resources for future generations. Partnerships are less likely to form in places with high levels of cultural or socioeconomic heterogeneity because having a large number of different policy preferences increases the costs of bargaining (Libecap 1989). However, if the costs and benefits of collaboration are distributed fairly around the community, individuals will be more willing to bear some of the costs.

Finally, partnership formation is likely to be affected by the type of industries and associated communities of interest in a particular area.

Extractive industries often possess a short-term outlook on resource management and generally resist any environmental policy initiatives. They are less likely to participate in a partnership, especially in the absence of an active environmental constituency threatening them with regulatory measures. Service industries, which frequently rely on maintenance of natural resources to attract visitors to their communities, are more likely to press for environmental policies. Most likely, partnerships will emerge when there is some mixture of these types of constituencies, since one function of partnerships is to resolve conflict between competing preferences for resource use.

Somewhat surprisingly, given the overall emphasis of IRC on the structure of institutions, neither the IAD nor political contracting framework says much about the types of higher-level institutions likely to facilitate the formation of local partnerships. One reason for this is that Ostrom focuses on common-pool resource (CPR) institutions that have emerged from virtually institution-free contexts in small-scale, resource-dependent communities (e.g., a small fishery, a small irrigation system) in many different countries. The situations confronting most watershed partnerships in the United States are normally much more complex. They occur within the context of American federalism and exist within a massively complex tapestry of institutions both within and across levels of the federal system. Watershed resources in the United States are not single-use resources; they are multiple-use resources with many different groups competing for appropriation rights. For these reasons, we know little about the institutional context in which watershed partnerships are likely to emerge.

Ostrom (1990) and her colleagues (Ostrom, Gardner, and Walker 1994) spend a great deal of time describing the characteristics of enduring CPR institutions (summarized in table 6.2); these factors may heavily influence the ongoing success of partnerships. In fact, many observers basically assume that collaborative partnerships exhibit Ostrom's criteria to a greater extent than command-and-control institutions and are superior institutions for that reason. Given the variance in partnership structures that we have observed and the research still needed on effectiveness, there is no guarantee the advocates are correct. Nevertheless, we expect partnerships to be more successful to the extent they do meet Ostrom's criteria. Furthermore, all of the hypotheses about partnership formation

Table 6.2
IRC hypotheses about enduring institutional structures

Individuals who benefit from partnership activities are clearly identified and included in collaborative process.

Benefits individuals receive from the collaborative process are commensurate with the contributions they make toward managing the resource.

Most individuals significantly affected by management decisions may participate in decision making either directly or through accountable representatives.

Monitors who actively audit stakeholder behavior are accountable to the members or are members themselves.

Stakeholders who violate rules are likely to be assessed graduated sanctions by other stakeholders or officials accountable to the stakeholders.

The partnership has procedures for resolving conflict in an efficient and low-cost manner.

The management decisions of the partnership are not significantly challenged or altered by existing government authorities.

stated in table 6.1 should also apply to partnership success, because the process of political contracting continues once the partnership is formed. Hence, table 6.2 essentially extends the number of hypotheses detailed in table 6.1 by describing specific features of institutional structure likely to contribute to partnership success over an extended period of time (adapted from Schlager 1995).

One of the main sources of transaction costs when dealing with watersheds is determining how to coordinate the behaviors of the many different stakeholder groups that use or affect watershed resources. Because they are generally fragmented into isolated subsystems based on statutory authority or political jurisdictions, command-and-control policies have difficulty coordinating multiple users. The inclusiveness of collaborative institutions reduces transaction costs by providing a forum for coordination.

Individuals are unlikely to bear the transaction costs of participation in watershed partnerships if they do not receive some benefit in return. As noted in chapter 5, one of the main benefits people derive from watershed management is protection of a resource they value. However, participants also receive benefits in the form of grant money, new knowledge, and new social and professional networks. Institutional structures providing rewards for participation are more likely to succeed.

Experimental studies of common-pool resource situations (Orbell and Dawes 1991; Ostrom, Gardner, and Walker 1994) and studies of procedural justice (Tyler and Blader 2000) have provided substantial evidence that people are more likely to cooperate when they participate in decisions, or at least feel their interests are adequately represented. In terms of monitoring and implementing a set of rules, Ostrom (1990) shows that compliance is more likely to occur when monitors and enforcers are trusted members of the community or viewed as appropriate representatives. Because people often make mistakes when attempting to cooperate or comply with a set of operational rules, sanctions should be graduated in the sense of starting with mild punishments and escalating to stronger punishments for repeat offenses. Light punishments, such as social disapproval from other stakeholders, serve as a signal to noncompliers to switch to cooperative behavior, giving those who make errors a chance to correct them. Heavier punishments for repeat offenders, such as being removed from the partnerships or subjected to the hammers of existing regulatory tools, are used to drive out inveterate defectors.

According to the IRC frameworks, watershed partnerships should also have some mechanism for resolving conflict between stakeholders, which generally manifests as differences in opinion over proposed management actions. Usually, the agreed-on set of collective choice rules provides this function, but at other times a professional mediator or facilitator may reduce the costs of conflict resolution. Once a watershed partnership succeeds in producing a management plan and a set of actions, it is important that external federal and state authorities provide their representatives to the partnership with the flexibility to implement the plans. Another way to provide justification from external governing authorities is to establish grant programs that provide money for implementation.

According to IRC frameworks, collaborative institutions with these particular structures are more likely to succeed by producing cooperation and improved water quality. Not all collaborative institutions embody every one of these institutional rules. The relative importance of each of the institutional rules is not well known and may change depending on other characteristics of the action situation. To complicate things further, measuring these institutional characteristics is extremely difficult. Thus, a host of empirical issues must be resolved before the full power of the IRC

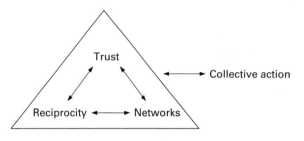

Figure 6.2
Reciprocal relationships between social capital (triangle) and collective action

framework is understood. Some of these issues are addressed in chapters 7 and 8, but many others are left for later research.

Social Capital Framework

Although social capital theory was initially developed by Putnam, Leonardi, and Nanetti (1993) and Coleman (1988), it has been elucidated most famously and exhaustively by Putnam's classic book, *Bowling Alone: The Collapse and Revival of American Community* (2000). Social capital is defined as the triad of trust, norms of reciprocity, and horizontal social networks. The social capital framework (SCF) predicts that each of the three elements reinforces the others in a "virtuous circle" and that together they foster collective action or civic-minded behavior (figure 6.2).

The vast majority of the social capital literature focuses on the effect of social capital upon civic engagement among the American general public. Civic engagement refers to collective behaviors facilitating a democratic and civil society, such as volunteering, philanthropy, participating in politics (e.g., voting or communicating with elected officials), and staying informed about current events. Applying the SCF to collaborative watershed management extends the scope of the theory in two ways. First, we are concerned with collective action among so-called policy elites (public officials and representatives of stakeholder organizations) rather than the general public. Second, the collective outcomes we wish to explain are negotiated agreements and their implementation rather than civic engagement.

The term *network* is used very broadly to mean any social arrangement that provides opportunities for "interpersonal communication and exchange, both formal and informal" (Putnam, Leonardi, and Nanetti 1993, 173). More specifically, social networks refer to membership in any type of voluntary association—from sports clubs to religious congregations. Putnam, Leonardi, and Nanetti (1993, 175) distinguish between horizontal and vertical networks. Horizontal networks involve "agents of equivalent status and power," whereas vertical networks link "unequal agents in asymmetric relations of hierarchy and dependence." Putnam argues that horizontal networks facilitate collective action indirectly through a number of important collateral benefits. First, participation in a network builds skills in communication, negotiation, compromise, and leadership. Second, existing networks often serve as templates for new organizations when the needs of a community grow or change. Third, networks build trust among participants by fostering cultural norms of cooperation and reciprocity and by imposing social sanctions on defectors. Another way to characterize networks is by their degree of connectivity, that is, the breadth and density of connections among actors in a network. Some social capital scholars treat all linkages among individuals and organizations as essentially equal, but Putnam (2000) views "bridging" relationships among people who are quite different from each other as more important than "bonding" relationships among people of the same nationality, ethnicity, or social class.

Turning now to the second concept in the triad, trust refers to confidence in people at large (known as generalized trust) or specific individuals (specific trust) to keep their promises, treat others fairly, and show some concern for others' welfare. Generalized trust is especially useful for initiating new relationships, whereas specific trust is necessary for maintaining existing relationships. Specific trust means believing that the members of one's network are likely to negotiate honestly, are worthy of respect, and are sufficiently honorable and competent to keep any promises previously made.

The third facet of Putnam's SCF is norms of reciprocity: a willingness to initiate and return favors and reward cooperative behavior. As with trust, both general and specific forms are useful. Reciprocity norms encourage individuals to apply themselves to public-minded initiatives, even when a purely rational cost-benefit approach would argue against involvement. Like institutional rational choice, social capital presupposes that people are "intendedly (or boundedly) rational," but SCF also assumes a heavy reliance on habits and norms to guide everyday behavior. Norms of reciprocity are congruent with long-term self-interest, because the benefits of repeated interactions generally outweigh short-term benefits of defection. However, expectations of reciprocity and trust that are built in the context of one interaction are often generalized to new interactions, which can accelerate the evolution of cooperation. For example, rather than evaluating the trustworthiness of every new acquaintance, people in communities with strong generalized social capital operate under the assumption that most people should be trusted most of the time unless there is a clear reason not to do so. In low-social-capital environments, the rule is to distrust people unless trust is clearly warranted.

Norm-driven behavior can be extremely efficient, because it reduces the transaction costs accompanying social exchange under pure rationality. Such costs include the time and money devoted to crafting enforceable contracts (services provided by attorneys, arbitrators, notary publics, credit bureaus), monitoring of agreements (auditors, regulators, police), and punishing defectors (judges, prison guards, probation officers). When trust and reciprocity norms are widely held within a community and few people take advantage of their neighbors' goodwill, cooperative behavior flourishes. As long as trust and reciprocity are the norm, they provide the "sociological WD-40" that lubricates the gears of collective action.

In general, the SCF can be construed as nested within Ostrom's (1999) version of IRC. They contain similar models of the individual: both assume that individuals are primarily self-interested, but recognize that it may be rational in the short term to bear the costs of collective action in the hope that it will provide long-term benefits. Both frameworks assume that people have limited capacity to process information, but do not suffer from systematically biased perceptions. And both treat norms of reciprocity and trust as part of what Ostrom would term community characteristics. An important difference, however, is that Putnam views norms of reciprocity and trust as a substitute for institutional rules in implementing agreements, whereas Ostrom views the keeping of promises as a product of good institutional rules (Ostrom 1999).

Table 6.3
Hypotheses regarding the effect of social capital on partnership outputs

SCF hypothesis 1: Consensus-based agreements should be more common and extensive in partnerships that exhibit high trust, strong norms of reciprocity, and extensive social networks.

SCF hypothesis 2: Project implementation should be more common and extensive in partnerships that exhibit high trust, strong norms of reciprocity, and extensive social networks.

Applying social capital theory to the study of collaborative watershed partnerships, we come up with the two general hypotheses listed in table 6.3. Social capital should contribute to both the making of agreements and the implementation of those agreements through restoration projects. More specifically, higher levels of trust, norms of reciprocity, and dense horizontal networks should contribute to both forms of collaborative outputs.

The Advocacy Coalition Framework

The advocacy coalition framework (ACF) is a policymaking framework developed by Sabatier and Jenkins-Smith (1993, 1999, 1988) to deal with "wicked" problems—those involving goal conflict, technical disputes, and multiple actors from several levels of government. It argues that actors from interest groups, agencies, research institutions, and legislatures may be grouped into advocacy coalitions whose members share a set of normative beliefs and perceptions of the world and act in concert to some degree in pursuit of their common policy objectives.

The ACF assumes that policymaking occurs primarily among specialists who regularly seek to influence policy within a policy subsystem, such as California water policy. A subsystem is characterized by both a functional dimension (e.g., water) and a territorial one (e.g., California) (Zafonte and Sabatier 1998). Historically, interaction has occurred primarily among specialists in a given functional area rather than among those in different functional areas at the same locale. In contrast, watershed partnerships emphasize the territorial component—a specific watershed—and integrate a number of functional domains involved in that watershed, such as water quality, flood control, endangered species, and national forest lands.

The ACF argues that creating new watershed partnerships will take time because people from different functional domains are not accustomed to working with each other and because they need to educate each other about the legal and political constraints of each policy domain. The subsystem perspective also suggests that maintaining local autonomy for the watershed subsystem will be difficult because each constituent functional agency possesses its own routes of accountability and appeal to state and federal agencies and their relevant legislative committees. In fact, most watershed partnerships contain members from functional subsystems dealing with water quality, flood control, agriculture or forestry, land use planning, and fish and wildlife. Partnerships represent an attempt to strengthen local integration across these functional areas while weakening hierarchical relationships within each functional domain.

The ACF seeks to explain policymaking within each watershed-defined, water-related subsystem. Policy is assumed to be dominated by specialists knowledgeable about that watershed, who can be grouped into two or more coalitions based on similar beliefs and some degree of coordinated behavior. Their behavior is affected by two sets of exogenous factors—one fairly stable, the other quite dynamic (see figure 6.3). Interaction, however, occurs primarily among actors within the subsystem. In addition, interaction among actors within the same coalition is assumed to be much more frequent than interaction among members of different coalitions.

The ACF differs from the IAD primarily in its model of the individual (Sabatier and Schlager 2000, Schlager 1995). While the IAD assumes self-interested actors rationally pursuing relatively simple material interests, the ACF assumes that normative beliefs must be empirically ascertained and does not a priori preclude the possibility of altruistic behavior. The ACF stresses the difficulty of changing normative beliefs and the tendency for actors to relate to the world through a set of perceptual filters composed of preexisting beliefs that are difficult to alter. Thus, actors from different coalitions are likely to perceive the same information in very different ways, leading to distrust. The ACF also borrows the key proposition of prospect theory (Quattrone and Tversky 1988):

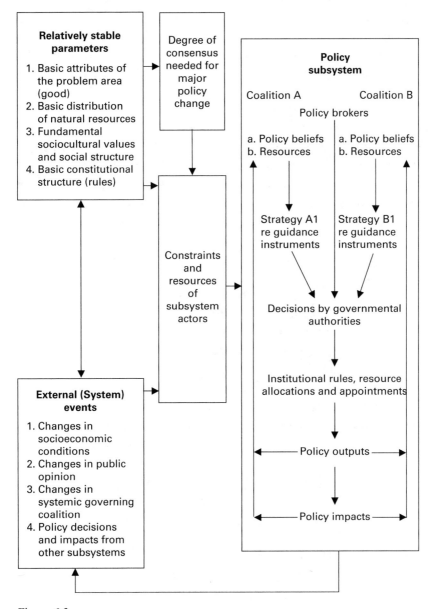

Figure 6.3
The advocacy coalition framework, 1998

actors value losses more than gains. The implication is that individuals remember defeats more than victories. These propositions interact to produce "the devil shift," the tendency for actors to view their opponents as less trustworthy, more evil, and more powerful than they probably are (Sabatier, Hunter, and McLaughlin 1987; Sabatier and Jenkins-Smith 1999). This in turn both cements relationships within coalitions and exacerbates conflict across coalitions. Perceptual filters also tend to screen out dissonant information and reaffirm conforming information, thus making belief change quite difficult. The ACF is thus more pessimistic than the IAD—or social capital theory, for that matter—about the likelihood that consensus-based negotiations in watershed partnerships will lead to policy agreements. The ACF's model of the individual is well suited to explain the escalation and continuation of policy conflict. As we shall see shortly, it requires further modification to account for de-escalation and agreement.

The ACF conceptualizes the belief systems of policy elites as a tripartite structure. At the deepest and broadest level are deep core beliefs. These involve very general normative and ontological assumptions about human nature, the relative priority of fundamental values such as liberty and equality, the relative priority of the welfare of different groups, the proper role of government versus markets in general (i.e., across all policy subsystems), and about who should participate in governmental decision making. The traditional left-right scales operate at the deep core level. Largely the product of childhood socialization, deep core beliefs are very difficult to change.

At the next level are policy core beliefs. These are applications of deep core beliefs to an entire policy subsystem, such as California water policy, and include such topics as the priority of different values, whose welfare counts, the relative authority of governments and markets, the proper roles of the general public, elected officials, civil servants, experts, and others and the relative seriousness and causes of policy problems in the subsystem as a whole. The general assumption is that policy elites are very knowledgeable about relationships within their policy subsystem and thus may be willing to adjust the application of certain deep core beliefs to that subsystem. For example, while conservatives generally have a strong preference for market solutions, some of them recognize significant market failure (e.g., externalities) in water pollution problems and thus are willing to support more governmental intervention in this policy area. Because policy core beliefs are subsystem-wide in scope and deal with fundamental policy choices, they are also very difficult to change.

The final level consists of secondary beliefs. Secondary beliefs are relatively narrow in scope (less than subsystem-wide) and address, for example, detailed rules and budgetary applications within a specific program, the seriousness and causes of problems in a specific locale, and public participation guidelines within a specific statute. Because secondary beliefs are narrower in scope than policy core beliefs, changing them requires less evidence and fewer agreements among subsystem actors and thus should be less difficult.

With respect to watershed partnerships, the ACF stresses the importance of the degree of belief conflict across coalitions. The greater the conflict, the less likely the partnership is to reach agreement on any plan, let alone engage in restoration projects. It also stresses the importance of information sources in belief change. Actors who rely solely on members of their own coalition are very unlikely to modify their beliefs significantly, while those who access sources from outside their own coalition are more susceptible to belief change, particularly on policy core issues. From this perspective, one of the major functions of a partnership is to gradually build trust among members from different coalitions, encouraging reliance on one another as trusted information sources. That, in turn, facilitates belief change and, eventually, the possibility of reaching agreement on the nature and seriousness of various problems, their causes, and the desirability of specific policy proposals. Face-to-face interaction over a considerable period of time is one of the best ways to reduce distrust and to soften the devil shift (for a somewhat similar argument, see Ostrom, Gardner, and Walker 1994).

The ACF argues that legislators, agency officials, interest group leaders, researchers, and intellectuals with similar policy core beliefs will form an advocacy coalition in an effort to coordinate their behavior and bring about changes in public policy. In any given policy subsystem, there may be two to five advocacy coalitions. Among members of a given coalition, trust is common and belief change is relatively easy on secondary beliefs. Given the devil shift, however, belief change across coalitions is hypothesized to be extremely difficult. Thus, there is a strong tendency for coalitions to be rather stable over periods of a decade or more. In fact, until recently, the ACF argued that major (policy core) policy change within a subsystem would occur only when significant perturbations from other policy areas or socioeconomic conditions changed the resources or the core beliefs of major actors and essentially led to the replacement of the previously dominant coalition by a minority coalition (Sabatier and Jenkins-Smith 1993).

Clearly, however, there are situations, such as Lake Tahoe in the 1980s (Sabatier and Pelkey 1990), in which coalitions that have been fighting for decades come to a negotiated agreement representing a substantial change from the status quo ante. In fact, the raison d'être of many multistakeholder partnerships is to craft agreements among actors who have been fighting for years. If the ACF is to be relevant to the study of watershed partnerships, then, it must be modified to identify the conditions under which, in the absence of a major "external perturbation," agreements involving policy core changes are crafted among previously warring coalitions.

Fortunately, a solution emerges by combining the hypotheses from the ACF concerning policy-oriented learning across coalitions (Sabatier and Jenkins-Smith 1988, Sabatier and Zafonte 2001) with the literature on alternative dispute resolution (ADR) (Bingham 1986; Carpenter and Kennedy 1988; O'Leary and Bingham 2003; Susskind, McKearnan, and Thomas-Larmer 1999; Ury 1993). This fusion is possible because many ADR theorists, particularly Carpenter and Kennedy (1988), use a model of the individual that stresses the role of perceptual filters and distrust in creating a spiral of escalating conflict. Both ACF and ADR start with a situation in which individuals in a dispute are grouped into coalitions consisting of individuals with similar beliefs and interests, often interpret the same piece of information in very different ways, distrust their opponents' ability to negotiate fairly and keep their promises, and distrust their opponents' ability to understand, let alone recognize as legitimate, their own goals and interests.

In such a situation, both the ADR literature and the ACF's discussion of the characteristics of professional fora necessary to create policy-oriented learning among scientists from different coalitions come to very similar prescriptions concerning the design of institutions for negotiating and implementing agreements:[2]

Incentive to negotiate seriously: A hurting stalemate.   The basic precondition to successful negotiations is a situation in which all parties to the dispute view a continuation of the status quo as unacceptable. The ACF refers to this as "a policy stalemate," while the ADR literature refers to "a hurting stalemate" (Zartman 1991). The assumption is that individuals satisfied with the status quo have little incentive to give up anything in negotiations. Thus, negotiating with them is probably a waste of time.

Composition.   Both frameworks stress the necessity of including representatives from all relevant groups of stakeholders, even those labeled "difficult" (so long as they represented a significant group of stakeholders). This assumes that, at least in the United States, there are so many venues of appeal for actors excluded from negotiations that it is better to include them from the start rather than waste time in negotiations likely to be nullified or circumvented by appeals from excluded stakeholders.

Leadership.   Sabatier and Zafonte (2001) argue that the chair of the professional forum called to resolve disputes among scientists from competing coalitions should be a respected neutral whose role is to remind participants of professional norms. The ADR literature stresses the importance of neutral and skilled mediators (Bingham 1986) and of facilitators skilled at running meetings.

Consensus decision rule.   This is the defining characteristic of much of the ADR literature (Carpenter and Kennedy 1988; Susskind, McKearnan, and Thomas-Larmer 1999). While not explicitly mentioned in Sabatier and Zafonte (2001), the basic logic behind consensus is the same as for inclusion: given the multitude of venues of appeal in the American political system, a dissatisfied party can wreck the implementation of any agreement. Therefore, this model advocates including them in the negotiations and granting them veto power.

Funding.   Because the ACF views most administrative agencies as belonging to coalitions, it assumes that funding for a consensus process should come from sources who are members of different coalitions (Sabatier and Zafonte 2001).

Duration and commitment.   Given the complexity of stakeholder negotiations and the time it takes to sort out technical issues—let alone find win-win solutions—a half-dozen meetings over a year or so is probably the minimum. In addition to agreeing to participate over an extended period of time, there should be continuity in the participation of representatives from a given organization. Turnover kills trust building because specific trust is a product of personal relationships. Finally, participants in a forum or partnership should be required to report regularly to their constituents, lest they independently agree to compromises that will ultimately prove unacceptable to their group.

The importance of empirical issues.   Both the ACF and ADR agree that purely normative issues, such as abortion, are not ripe for negotiation because there is virtually no prospect of changing an opponent's views. Thus, a substantial portion of the conflict must deal with empirical issues—primarily the seriousness and causes of the problem—which, with time and effort, can be at least partially resolved by stakeholders from different coalitions.

The importance of building trust.   Both literatures assume that negotiations begin with massive distrust between opponents. A necessary condition for reaching agreement is that participants come to trust their opponents to listen carefully to their views, look for mutually acceptable compromises, and keep their promises. This takes time, effort, and carefully crafted process rules promoting fair and respectful treatment of all participants.

Alternative venues.   While the American political system generally provides multiple venues of appeal to dissatisfied stakeholders, agreements are more likely to occur and to be implemented when alternative venues are relatively few in number or relatively unappealing. In the ADR literature (Ury 1993), this is known as BATNA (Best Alternative to a Negotiated Agreement). Stakeholders are more likely to negotiate seriously if their alternatives to the stakeholder negotiation are relatively unattractive.

The hypotheses from both the traditional ACF and the recent revisions inspired by the ADR literature are summarized in table 6.4.

Conclusions

In chapter 1, we presented a rather simple flow diagram that seeks to explain the formation and success of watershed collaboratives with five sets of variables: ecological and socioeconomic context, process rules, civic community, policy outputs, and impacts on watershed health. Throughout the book, we use that flow diagram to guide and organize our inquiry.

Within that context, this chapter has three objectives. First, we have sought to relate the elements in the flow diagram to broader theoretical frameworks in the social sciences. In particular, we have improved the sense of causal process in the flow diagram by relating it to the some-

Table 6.4
ACF hypotheses about reaching effective negotiated agreements

---

Hypotheses from the original ACF

Agreements are less likely when there is intense policy core conflict across coalitions.

Agreements are more likely when there exists a professional forum to help resolve technical disputes among experts from different coalitions.

Agreements become more likely when participants begin seriously considering information provided by members of opposing coalitions.

Hypotheses from the merger of ACF and ADR

Agreements are more likely when there is "a hurting stalemate," that is, when all major stakeholders regard the status quo as unacceptable.

The implementation of agreements is more likely when all major stakeholders are included in the negotiations.

The implementation of agreements is more likely when there is a consensus decision rule.

Agreements are more likely when there is a respected, knowledgeable, and relatively neutral person to lead the negotiations.

Agreements are more likely when key stakeholders commit at least a year to the negotiations, stay personally involved (there is no turnover), and report regularly to their constituents.

Agreements are more likely when some of the major conflicts concern empirical topics.

Agreements are more likely to occur and to be implemented when most stakeholders trust each other to treat others' concerns seriously and to keep agreements.

Agreements are more likely to be reached and implemented when more than one coalition provides funding.

---

what different models of the individual found in institutional rational choice, social capital, and the advocacy coalition framework. In our view, this is a critical improvement. Understanding collective human behavior—which is, after all, what watershed collaboratives are all about—requires a model of how individual human beings make decisions. Likewise, macrolevel aspects of these theoretical frameworks, such as the multiple levels of action in the IAD and the concept of policy subsystems in the ACF, contribute to our understanding of the difficulties that watershed collaborative face and the strategies available to meet these challenges. In short, the first purpose of this chapter is to use broader theoretical frameworks to flesh out on our rudimentary flow diagram.

Second, by relating our findings regarding watershed collaboratives to broader bodies of theory, we hope to make those findings of interest to scholars and practitioners who do not care about watershed collaboratives. For example, the findings in chapter 8 suggest that there is a considerable halo effect from perceptions of trust in a partnership to perceptions of partnership impacts. And, in chapter 7 we will see that collaborative partnerships in the National Estuaries Program improved actors' perceptions of the fairness of the process, the influence of opponents, and actors' willingness to listen to adversaries. There is certainly a plausible argument that these findings might also apply to collaborative processes in, say, urban redevelopment or mental health services (Ogu 2000), and possibly to the common property resource problems that Ostrom has studied so extensively.

The third purpose of this chapter is to present the conceptual foundations underlying the arguments made in chapters 7 and 8. That way, we can focus in those empirical chapters on operationalizing specific variables and explaining the specific quantitative techniques employed and the results of those specific analyses. It should also be clear that there are many aspects of the theoretical frameworks that we simply do not have the data or time to explore in chapters 7 and 8.

Given these objectives, how can we compare the theoretical frameworks discussed in this chapter?

First, they differ in their scope and what they are seeking to explain. The most elaborated and widely used frameworks are those derived from institutional rational choice—Ostrom's IAD and Lubell's political contracting approach. Putnam's social capital approach is much less extensively developed (at least for our purposes) than either IRC or the ACF of Sabatier and Jenkins-Smith. The IRC frameworks deal with both the formation and performance of watershed partnerships, while social capital is rather amorphous in its scope, and the ACF focuses on factors affecting the reaching and implementing of agreements.

Second, the frameworks all agree that the development of trust is critical to the performance of watershed partnerships, but the ACF views this as much more difficult than the other two. IAD tends to view trust as the product of institutional rules, while social capital views trust primarily as a social norm that substitutes for institutional rules.

Third, the most important difference among the frameworks concerns their models of the individual. Both IRC and social capital view individuals as primarily self-interested and boundedly rational. Both view learning processes as critical to overcoming information limitations but see no systematic barriers to such learning. In contrast, the ACF focuses on the role of perceptual filters and the devil shift in systematically inhibiting learning (belief change) from adversaries. The ACF is also much more concerned with belief change, particularly on relatively technical issues like the severity and causes of policy problems, and its assumed importance in reaching policy agreements. The recent borrowing from the ADR literature has broadened the scope of belief change and conflict resolution to all stakeholders, as well as clarifying and extending the conditions conducive to reaching and implementing agreements.

The next two chapters explore how many of the ideas from these frameworks have been used to understand the behavior of watershed collaboratives.

Notes

1. A theoretical framework identifies sets of variables and the general relationships among them. It is generally broader in scope, but less detailed, than a theory and certainly than a model of a specific situation (Ostrom 1999). In our view, IAD, the ACF, and TCE are all quite detailed theoretical frameworks that some might regard as theories. Ostrom argues that IAD in general is a framework, but its application to common pool resource situations is sufficiently detailed and precise to constitute a theory. We prefer to take a conservative view, reserving the term *theory* for, Newtonian mechanics, the neo-Darwinian synthesis in biology, and neoclassical microeconomics, among others.

2. This really is a case of parallel discovery. Pelkey introduced Sabatier to the ADR literature in approximately 1999 or 2000, shortly after they began working together on the Watershed Partnership Project. But Sabatier and Zafonte had laid out their basic arguments for successful professional fora in papers delivered in Rotterdam in summer 1995 and at the AAAS meetings in Seattle in February 1997. They were eventually published in Sabatier and Zafonte (2001).

7

Do Watershed Partnerships Enhance Beliefs Conducive to Collective Action?

Mark Lubell

Our dynamic framework for watershed management argues that one consequence of collaborative watershed management is changes in the civic community in a particular watershed. One important aspect of civic community is collective action beliefs: beliefs about the nature of watershed problems (e.g., problem severity, diffuseness, and uncertainty) and institutional performance (e.g., conflict resolution, trust among stakeholders, and perceived fairness). Collective action beliefs reflect incentives to cooperate in bearing the costs of cooperation and therefore directly influence the level of cooperation and ultimately the effectiveness of watershed management. This chapter compares the beliefs of stakeholders participating in the U.S. EPA's National Estuary Program (NEP) to stakeholders from estuaries without the NEP, which are governed by traditional regulatory processes.[1] The NEP is the leading national example of a coastal watershed partnership; thus, this study represents a quasi-experimental design for testing the results of collaborative processes.

The concept of collective action beliefs combines insights from transaction cost economics (Eggertsson 1990, Libecap 1989, North 1990, Ostrom 1990, Weber 1998) with Sabatier and Jenkin-Smith's (1993) advocacy coalition framework (ACF). Transaction cost economics (TCE) maintains that cooperation is forthcoming when benefits outweigh transaction costs (information, bargaining, monitoring, and enforcement costs) of negotiating and enforcing collective agreements in the context of a watershed policy process. The transaction costs of collective action are reduced when there is a good match between the rules and practices of watershed policy and the characteristics of the watershed.

While TCE focuses on the structure of policy institutions, the ACF focuses on stakeholder beliefs. According to the ACF, beliefs guide stakeholders in assigning problem priorities, understanding causal relationships, and evaluating policies. In particular, the ACF states that more normative beliefs about how public policy should be made—such as environmentalism, views on public participation, and the role of property rights—influence stakeholders' perceptions of estuary problems and institutional performance.

This theoretical synthesis provides two criteria to assess the ability of watershed partnerships to increase the likelihood of cooperation and, ultimately, policy effectiveness. First, we examine whether NEP stakeholders hold collective action beliefs that are more supportive of cooperation than the beliefs of non-NEP stakeholders. If the NEP reduces the transaction costs of cooperation relative to traditional watershed management institutions, then NEP stakeholders should have more favorable beliefs. For example, the literature on social capital argues that trust reduces the costs of monitoring and enforcing collaborative agreements. In the context of watershed management, trust refers to a belief by one stakeholder that other stakeholders will fulfill the promises and obligations they have made. We demonstrate that levels of trust, along with other important collective action beliefs, are higher among NEP stakeholders.

Second, we examine whether watershed partnerships reduce disagreement among stakeholders—what Lubell (2000b; see also Kenney and Lord 1999) calls "cognitive conflict" and Sabatier, Hunter, and McLaughlin (1987) call the "devil-shift." Stakeholder disagreements often occur when policy beliefs lead to divergent perceptions of the watershed.[2] For example, disagreements between environmental and economic development interests about the severity of environmental problems often impede cooperation. In particular, we show that watershed partnerships reduce disagreement regarding policy processes, but not regarding the definition of environmental problems. These findings suggest collaborative processes are best considered an example of the science of "muddling through" (Lindblom 1959), where agreement on policies occurs without agreement on problem parameters.

The data come from a combined mail and telephone survey of 1,198 stakeholders from twenty estuaries with the NEP and ten estuaries without the NEP, providing a comparative perspective superior to research designs that study only watershed partnerships, and not watersheds without partnerships. For example, Yaffee et al.'s (1996) finding that 74 percent of ecosystem management efforts have improved stakeholder communication would not make an impressive case if 90 percent of the ecosystems without an ecosystem management program also had improved stakeholder cooperation.

However, this strategy requires a critical causal assumption: differences between NEP and non-NEP stakeholders are attributable to the presence or absence of the NEP. Clearly, the opposite case is possible: the NEP exists in a particular estuary because collective action beliefs already supported cooperation and stakeholder disagreement was minimal. There are several reasons we do not pay more attention to this causality problem in the context of this chapter.

First, personal interviews with NEP stakeholders suggest the NEP program has an independent causal effect on stakeholder beliefs. Many stakeholders noted how the NEP increased their knowledge of environmental problems and their trust and communication with other stakeholders. Second, a previous study (Lubell 2000a) found no evidence of selection bias. This could be because the geographic distribution of the NEP programs has as much to do with pork barrel politics as placing the NEP in estuaries where the conditions for collective action are best developed. Third, even if the NEP is not the direct causal link (i.e., stakeholders' experience in the collaborative process in and of itself does not change beliefs), any differences between NEP and non-NEP stakeholders at the very least represent different levels of progress in the evolution of cooperation. In this case, the NEP most likely plays an indirect role by providing an incentive for stakeholders to organize in order to secure the acceptance of their estuary into the program.[3]

In the next section, we discuss watershed management as a collective action problem and the role of beliefs about transaction costs, policy beliefs, and watershed policies in influencing cooperation. Then we present regression analyses using several key collective action beliefs related to benefits and transaction costs as dependent variables to investigate whether the NEP changes beliefs in ways that enhance the level of stakeholder cooperation.

Transaction Costs, Watershed Institutions, and Policy Beliefs

The transaction cost approach views watershed management as a collective action problem. Because watershed resources are nonexcludable, they are subject to the same collective dilemmas that plague other common pool resources: overuse of ecosystem resources (the flow problem) and underinvestment in natural capital (the stock problem; see Ostrom 1990).[4] Additional economic losses are incurred as a result of conflict between stakeholders as they attempt to secure property rights to watershed resources (Libecap 1989). For example, consider the high costs of environmental litigation under the Endangered Species Act and many permitting processes within the U.S. EPA, violent confrontations between Native American lobster fishers and Canadian fisheries authorities, direct action tactics in places like Vail, Colorado, and death threats levied by wise-use groups against environmentalists and natural resource managers. Hence, the welfare gains available from solving watershed problems include both protecting natural resources and reducing the costs of stakeholder conflict (Cheung 1970, Gordon 1954, Ostrom 1990).

Solving watershed collective action problems requires stakeholder cooperation. Watershed management is successful when potential benefits outweigh the transaction costs of cooperation. The welfare gains available from solving underlying collective action problems (such as reducing resource overexploitation and conflict and preserving natural capital) are the main benefits of cooperation. Transaction costs include the costs of searching for mutually beneficial policies, bargaining over which of those policies are chosen, and monitoring and enforcing the resulting political agreement (Heckathorn and Maser 1987, North 1990). When the net benefits—benefits minus transaction costs—of watershed management are positive, cooperation between stakeholders should be forthcoming and collective action problems should be alleviated.

From this perspective, the primary advantage of watershed partnerships is to provide an alternative policy institution that reduces the transaction costs of cooperation in comparison to the traditional command-and-control model. Transaction costs are minimized when the rules and practices of a policy institution are congruent with the type of collective action problem at hand. Hence, collaborative watershed partnerships should reduce transaction costs to the extent they are better suited than the command-and-control model to solving the complex, diffuse, and boundary-spanning nature of problems like nonpoint source pollution, habitat destruction, and biodiversity. In the next sections we discuss how these changes in transaction costs might be reflected in the collective action beliefs of stakeholders.

Beliefs about Benefits and Transaction Costs

In the following sections, we identify specific collective action beliefs related to the perceived benefits and transaction costs in a watershed and state hypotheses about how those beliefs should differ in watersheds with and without a watershed partnership. Because we use the NEP as an example of a watershed partnership, these hypotheses will receive empirical testing by examining differences in collective action beliefs between NEP and non-NEP stakeholders.

Beliefs about Watershed Problem Characteristics

Since one of the main benefits of collective action is solving environmental problems, stakeholders who believe problems are severe are more likely to cooperate. If stakeholders do not believe environmental problems are severe, then the benefits of collaboration appear low, and they are not likely to support costly environmental policies. Thus, to the extent watershed partnerships increase the salience of environmental problems in a watershed, NEP stakeholders will believe watershed problems are more severe.[5]

Another important belief about watershed problems is problem diffusion—the number, diversity, and geographic dispersion of human activities causing a particular environmental impact. Diffuse problems affect the transaction costs of watershed management in ways similar to how migratory fish species increase the costs of fisheries management (Schlager, Blomquist, and Tang 1994). The inability of the National Pollution Discharge Elimination System's permitting system to handle nonpoint sources of pollution is a case in point. Nonpoint pollution comes from heterogeneous, geographically diffuse sources spread throughout the population, greatly raising the transaction costs of monitoring and enforcing traditional policies. Proponents of watershed partnerships argue that collaborative processes, by providing incentives for voluntary action and information about best management practices, have a comparative advantage over traditional watershed policies for solving diffuse problems. Consistent with this comparative advantage, NEP stakeholders will believe problems are more diffuse, which leads to greater support for partnership policies.

Finally the adequacy of scientific knowledge about watershed problems is related to transaction costs. Because transaction costs are a function of uncertainty, they are high when stakeholders perceive scientific knowledge as inadequate. The highly interconnected nature of watersheds challenges scientific knowledge because changes in one aspect of an ecosystem have complex, delayed, and serious influences on other aspects of the system (Costanza et al. 1997). General uncertainty about causes and consequences of environmental problems increases the difficulty of allocating the costs and benefits of collective action. Consequently, watershed partnerships like the NEP spend a great deal of time searching for scientific information and commissioning studies on specific watershed problems. To the extent these research efforts are successful, NEP stakeholders should be more likely than non-NEP stakeholders to believe scientific knowledge is adequate.

Beliefs about Institutional Performance

In addition to beliefs about problem characteristics, beliefs about institutional performance also affect cooperation. In this chapter, institutional performance broadly refers to the ability of collaborative processes to improve the relationships between stakeholders and thus reduce the transaction costs of collective decision making. We focus on three basic beliefs about institutional performance here: conflict resolution, trust, and fairness.

Since stakeholder conflict is one of the main economic losses of shared resource situations, one of the main benefits of policy institutions is their ability to resolve conflict. Proponents argue that collaborative processes resolve conflict between watershed stakeholders without resorting to outside legal or administrative arenas. NEP stakeholders therefore should be more likely than non-NEP stakeholders to believe conflict resolution is possible.

The amount of trust between stakeholders is another important belief affecting transaction costs and policy effectiveness (see chapter 4). Research on social capital demonstrates that trust, networks of civic engagement, and norms of reciprocity are critical resources for sustaining cooperation (Coleman 1990; Putnam, Leonardi, and Nanetti 1993; Taylor and Singleton 1993). High levels of trust reduce transaction costs by reducing uncertainty about stakeholder motivations and behavior. From this perspective, trust reflects self-interest: a trustworthy partner is one who can be expected to behave in a manner beneficial to the person initiating an exchange.[6] Scheberle (1997) documents the importance of trust for implementing environmental policies that span levels of the fragmented federalist system, where implementation requires bargains and coalition building between multiple stakeholders. By providing an arena for repeated social interaction, the NEP should lead to higher levels of trust.

However, stakeholders are not willing to participate in a collaborative institution if they believe the costs and benefits of collective action are not distributed fairly. Thus, stakeholders who think their interests are not adequately represented in the decision-making process, or who believe that their opponents control the process and outcome of decision making, are less likely to cooperate. One of the most common complaints environmental groups levy against watershed partnerships is that they represent a compromise to economic interests, allowing them greater local control of policy outputs. Of course, economic interests accuse environmental interests of controlling the process. Conversely, proponents of watershed partnerships argue that the inclusive nature of collaboration within watershed partnerships should reduce the tendency of one interest to dominate decision making. Thus, NEP stakeholders should believe policies are fairer and less subject to the domination of a particular narrow interest than stakeholders in non-NEP partnerships.

In sum, if watershed partnerships reduce the transaction costs of watershed management, they should influence collective action beliefs in ways that increase support for cooperation. The testable hypotheses state that in comparison to stakeholders in watersheds without the NEP, stakeholders in watersheds with the NEP should believe that environmental problems are more severe and diffuse, scientific knowledge is more adequate, conflict resolution is more successful, other stakeholders are more trustworthy, and decision making is fairer. These differences in collective action beliefs would lead to an increase in support for cooperation, which should increase the performance of watershed institutions.

Policy Beliefs and Stakeholder Disagreement

The formation of collective action beliefs is not affected exclusively by the benefits and transaction costs of collective action in the watershed. Sabatier and Jenkin-Smith's ACF argues that more abstract policy beliefs about how environmental policy should be made will constrain the formation of secondary beliefs about specific policy solutions within the watershed. When forming secondary beliefs, people use information processing strategies that give greater weight to information bits consistent with their policy beliefs and less weight to inconsistent information (Lubell 2000a). Stakeholder disagreement occurs when people with varying policy beliefs have differing secondary beliefs related to the benefits and transaction costs of collective action within the watershed. Lubell (2000a, 2000b) finds three policy beliefs to be particularly important for generating stakeholder disagreement within the NEP:

Environmentalism—preference for environmental protection over economic development and a general belief in the value of biodiversity

Conservatism—preference for private property rights and a belief that the market is superior to government for determining allocation of natural resources

Inclusiveness—belief that public participation in policy decisions should be maximized

The clash between environmentalism and conservatism produces the greatest disagreement. Environmentalists think problems are severe and diffuse and that economic interests exert undue control over watershed policies. Conservatives think environmental problems are less severe and more concentrated (i.e., somebody else must be responsible), and that environmental interests exert undue control. As stakeholders express more extreme beliefs on either side of the environment–property rights debate, they are much less likely to trust stakeholders with different perspectives. The existence of starkly divergent beliefs reduces the likelihood of consensus and collective action. When stakeholders cannot agree on fundamental issues such as the severity or causes of environmental problems or the fairness of the decision-making process, it is unlikely they will be able to sustain cooperation.

Inclusiveness somewhat reduces negative perceptions of institutional performance. As stakeholders' commitment to participation increases, they are more likely to believe watershed policies are fair and less likely to believe any single advocacy coalition has undue influence.

One goal of watershed partnerships is to reduce disagreement by encouraging interaction between advocacy coalitions that are typically in direct opposition. Instead of trying to convince an administrator or judge that their particular viewpoint is right, collaborative processes facilitate understanding of divergent viewpoints. The exposure to alternative viewpoints should reduce the motivation of stakeholders to use their policy beliefs as guides for information processing. Instead, they should evaluate information about the watershed in a more even-handed manner in an effort to discover an optimal, or at least mutually beneficial, solution to watershed problems. Moreover, the emphasis on collaborative processes within watershed partnerships should encourage stakeholders to abandon their traditional policy positions in favor of a more common vision. There should be fewer differences between stakeholders with competing beliefs in terms of how they view critical issues like problem severity, fairness, trust, and interest group influence. The testable hypothesis is that for NEP stakeholders, policy beliefs should have less of an effect on the formation of secondary beliefs.

To the extent watershed partnerships alleviate stakeholder disagreement, they may reduce transaction costs and facilitate cooperation. However, the ability of watershed partnerships to reduce disagreement might be substantially greater for beliefs about institutional performance relative to beliefs about environmental problems. Proponents of collaborative processes often argue that the negotiation process should create a common understanding of problem characteristics and policy means and objectives. At the same time, critics of collaborative processes argue that insistence on agreement might lead to lowest-common-denominator decisions. But according to Lindblom's (1959) science of muddling through, the test of a good policy is not agreement on means and objectives. Rather, there is often agreement on a particular policy because that policy serves different ends for different actors. This suggests stakeholders in watershed partnerships may often agree to disagree on the outlines of environmental problems, but still find common ground through participation in the collaborative process as a mechanism of conflict resolution.[7]

Research Design and Methods

To test the effects of watershed partnerships on collective action beliefs and stakeholder disagreement, we use survey data of 1,198 stakeholders from twenty estuaries with the U.S. Environmental Protection Agency's NEP and ten estuaries without the NEP. The NEP data combine a mail survey sent to a sample of 1,668 estuary stakeholders and a follow-up telephone survey of 796 mail survey nonrespondents from twelve of the original twenty NEP sites (see appendix 7B). The mail survey generated 501 usable responses (30 percent response rate), and the follow-up telephone survey generated 405 responses (50 percent response rate), for a combined mail-phone total of 906 NEP respondents (54 percent response rate for initial sample of 1,668).[8] The non-NEP data consist of telephone interviews from a sample of 466 estuary stakeholders, which generated 312 usable interviews, for a response rate of 65 percent (see appendix 7B for the complete list of estuaries and response rates).[9]

We generated the NEP sample universe by combining lists of contacts provided by U.S. EPA's Office of Wetlands, Oceans and Watersheds with lists of stakeholders provided by individual NEP directors. The NEP stakeholders were generally individuals directly involved with the Management Conferences convened for each NEP. Generating the non-NEP sample was considerably more difficult because there were no existing lists of stakeholders. Hence, we generated lists by searching the Internet for active projects and interest groups in the particular estuary and using the National Wildlife Federation's 1998 *Conservation Directory* to find additional stakeholders. We then called the initial list of contacts generated by the search process and asked them to identify additional stakeholders active in the estuary, for a total baseline sample population of 340 contacts. The telephone survey company then used a snowball procedure, which asked the original 340 contacts for more names, to generate 126 more potential respondents, for a total of 466 potential non-NEP respondents.

To demonstrate the survey respondents are representative of a wide range of estuary stakeholders, table 7.1 presents a cross-tabulation of respondents according to stakeholder type and location in the federal system. As can be seen, 57 percent of the sample are government representatives (mostly from administrative agencies), 12 percent environ-

Table 7.1
Cross-tabulation of stakeholder type by federal level

Federal Level	Government	Environmental group	Business group	Research and education	Other	Total
National	134 (11.6%)	16 (1.4%)	19 (1.7%)	23 (2.0%)	22 (1.9%)	214 (18.6%)
State	229 (19.9%)	43 (3.7%)	26 (2.3%)	32 (2.8%)	47 (4.1%)	377 (32.7%)
Regional	94 (8.2%)	37 (3.2%)	27 (2.3%)	14 (1.2%)	46 (3.9%)	217 (18.8%)
Local	170 (14.8%)	39 (3.4%)	28 (2.4%)	3 (0.3%)	54 (4.7%)	294 (25.5%)
Other	16 (1.4%)	5 (0.4%)	10 (0.9%)	6 (0.5%)	13 (1.1%)	50 (4.3%)
Total	643 (56.8%)	140 (12.1%)	110 (9.5%)	78 (6.8%)	181 (15.7%)	1,152 (100%)

Note: Cell entries are total number of respondents from each category of stakeholder type and federal level, with percentages of valid sample ($N = 1,152$) in parentheses.

mental groups, 10 percent business groups, 7 percent research, and 16 percent other types such as citizens at large and consultants.[10] Clearly, estuary politics is heavily devoted to intergovernmental coordination, but interest groups from both sides of the environment-economy debate and researchers are involved as well. The small proportion of nongovernmental actors does not mean they are unimportant; although they constitute a minority of the sample, many individuals represent much larger groups.

Estuary politics involves stakeholders from all governmental levels. Overall, state (33 percent) and local (26 percent) stakeholders are the most active players. This makes sense given the central role of state agencies in the NEP process and the overall role of states in protecting ecosystems within their boundaries. Similarly, local government actors consistently play an important role in estuary politics because they control land use; are usually the main operators of drinking, storm-, and wastewater treatment facilities; and are always on the lookout for environmental funding from higher levels of the federal system. However, the federal government is also represented, reflecting the facts that the NEP is a U.S. EPA initiative, and many different federal agencies have jurisdiction over different aspects of estuarine systems. Environmental and business groups are also most likely to come from lower organizational levels since estuary politics involves primarily local issues that frequently fall beneath the radar scope of national interest groups.

Before empirically testing the ability of the NEP to change collective action beliefs and moderate disagreement, we will briefly discuss the choice of estuaries in the study. We attempted to include all twenty-eight NEP estuaries in the study, but only twenty agreed to participate. Fortunately, those twenty estuaries are well distributed geographically and chronologically across the five cohorts (Tier I through Tier V) of the NEP program.

We used geographic proximity as the main criterion to select non-NEP estuaries, seeking at least one non-NEP estuary from each of the regions represented by NEP estuaries. Matching on regions minimizes the potential biases associated with differences in environmental problems and political cultures. For example, Pacific Northwest estuaries face problems with logging, endangered species, and hydrological alteration. Gulf of Mexico estuaries face problems of emerging development, disappearing wetlands, and the decline of gulf fisheries. Furthermore, environmental values are more salient in the Northwest than in the Southeast. The secondary criterion used was population density. Even if estuaries face the same variety of environmental problems within a region, the severity of these problems is exacerbated by the intensity of human settlement.

Unfortunately, the geographic distribution of NEP estuaries makes it impossible to choose estuaries that are identical on all characteristics except the presence or absence of the NEP. The U.S. EPA's selection process tends to focus on nationally visible estuaries where population pressure is threatening the environmental and economic values of the ecosystem. Hence, NEP estuaries are, on average, larger, more densely populated, and richer, with more environmental problems, more urban land use, and more agriculture than non-NEP estuaries. In most regions, the most developed and best defined estuaries are already part of the NEP, leaving only less developed areas for comparison.

To account for these differences, the models below include several estuary-level characteristics as control variables: 1990 population density, percentage of agricultural land use, and total watershed size (in square miles). These are some of the same estuary characteristics used in the treatment effects regression model discussed in Lubell (2000a). Here, we choose the alternative strategy of directly including them in linear regression models. Not only does this strategy increase confidence in the current findings, it also serves as an additional analysis to compare with the treatment effects models from Lubell (2000a). One complication exists: the estuary-level variables spread a single observation across multiple units of analysis, thus creating the possibility of correlated error terms between respondents within the same estuary. Hence, all results report Huber-White robust standard errors and allow for correlation between the error terms of respondents from the same estuary (Huber 1967; StataCorp 1999; White 1980, 1982).

Does the NEP Change Collective Action Beliefs?

The first test involves using linear regression to estimate the influence of several independent variables to explain variation in the benefits and costs of collective action. The independent variables are (1) a dummy variable coded 0 for non-NEP estuaries and 1 for NEP estuaries, (2) three policy beliefs of environmentalism, inclusiveness and conservatism, and (3) the estuary-level control variables. Seven dependent variables represent collective action beliefs: problem severity, problem diffusion, scientific knowledge, external conflict resolution, trust, fairness, and economic interest domination (see appendix 7A for the exact wording of questions). To reiterate, beliefs about attributes of watershed problems are severity, problem diffusion, and scientific knowledge. Beliefs about institutional performance are conflict resolution, trust, overall fairness, and domination by economic interests.[11]

If the NEP reduces transaction costs, then the regression coefficient for the NEP dummy in each model should be statistically significant and in a direction that increases the likelihood of cooperation. The NEP dummy coefficient should be positive for problem severity, scientific knowledge, problem diffusion, trust, and fairness and negative for external conflict resolution and economic interest domination. This analysis also demonstrates the incidence of stakeholder disagreement due to differences between stakeholders in terms of their policy beliefs. In particular, stakeholders' commitments to environmental and conservative values should affect beliefs about the benefits and transaction costs of collective action in opposite directions, especially for perceptions of estuary problems and economic domination of the policy process. A commitment to inclusiveness should positively affect perceptions of institutional performance, reflecting a faith in the ability of participatory decision making to resolve conflict among competing interests.

Table 7.2 presents the results of these regressions.[12] Most important, the NEP dummy is statistically significant and in the expected direction in six of the seven models. The NEP increases the expected value of scientific knowledge by 5 percent and problem diffusion by 9 percent. At the same time, the NEP reduces the belief that conflict must be moved outside the estuary by 15 percent and that economic interests dominate by 15 percent, while increasing stakeholder trust by 6 percent and overall fairness perceptions by 12 percent. The NEP does not appear to have an effect on perceptions of problem severity. This is most likely due to the fact that both problem severity and the presence of the NEP are partly affected by broader estuary characteristics like watershed size. Given the hypothesized relationship of these collective action beliefs to overall levels of cooperation (see chapter 8), these differences suggest the NEP increases support for estuary policies and subsequent policy effectiveness.

The considerable effects of the NEP on indicators of institutional performance like fairness, conflict resolution, and interest domination corroborate Yaffee et al.'s (1996) finding that the most obvious effect of ecosystem management is improved communication and cooperation. This is not surprising given that the NEP provides a new forum for stakeholder interaction and dialogue and emphasizes consensus. However, the NEP also has a strong influence on perceptions of problem diffusion, which reflects the comparative advantage of the NEP for solving diffuse problems like nonpoint source pollution. The great amount of information generated by the NEP not only increases overall scientific knowledge, but apparently persuades (or reveals to) stakeholders that watershed problems are more complex than point source discharges. Changing beliefs about problem diffusion in a way that is more consistent with the governing style of watershed partnerships should in-

Table 7.2
Does the NEP change collective action beliefs?

	Dependent variables: Beliefs about estuary problems			Dependent variables: Beliefs about institutional performance			
	Problem severity	Scientific knowledge	Problem diffusion	External conflict resolution	Trust	Fairness	Interest domination
Independent variables							
NEP institution	.006	.046	.086	-.151	.055	.116	-.152
	(.047)	(.018)*	(.037)*	(.024)*	(.021)*	(.021)*	(.029)*
Inclusiveness	.075	.047	.137	-.130	.133	.114	-.070
	(.027)*	(.035)	(.029)*	(.046)*	(.030)*	(.040)*	(.036)**
Environmentalism	.169	.007	.191	.082	-.043	.009	.251
	(.032)*	(.026)	(.038)*	(.034)*	(.029)	(.031)	(.046)*
Conservatism	-.100	-.065	-.180	-.043	.007	-.022	-.126
	(.046)*	(.033)**	(.039)*	(.052)	(.028)	(.033)	(.049)*
Watershed control variables							
1990 population density	.0001	.0001	.0001	-.0001	-.0001	-.0001	<.0001
	(.0001)	(.0001)	(.0001)	(.0001)	(.0001)	(.0001)	(.0001)
% agricultural land	.0012	.0018	.00014	.0015	-.0001	.0009	.0023
	(.0015)	(.0008)*	(.0011)	(.0012)	(.0008)	(.0007)	(.0015)
Total watershed area (miles²)	.0004	-.0005	.0005	.0007	-.0003	-.0004	.0001
	(.0004)	(.0001)*	(.0002)*	(.0001)*	(.0001)*	(.0001)*	(.0002)
Constant	.404	.498	.382	.624	.510	.465	.477
	(.052)*	(.044)*	(.047)*	(.049)*	(.044)*	(.047)*	(.042)*
Model fit	$F = 6.70$*	$F = 11.94$*	$F = 12.84$*	$F = 11.93$*	$F = 5.44$*	$F = 7.73$*	$F = 12.25$
	$R^2 = .079$	$R^2 = .040$	$R^2 = .131$	$R^2 = .080$	$R^2 = .035$	$R^2 = .072$	$R^2 = .117$

Note: Cell entries are unstandardized regression coefficients; robust standard errors are in parentheses. Hypothesis tests of coefficient = 0, * $p < .05$, ** $p < .10$.

crease the likelihood of the NEP becoming a stable, self-perpetuating institution.

Stakeholder disagreement is also apparent. Moving across the range of the environmentalism scale significantly increases beliefs about problem severity by 17 percent and problem diffusion by 19 percent, while conservatism decreases the same beliefs by 10 percent and 18 percent, respectively. Similarly, environmentalism increases the belief that economic interests dominate decision making by 25 percent, while conservatism decreases the same belief by 13 percent. These different perceptions reflect the policy preferences of conflicting advocacy coalitions. Environmentalists emphasize problem severity because serious problems receive more public attention and government resources. Conservatives downplay severity to avoid the restrictions and economic costs of environmental regulations. If environmentalists can convince decision makers that economic interests dominate the policy arena, they may be able to gain more power for themselves. Of course, economic interests will disagree because they do not want to give up power. These divergent beliefs reflect the traditional battle lines of environmental conflicts and pose major barriers to collaboration.

The analyses also demonstrate the moderating influence of inclusiveness. Inclusiveness increases trust by 13 percent and fairness by 11 percent, while reducing the perception that conflict will be moved outside the estuary by 13 percent and that economic interests dominate by 7 percent. People who place faith in public participation are more optimistic about institutional performance, perhaps reflecting a faith in democratic processes to reduce conflict in a fair manner and build social capital among conflicting interests. Interestingly, inclusiveness also increases beliefs about problem severity by 8 percent and problem diffusion by 14 percent. Stakeholders' beliefs about estuary problems are consistent with their perspective on the breadth of public participation.[13] Broad public participation is more effective for diffuse problems; hence, stakeholders who believe estuary decision making should be participatory also think more people are involved in producing the problem and the problem is more severe.

Judged in terms of its ability to change collective action beliefs in ways that facilitate cooperation, the NEP appears to be an effective program. Assuming collective action beliefs reflect the benefits and transaction costs of cooperation with a moderate degree of accuracy, these belief changes are evidence that the NEP does reduce the transaction costs of watershed management. In the next section, we analyze whether or not the NEP has the additional effect of alleviating stakeholder disagreement, which is still clearly present in the above analyses.

Does the NEP Moderate Stakeholder Disagreement?

To analyze the effect of the NEP on stakeholder conflict, we added two interaction terms to the seven regression equations presented: NEP*Environmentalism and NEP*Conservatism.[14] If the regression coefficients for these interaction terms are significant, then the marginal effects of the policy beliefs on collective action beliefs are conditional on the presence or absence of the NEP. To assess the significance of the interaction terms, we first computed all seven regression equations with both interaction terms. To avoid potential problems of multicollinearity, we then dropped any insignificant interaction terms and recomputed the regressions, retaining only the significant interactions. We found significant interaction terms for three of the key collective action beliefs: trust, fairness, and interest domination. Table 7.3 presents the final results of these analyses.

If the NEP completely eliminates stakeholder disagreement, then the interaction terms should reduce the effects of environmentalism and conservatism to zero for NEP stakeholders.[15] This would provide evidence that NEP stakeholders are more likely to form their collective action beliefs using relevant information they encounter while participating in the partnership and processing that information in an evenhanded manner. In contrast, policy beliefs will still have a greater effect on the collective action beliefs of non-NEP stakeholders, leading to divergent perceptions. Non-NEP stakeholders would continue to process information in a biased manner, giving more weight to information consistent with their policy beliefs.

To better visualize the results for all models, figure 7.1 presents the marginal effects of environmentalism and conservatism for NEP and non-NEP stakeholders for all three collective action beliefs with significant interactions. If the NEP reduces disagreement, then the marginal effects of policy beliefs among NEP stakeholders should be close to

Table 7.3
Does the NEP moderate cognitive conflict?

	Dependent variables		
	Trust	Fairness	Interest domination
Independent variables			
NEP institution	−.117	−.044	.088
	(.068)**	(.052)	(.054)
Inclusiveness	.133	.118	−.077
	(.029)*	(.040)*	(.035)*
Environmentalism	−.179	−.161	.506
	(.067)*	(.090)*	(.046)*
Conservatism	−.086	−.021	−.128
	(.030)*	(.032)	(.049)*
Interactions			
NEP*Environmentalism	.176	.220	−.328
	(.067)*	(.091)*	(.069)*
NEP*Conservatism	.121	—	—
	(.045)*		
Constant	.641	.589	.292
	(.071)*	(.077)*	(.053)
Model fit	$F = 11.23$*	$F = 8.34$*	$F = 33.02$*
	$R^2 = .042$	$R^2 = .080$	$R^2 = .127$

Note: Cell entries are unstandardized regression coefficients; standard errors are in parentheses. Hypothesis tests of slope coefficient = 0, $*p < .05$, $**p < .10$. The table does not report slope coefficients for watershed control variables, but they were included in the estimation procedure.

zero. Starting with trust, in NEP estuaries, the marginal effect of environmentalism on trust within the NEP equals −0.3 percent (significant, positive NEP*Environmentalism interaction), while the marginal effect of conservatism on trust within the NEP equals 3.5 percent (significant, positive NEP*Conservatism interaction). In non-NEP estuaries, the marginal effect of environmentalism on trust is −17.9 percent, and the marginal effect of conservatism equals −8.6 percent. The trust equation demonstrates the first interesting effect: the NEP appears to reduce the tendency of stakeholders with strong policy beliefs to distrust other estuary stakeholders and even leads to greater trust among conservatives. In non-NEP estuaries, as stakeholders' commitments to both these values increase, they are less likely to trust other stakeholders. The traditional

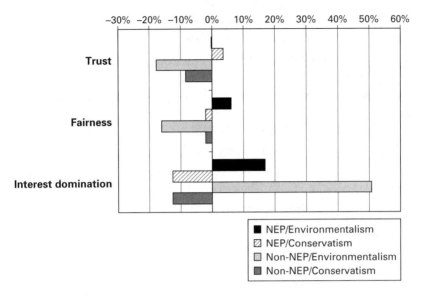

Figure 7.1
Marginal effects of policy core beliefs in NEP versus non-NEP estuaries

lines of conflict are clearly apparent in non-NEP estuaries. However, as envisioned by proponents of collaboration, the NEP appears to diminish barriers to the accumulation of social capital.

Similar reductions in disagreement are seen for both measures of fairness, especially for environmentalism. The marginal effect of environmentalism in non-NEP estuaries equals −16.1 percent, while in NEP estuaries the marginal effect of environmentalism is 5.9 percent. Environmentalists, in other words, feel their interests are better represented in the NEP. The pattern for interest domination substantiates this conclusion. The strong positive effect (50.6 percent) of environmentalism on beliefs about economic interest domination in non-NEP estuaries is greatly reduced in NEP estuaries (16.8 percent). Environmentalists continue to think economic interests have undue influence over NEP policies, reflecting a reluctance to give economic interests any claim over estuary resources. But the effect is much more apparent among non-NEP stakeholders, where moving across the range of the environmentalism scale increases perceptions of economic interest domination by 50.6 percent, by far the largest effect in any of the models. The NEP*-Conservatism interaction effects are not significant for either measure of fairness. In both NEP and non-NEP estuaries, conservatives are more likely to think environmental policies are unfair, while at the same time believing that economic interests do not dominate policymaking.

In terms of its ability to reduce disagreement, the NEP appears to have several positive consequences. It reduces the tendency of strong ideologues to distrust stakeholders from conflicting advocacy coalitions. Environmentalists in particular are more likely to feel their interests are represented and less likely to believe their opponents dominate the process. The positive effects of the NEP on the possibility of collective action are most evident in terms of perceptions of institutional performance. This is consistent with the baseline findings that show the NEP causes the most favorable changes in beliefs about fairness, trust, and conflict resolution.

However, the NEP does not eliminate all disagreement. Especially with respect to problem diffusion and problem severity, conservatives and environmentalists have competing beliefs regardless of institutional structure. They may agree that collaborative processes are superior to adversarial institutions for solving environmental conflicts, but they are still bringing their differences of opinion regarding problem characteristics to the negotiating table.

From the consensus or belief system perspective, resolving these differences may be necessary for successful policy implementation. However, as the strategy of muddling through argues, reaching agreement on a policy solution does not require agreement on causes and consequences (Lindblom 1959). Thus, the ability of the NEP to reduce disagreement about institutional performance suggests that consensus should be defined as agreement on the process of resolving conflict and choosing policies despite continuing disagreement over problem characteristics.

Conditional Effects of the NEP

Interaction effects cut both ways. Not only are the marginal effects of policy beliefs conditional on the presence or absence of the NEP, the marginal effect of the NEP on collective action beliefs is conditional on policy beliefs.[16] Figures 7.2 and 7.3 display the marginal effect of the NEP on collective action beliefs moving across the range of environmentalism and conservatism, respectively, holding the other relevant policy belief at the mean level in the sample. Lines with a positive (negative)

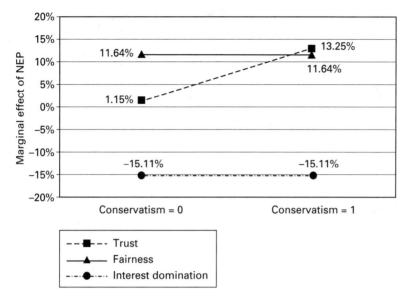

Figure 7.2
Marginal effect of the NEP as a function of conservatism

slope indicate the NEP has a more positive (negative) effect among stakeholders committed to a particular policy belief; flat lines indicate no
interaction.

Examining the interactions between the NEP, environmentalism, and
conservatism reveals that the positive effects of the NEP reported in table
7.1 are in reality concentrated among stakeholders with certain policy
beliefs. Indeed, for some stakeholders, the NEP may actually change collective action beliefs in ways that reduce the likelihood of collective
action.

Moving across the range of conservatism increases the marginal effect
of the NEP on trust from 1.2 percent to 13.3 percent. The ability of the
NEP to build trust is actually more pronounced among more conservative stakeholders, confirming the ability of the NEP to build social capital
between conflicting advocacy coalitions. Conservatism does not influence
the marginal effect of the NEP on either interest domination (−15.1 percent) or procedural fairness (11.6 percent), holding environmentalism at
the mean.

The ability of the NEP to change attitudes in ways that enhance collective action is most pronounced among strong environmentalists. As seen

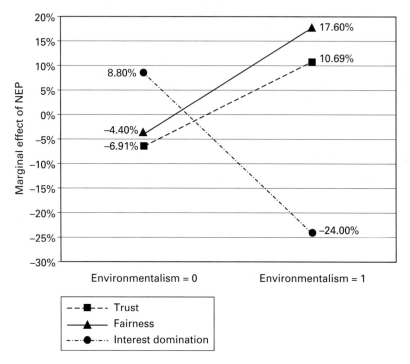

Figure 7.3
Marginal effect of the NEP as a function of environmentalism

in figure 7.3, moving across the range of environmentalism increases the marginal effect of the NEP on trust from −6.9 percent to 10.7 percent and fairness from −4.4 percent to 17.6 percent, while decreasing beliefs about economic interest domination from 8.8 percent to −24 percent. As with strong conservatives, the NEP does a better job of building social capital among strong environmentalists. The effects of the NEP on fairness considerations are particularly interesting. Strong environmentalists think their interests are better represented and economic interests are less dominant in the NEP relative to traditional watershed management. Supporters of economic development, on the other hand, are less likely to think estuary policies are fair. For environmentalists, the NEP represents a superior venue for achieving their policy preferences, which is hardly surprising given the environmental mission of the U.S. EPA.

These analyses of the conditional effects of the NEP highlight an important theoretical advancement in the study of collective action, beliefs, and institutions. Institutions and beliefs cannot be considered independent of one another; the performance of institutions depends on the beliefs of the actors involved. Stakeholders' beliefs determine how they process the information generated by the institution and how they evaluate policy institutions. For example, the NEP does a better job of improving fairness evaluations among strong environmentalists. This suggests that different types of institutions will be more or less successful in solving collective-action problems when applied to different beliefs.

At the same time, the functioning of belief systems depends on institutional structures. In particular, the relationship between policy beliefs and collective action beliefs changes in different institutional settings. For example, in watershed management, the relationships between trust and the policy beliefs of conservatism and environmentalism are different in NEP versus non-NEP estuaries. The collaborative process of the NEP appears to reduce the constraining influence of policy beliefs on the formation of secondary, collective action beliefs. Beliefs and institutional structures are interconnected components of the overall system of governance.

Conclusion: Watershed Management and the Possibility of Cooperation

The analyses in this chapter demonstrate that watershed partnerships like the NEP affect the beliefs of stakeholders in ways that increase the likelihood of cooperation, which in theory is ultimately linked to policy effectiveness. In comparison to non-NEP stakeholders, the average NEP stakeholder believes estuary problems are more diffuse, estuary policies are fairer and better at conflict resolution, scientific knowledge is more adequate, and other stakeholders more trustworthy. These changes in collective action beliefs are consistent with the hypothesis that the NEP increases the benefits and decreases the transaction costs of watershed management. The findings corroborate proponents' claims that collaborative watershed management is better suited to complex watershed collective action problems than traditional command-and-control policies.

The NEP also reduces disagreement with regard to beliefs about institutional performance. Strong commitments to either environmentalism or conservatism are much less likely to generate distrust among NEP stakeholders than among non-NEP stakeholders. Environmentalists in particular appear to believe their interests are better represented and policy decision making less dominated by economic interests within the

NEP. As stakeholders' commitment to environmental values increases, the NEP becomes a more attractive governance institution. While one possible interpretation of this finding is that the NEP is captured by environmental interests, even strong conservatives think the NEP improves the overall level of fairness as long as they have an average level of environmentalism. Only among strong antienvironmentalists does the NEP have a negative effect on perceptions of fairness, reflecting the tendency of some economic interests to oppose any environmental policy, whether new or traditional.

In general, the NEP appears to have the strongest effects on beliefs about institutional performance. The NEP builds social capital and resolves conflict between competing advocacy coalitions and is perceived as fairer than traditional watershed management institutions. At the same time, disagreement over institutional processes is less apparent in NEP estuaries. This generalization is not surprising because the most immediate policy change due to the NEP is providing a new venue for stakeholder interaction. Because environmental outcomes are often a longer-term process, changing beliefs about characteristics of watershed problems is also more difficult.

One policy implication of the NEP's strong effect on beliefs about institutional performance is that collaborative processes should be evaluated from the perspective of muddling through (Lindblom 1959). The success of NEP policies may not depend on complete agreement between stakeholders on the characteristics of environmental problems or the means and objectives of watershed policies. Rather, the success of watershed partnerships and other collaborative institutions should be judged with respect to the ability of stakeholders to agree on the legitimacy of the collaborative process. Effective collaborative processes do not always eliminate disagreements; rather, they find acceptable ways to make collective decisions despite disagreements. From this perspective, the advantage of watershed partnerships over traditional command-and-control institutions lies in their ability to reduce the real or perceived transaction costs of collective choice.

The limitations of evaluating watershed partnerships using belief criteria deserve reiteration. Belief change is a necessary but not sufficient step in the evolution of cooperation. Because expressing beliefs involves minimal costs to an individual, there is no guarantee that belief change is followed by behavioral change. Consequently, belief change may be short term or fluctuate over time. Actual changes in policy outputs and environmental outcomes are even further down the chain of causal linkages that lead to the successful resolution of environmental conflicts. The challenge facing watershed partnerships is to use belief change as a foundation for building sustainable institutions that structure the behavior of succeeding generations of policymakers, stakeholders, and citizens, while surviving fluctuations in political, economic, and ecological fortunes. While the ability of watershed partnerships to change beliefs justifies continuing these policy experiments, the experiments will fail if belief changes do not lead to changes in behavior and environmental outcomes. Chapter 8 explores whether there is at least a short-term link between beliefs like trust and actual agreements and watershed projects.

The challenge facing research on watershed partnerships is to discover valid and reliable methods for measuring behavioral, policy, and environmental changes over time to more comprehensively evaluate the impact of various institutional arrangements. This chapter's analysis constitutes a significant improvement over analyses that rely on only qualitative data. While case study work is invaluable to developing hypotheses, testing those hypotheses in a comparative perspective requires quantitative data that can be generalized across different watershed settings. In addition, the sort of conditional analyses conducted in this chapter— where, for example, NEPs had a greater impact on moderating the beliefs of environmentalists than conservatives—would be extraordinarily difficult with qualitative data alone.

Appendix 7A: Question Wording and Variable Construction

Unless otherwise noted, all variables are measured on a disagree-agree scale with integer response values ranging between $[0, 10]$, with $0 =$ strongly disagree and $10 =$ strongly agree. Specific value labels are included in the descriptions below if needed. For some questions (e.g., problem severity), respondents were asked to evaluate seven specific estuary issues and provide an overall evaluation as well; this analysis uses the overall evaluations. Question wording was slightly different for non-NEP and NEP respondents to reflect participation in different collective choice arenas. For purposes of analysis all variables were linearly transformed to a $[0, 1]$ range.

Dependent Variables Measure Collective Action Beliefs

Problem severity: Concerning the overall health of your estuary, do you think the problems associated with each issue listed below are very severe, not severe, or somewhere in between? 0 = The problems are not severe; 10 = The problems are very severe.

Science: On average, do you perceive the level of scientific understanding about the causes and causes of problems in your estuary to be very inadequate, very adequate, or somewhere in between? 0 = Scientific understanding is very inadequate; 10 = Scientific understanding is very adequate.

Problem diffusion: Would you say that a full resolution of the problem would require changes in the activities or behavior of a small number of citizens and businesses, would it require changes of almost everyone in the estuary, or somewhere in between? 0 = Only a small number would need to change; 10 = Almost everybody would need to change.

External conflict resolution: When conflicts arise, do you think that you can resolve conflicts to the satisfaction of your organization with the partnership, or do you think your organization will need to shift the dispute to courts, political, or other administrative arenas? 0 = Resolve conflict inside partnership; 10 = Shift disputes outside partnership.

Trust: Thinking about the range of contacts you have had with other stakeholders, do you completely trust these stakeholders to fulfill the promises and obligations made on each issue in the context of the partnership, completely distrust them, or somewhere in between? 0 = Completely distrust; 10 = Completely trust.

Procedural fairness (alpha = .76):

1. Overall, the decision-making process in the partnership is fair to all stakeholders. Disagree/Agree.

2. My organization's interests and concerns are adequately represented in the partnership. Disagree/Agree.

Economic domination: Economic interest groups have an undue influence on partnership decisions. Disagree/Agree.

Independent Variables Measuring Policy Beliefs

Environmentalism: In general, how would you describe your policy orientation on estuary issues when trade-offs between environmental protection and economic development are important? 1–7 scale; 1 = prodevelopment; 7 = proenvironment.

Government role (alpha = .70):

1. Preserving the rights of individual citizens is more important than protecting the environment. Disagree/Agree.

2. In general, government agencies and regulations intrude too much on the daily lives of private citizens. Disagree/Agree.

Inclusiveness: Maximizing the scope of public participation in environmental policy improves policy effectiveness. Disagree/Agree.

Appendix 7B: Survey Response Rates by Estuary and Instrument Type

Estuary	Mail	Telephone follow-up	Total response rate
NEP estuaries			
Albemarle-Pamlico, N.C.	20/101 (20%)	35/81 (43%)	55/101 (54%)
Barataria-Terrebonne, La.	24/77 (31%)	NA	24/77 (31%)
Barnegat Bay, N.J.	34/115 (30%)	37/81 (46%)	71/115 (62%)
Casco Bay, Me.	17/42 (40%)	14/25 (56%)	31/42 (73%)
Charlotte Harbor, Fla.	40/137 (29%)	57/97 (59%)	97/137 (71%)
Corpus Christi, Tex.	45/141 (32%)	57/96 (59%)	102/141 (73%)
Delaware inland bays, Del.	28/92 (30%)	27/64 (42%)	55/92 (60%)
Galveston Bay, Tex.	10/40 (25%)	NA	10/40 (25%)
Long Island Sound, N.Y.	22/101 (22%)	33/79 (42%)	55/101 (55%)
Lower Columbia River, Wash./Ore.	23/65 (35%)	21/42 (50%)	44/65 (68%)
Maryland coastal bays, Md.	27/100 (27%)	29/73 (39%)	56/100 (56%)
Mobile Bay, Ala.	33/105 (31%)	33/72 (46%)	66/105 (62%)
Narragansett Bay, Mass., R.I.	13/32 (41%)	NA	13/32 (41%)
New Hampshire estuaries, N.H.	26/73 (36%)	33/47 (70%)	59/73 (80%)
N.Y./N.J. harbor	14/42 (33%)	NA	14/42 (33%)
Peconic Bays, N.Y.	19/111 (17%)	NA	19/111 (17%)
Puget Sound, Wash.	6/25 (24%)	NA	6/25 (24%)
San Francisco Bay, Calif.	25/73 (34%)	NA	25/73 (34%)
Tillamook Bay, Ore.	28/96 (29%)	NA	28/96 (29%)
Tampa Bay, Fla.	32/100 (32%)	29/68 (43%)	61/100 (61%)
Unknown (ID tag removed)	15		
Total	501/1,668 (29%)	405/825 (51%)	906/1,668 (54%)

Estuary	Mail	Telephone follow-up	Total response rate
Non-NEP estuaries			
Apalachicola Bay estuary	17/22 (77%)	16/18 (89%)	33/40 (83%)
Atchafalaya Bay estuary	20/23 (87%)	9/16 (56%)	29/39 (74%)
Cape Fear River estuary	19/34 (56%)	10/16 (63%)	29/50 (78%)
Gray's Harbor estuary	24/35 (69%)	5/6 (83%)	29/41 (71%)
Lower Saint John's River estuary	26/39 (67%)	10/19 (53%)	36/58 (62%)
Martha's Vineyard estuary	14/31 (45%)	5/10 (50%)	19/41 (47%)
Penobscot Bay estuary	22/42 (52%)	6/10 (60%)	28/52 (54%)
Pensacola Bay estuary	25/26 (96%)	16/21 (76%)	41/47 (87%)
Saco Bay estuary	26/42 (62%)	9/9 (100%)	35/51 (69%)
St. Andrew's Bay estuary	28/49 (57%)	5/8 (63%)	33/57 (59%)
Total	221/343 (64%)	91/133 (69%)	312/476 (65%)

Note: Entries in cells are surveys completed divided by total sample number in each estuary, for each type of survey instrument. NEP survey respondents consist of original mail targets, plus a telephone survey follow-up of mail survey nonrespondents. NA indicates estuaries that did not receive a telephone follow-up. Non-NEP telephone survey respondents include original seed lists of stakeholders identified by the author and "snowball" list of additional stakeholders identified by seeds. Response percentages are in parentheses. Response rates include respondents who were ineligible because they were not active in the estuary in the twelve months preceding the survey or had incorrect contact information. Ineligible respondents constitute the bulk of nonrespondents; hence, the refusal rate is substantially lower than the response rates reported above.

Notes

1. Established under Section 320 of the 1987 Clean Water Act Amendments, the NEP is a model for watershed partnerships. States nominate estuaries for inclusion into the NEP; there are currently twenty-eight NEP estuaries around the country. For estuaries that meet U.S. EPA criteria, the EPA signs an agreement with the nominating states authorizing the formation of a Management Conference, which includes private and public stakeholders from all levels of the federal system. The Management Conference is a collaborative three- to five-planning process that brings all these actors together to produce a Comprehensive Conservation Management Plan (CCMP). The CCMP identifies estuary problems, the

policy actions needed to address those problems, and in many cases the public and private stakeholders who are expected to implement the policies. There is usually an extensive period of fact finding involving factors of concern to different stakeholders. The decision rules tend to be relatively consensual. Face-to-face negotiations normally take several years to negotiate the overall plan. But implementation of specific aspects of the CCMP is normally left to specific member agencies.

2. Ostrom (1999) defines the action arena as "the social space where individuals interact, exchange goods and services, solve problems, dominate one another, or fight (among the many things that individuals do in an action arena)." Action arenas are further subdivided into action situations and actors. Taken together, I argue that the characteristics of the action arena determine the benefits and transaction costs of collective action. For the purposes of watershed management, the watershed and its associated ecological characteristics, institutions, and multiple stakeholders constitute the action arena.

3. Of course, it is clearly important to understand the causal processes involved as completely as possible, and I am not trying to evade the issue. In reality, I believe the NEP plays both an indirect and direct role in the evolution of cooperation within estuaries. The indirect role is providing an incentive to cooperate in order to pursue a successful NEP nomination. But once the Management Conference is in place, the resulting money, studies, meetings, and policies most likely accelerate the evolution of cooperation to an even greater degree. Completely establishing every step of the causal process is beyond the scope of this chapter, and maybe even beyond the scope of our research design.

4. Ecological economists identify two types of resources in estuaries (and ecosystems in general) that affect human welfare: natural capital and ecosystem services (Costanza et al. 1997). Natural capital is the stock of natural processes in the estuary such as hydrological dynamics, wildlife habitat, and energy exchange systems. Ecosystem services are the flows of resource units produced by natural capital, such as drinking water or fish, which people consume.

5. Note that I am assuming beliefs about problem severity are related to the collective outcomes that would occur in the absence of successful policies. If stakeholders view problem severity as an indicator of institutional performance, then watershed partnerships that make people think problems are worse would actually decrease cooperation.

In fact, results from a previous analysis showed problem severity did not have a significant effect on attitudinal support in either direction. It is probably the case that questions about problem severity elicit thoughts about the baseline problem among some stakeholders and thoughts about institutional performance among others. Hence, there would be a tendency for these two types of question answers to cancel each other out on average. Given the centrality of the problem severity concept in many theoretical frameworks, further research should disentangle these two possibilities.

6. In fact, all collective action beliefs are reflections of self-interest because they act as heuristics for tracking the benefits and transaction costs of collective

action. I assume people will engage in collective action only when the feel that benefits outweigh costs. However, it is not always the case that a particular stakeholder's collective action beliefs are always accurate monitors of watershed characteristics. Collective action beliefs are subject to persuasion and mistakes, and influenced by stakeholders' basic ideological viewpoints. However, the process of policy learning would assume that as stakeholders gain more experience in a particular collective action arena, their beliefs would become more accurate monitors of benefits and transaction costs.

7. In a sense, this idea is similar to the one that the strength of democracy is not its ability to make all think the same thing. Rather, the strength of democracy is that people agree on the legitimacy of a set of processes for resolving differences in opinion. For example, after the resolution of a court case, the plaintiff and the defendant probably still do not agree on who is right and who is wrong, but both are willing to accept the judge's decision. Similarly, after the 2000 presidential election, most Democrats probably do not agree that George W. Bush is the best choice. However, many are still willing to accept the outcome of the election as legitimate, despite the Florida fiasco.

8. The combination of mail and telephone surveys raises the possibility of instrumentation bias. Fortunately, the differences in means between telephone and survey respondents are not significant for most of the variables, so there is little evidence of instrumentation bias.

9. Overall, the response rate compares favorably to surveys of watershed partnerships conducted by other researchers: 51 percent by Wooley and McGinnis (1999) and 41 percent by Johnson and Campbell (1999).

10. The budget for the telephone survey required me to collapse the number of categories used to identify stakeholder types and position within the federal system. Results from the NEP mail survey present a more detailed picture: 60 percent government officials (mostly from administrative agencies), 11 percent environmental groups, 7 percent marine recreation/fisheries/forestry/agriculture, 5 percent business and real estate, 9.5 percent university/education, and 7.5 percent other. For levels of the federal system, there were 17 percent national, 10 percent subnational, 28 percent state, 17 percent substate, and 28 percent local (county, municipality, special district). Similarly, there is little variation in response rate across stakeholder type, with the exception of environmental groups, which are slightly more likely to respond. Overall, the more detailed data confirm my evaluation that the sample population is a good representation of the stakeholders active in estuary policymaking. Whether the representation of actor types is "fair" from a normative standpoint is beyond the scope of this chapter, although the approximately equal balance of environmental groups and business groups seems promising.

11. All measures of beliefs, including the dependent variables, are linearly rescaled to a continuous $[0, 1]$ range. For the beliefs originally measured on a $[0, 10]$ scale, this means dividing the original measurement by ten. This transformation does not change the statistical relationship between the variables, but it

does provide a convenient way to compare regression coefficients among different variables without using confusing standardized coefficients. When multiplied by 100, the ordinary-least-squares regression coefficients for the belief variables are interpreted as the change in the expected value (expressed as a percentage of the range of the dependent variable in the sample) of the dependent variables moving across the entire range of the relevant independent variable. For example, if the expected value of trust equals .497 when the NEP dummy and all policy beliefs equal zero and the slope coefficient for the NEP dummy equals .050, then ceteris paribus, the expected value of trust when the NEP dummy equals 1 will be .547 (an absolute change of 5 percentage points). For brevity, I will discuss the effects of the independent variables in terms of absolute percentage point change, not to be confused with percentage change.

For readers unfamiliar with regression analysis, the precise numerical interpretation of the regression coefficient is not essential. Regression coefficients merely symbolize the causal relationship between two variables, which could be positive, negative, or nonexistent. A positive regression coefficient means that as the independent variable increases in value, the dependent variable will also increase in value. A negative coefficient means that as the independent variable increases in value, the dependent variable decreases in value. If a regression coefficient is statistically significant, that means we can be confident the causal relationship exists for all estuary stakeholders. Hence, to assess the validity of my hypotheses, the more casual reader need only examine the sign and significance of each regression coefficient.

12. The largest weakness of these models is the low goodness of fit (R2). Clearly, collective action beliefs are not only a function of institutional structure and policy values. A variety of experiences within a particular watershed management institution, such as the behavior of other stakeholders, also will affect collective action beliefs. Unfortunately, measuring some of these factors is extremely difficult without direct observational data of many interactions in each estuary, which was beyond the scope of this project. The possibility of missing variables combined with the random measurement error typical of survey instruments reduced the overall explanatory power of the models. More complete models of collective action beliefs await further innovations in measurement. However, the models here represent tests of specific hypotheses, and largely support the theoretical arguments.

13. There is certainly a case to be made for reciprocal causation here. Stakeholders may believe public participation should be broad because problems are diffuse and serious. If problems were not diffuse and serious, maybe they could be handled quickly by a small group of experts. I do not currently have the data required to examine the dynamics of this relationship in more detail.

14. The interaction terms are the product of the NEP dummy times the relevant policy belief scale.

15. To compute the effect of a particular policy belief in the NEP, the regression coefficient for that policy belief must be added to the regression coefficient of the relevant interaction term. In contrast, the effect of a policy belief among

non-NEP stakeholders is simply the regression coefficient for the policy belief alone. For example, the effect of environmentalism on trust for NEP stakeholders is $(-.179 + .176 = -.003$, or $-.3$ percent), and for non-NEP stakeholders the effect is $-.179$ (or -17.9 percent).

16. The marginal effect of the NEP in each equation is simply the first derivative with respect to NEP. For example, the marginal effect of conservatism on trust equals $(-.117 + .176*\text{environmentalism} + .121*\text{conservatism})$.

8

Are Trust and Social Capital the Keys to Success? Watershed Partnerships in California and Washington

William D. Leach and Paul A. Sabatier

This chapter seeks to explain variation in the success of watershed partnerships, focusing on the roles of social capital and interpersonal trust. Of particular interest is the supposedly reciprocal (two-way) relationship between trust or social capital, on the one hand, and success, on the other. Conclusions are drawn from a quantitative analysis of seventy-six partnerships sampled randomly from California and Washington State.

As discussed in chapter 1, watershed partnerships consist of representatives from private interest groups, local public agencies, state or federal agencies, and researchers who convene about once a month to discuss the management of a river, stream, or watershed. Unlike the collaborative engagement processes discussed in chapters 4 and 5, partnerships are intended to last several years, if not indefinitely, and the specific issues discussed may change from year to year, as one issue is resolved or tabled and others come to the fore. This chapter examines three aspects of success, reflecting the main outputs and outcomes that partnerships pursue: (1) the extent of agreement achieved by the partnership, which can range from simply agreeing on an agenda to agreeing on a comprehensive management plan with goals, principles, and lists of restoration and other implementing projects; (2) the actual implementation of restoration and other projects by members of the partnership; and (3) the perceived outcomes of the partnership on watershed problems deemed important by the stakeholders. The last is a surrogate for actual outcomes, which, as explained in chapter 1, are extremely difficult to measure.

Chapter 6 explained how several theoretical frameworks have pointed to trust and social capital as two of the most important precursors to partnership success. Both are multifaceted concepts. A trustworthy person is someone who keeps promises and agreements, tries to take others' welfare into account when making decisions, and offers and returns favors. Trust is essential for agreements among stakeholders whose interests, values, and perceptions are often in direct conflict. Trust involves knowing that one's fellow stakeholders are likely to negotiate honestly, are worthy of respect, and are sufficiently honorable and competent to keep any promises they make.

Under the rubric of social capital, developed by Putnam and his colleagues (1993, 2000) and Coleman (1988) come norms of reciprocity (that one should return favors) and extensive social networks. Cultural norms that encourage reciprocity provide the foundation for agreements born of compromise. Individuals who develop dense social networks tend to acquire better negotiation and leadership skills plus a wealth of personal contacts to whom they can turn for advice or material assistance.

One of the most challenging questions for empirical research on watershed partnerships is the supposedly reciprocal relationship between trust and success or between social capital and success. Putnam, Leonardi, and Nanetti (1993) assume that trust within a partnership facilitates agreements and that agreements help build trust. In theory, the salutary effect of trust is reciprocal, because each agreement or restoration project confirms the trustworthiness of other members of the partnership. For example, agreements demonstrate that fellow stakeholders negotiate in good faith and are willing to compromise. Successful project implementation demonstrates that stakeholders honor their commitments and work competently. Similarly, success spawns further social capital when acts of reciprocity reinforce norms of reciprocity, and when small but visible accomplishments encourage new stakeholders to join the partnership and current participants to redouble their efforts.

Applied to watershed partnerships, the hypothesized reciprocal relationship is depicted in figure 8.1. The first tangible output of a successful partnership, an agreement, is a product of the various characteristics of the partnership process and its environmental and social context, as well as the existing level of social capital and trust. Process and context also influence the amount of trust and social capital. Having reached an agreement, a partnership can then seek to implement it through one or more restoration projects. Trust and social capital, as well as context

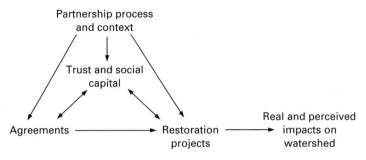

Figure 8.1
Hypothesized relationships between partnership characteristics, outputs, and outcomes

and process, again influence the stakeholders' ability to successfully carry out such projects. Finally, restoration projects (if well designed and well executed) lead to positive effects on watershed conditions—the ultimate goal of any partnership. Double-headed arrows in Figure 8.1 represent the reciprocal relationships between trust and social capital and the two partnership outputs.

If it can be shown that highly successful partnerships have high levels of social capital and trust, then the next question becomes, "Did trust and social capital lead to success, or did success lead to trust and social capital?" This is the central question of the chapter. After introducing the study of seventy-six partnerships in California and Washington and describing measures for each of the concepts in Figure 8.1, a one-way linear regression model is developed for each partnership output and outcome, using data on partnership process and context as explanatory variables. The results are then compared to models in which trust, social capital, and success are treated as reciprocal.

The results indicate that both trust and social capital are important for promoting agreements within watershed partnerships. However, trust is a catalyst for agreements mainly among partnerships older than three years. Younger partnerships frequently overcome high levels of distrust to reach agreements in crisis situations, such as flooding. The effect of trust and social capital on partnership agreements appears to be one way, not reciprocal. Neither trust nor social capital explains the implementation of restoration projects, except to the extent these variables promote agreements, which then lead to projects. Finally, the data reveal evidence of a halo effect, in which high levels of interpersonal trust and social capital inflate stakeholders' perceptions of their partnership's impact on watershed conditions.

Research Methods

Quantitative case studies of seventy-six randomly sampled watershed partnerships in California and Washington were compiled between 1999 and 2003 (Leach, Pelkey, and Sabatier 2002). These two states were selected to include one state with institutional mechanisms for funding and assisting watershed partnerships (Washington)[1] and one state that had not formally recognized collaborative approaches to watershed management (California).[2] The two states were also attractive because of their large numbers of partnerships to study and their relative proximity to the researchers based at the University of California, Davis, in northern California.

The field research began with an effort to identify all partnerships in California that were active at any point between 1995 and 2001, including partnerships that are now defunct.[3] To be included in the sampling frame, a partnership needed to meet at least four times per year and needed to focus on managing one or more streams, rivers, or watersheds. To ensure an adequate diversity of stakeholders, each partnership needed to include (1) at least one state or federal official; (2) at least one representative of local government—either a general-purpose city or county, or a special district (such as water or school district); and (3) at least two opposing interests, such as a resource user and either a regulating agency or environmental group.

The search revealed a population of 150 partnerships in California, from which 47 were randomly sampled with geographic stratification, such that no more than two partnerships were selected from a single watershed (table 8.1).[4] In Washington, we randomly selected 25 watersheds and sampled 1 to 2 partnerships from each, totaling 29 partnerships.[5] Because the selection process was random and the sample size is relatively large, the overall results should be representative of watershed partnerships in the two states.

The sample includes twelve partnerships that had disbanded by the time of our study. Four of these disbanded because they achieved their main objectives. The other eight disbanded after their negotiations ended in stalemate.

For each selected partnership, we (1) interviewed three to six key participants, including the partnership's coordinator-facilitator plus at least one key participant from a proenvironment perspective and at least one participant from a prodevelopment perspective; (2) analyzed relevant documents such as watershed plans and meeting minutes; and (3) mailed a survey to all participants sufficiently knowledgeable about the partnership to complete at least part of the questionnaire, plus several knowledgeable nonparticipant observers.

For the survey, the names of the participants and knowledgeable observers were obtained during the interviews. The smallest partnership had six survey recipients, and the largest had over a hundred. The resulting data set includes 315 interviews and 1,625 surveys (out of 2,498, for a response rate of 65 percent). Response rates for individual partnerships ranged from 45 percent to 88 percent.

Half of all survey respondents are government employees, with 12 percent representing federal agencies, 14 percent state agencies, and 25 percent local agencies. Indian tribes constitute 2 percent of respondents, private sector resource users 18 percent, environmental advocates 15 percent, facilitators or technical consultants 6 percent, and other stakeholders 8 percent.

Measures of Partnership Success

Drawing on the survey and interview data, we can construct measures for each of the three partnership outputs and outcomes from Figure 8.1:

- The level of agreement reached
- Restoration projects (implementation of agreements)
- Perceived effects on environmental and social conditions in the watershed (given that it is almost impossible to measure actual impacts).

Agreements The classic benchmark of success for environmental disputes is consensus on substantive issues. The level of agreement was measured using interviews and relevant documents to determine whether each partnership had achieved the following levels of agreement, which form an ordinal five-point scale:

Table 8.1
Randomly sampled partnerships

California (n = 47)
Alameda Creek Watershed Program Steering Committee
Alhambra Creek Watershed Management Committee
American River Watershed Group
Battle Creek Watershed Conservancy
Big Chico Creek Watershed Alliance
Butte Creek Watershed Conservancy
Cache Creek Stakeholders Group
Carmel River Watershed Council
Central Sierra Watershed Committee
Cherokee Watershed Group
Cosumnes River Task Force CRMP
Dos Palmas Cooperative Management Committee
Dry Creek CRMP
Eel River Watershed Improvement Group
Garcia River Watershed Advisory Group
Goose Lake Fishes Working Group
Gualala River Watershed Council
Klamath River Fisheries Task Force
Los Angeles and San Gabriel Rivers Watershed Council
Lower Stony Creek Task Force and Technical Team
Marin Coastal Watershed Enhancement Project
Mokelumne River Watershed Group
Morro Bay National Estuary Program
Navarro River Watershed Advisory Group
Northern Klamath Bioregional Group
Oakhurst River Parkway Partnership
Panoche/Silver Creek CRMP
Pescadero-Butano Creek CRMP
Pine Creek CRMP
Russian River Watershed Council
Sacramento River Fisheries and Habitat Restoration
San Francisquito Creek CRMP
San Joaquin River Management Program
San Joaquin Valley Conservation Partnership
San Juan Creek Feasibility Study Management Team
Santa Ana River Watershed Group
Scott River Watershed Council
Shasta-Tehama Bioregional Council
Smithneck Creek CRMP

Table 8.1
(continued)

Sonoma Marin Animal Waste Committee
South Fork Dialogue
South Fork Trinity River CRMP
Stanislaus Stakeholders
Tuolumne River TAC
Upper Salinas Watershed CRMP
Watsonville Sloughs Water Resources Program
Yuba Watershed Council

Washington ($n = 29$)
Cedar River Council
Chehalis Basin Partnership
Clean Water District
Douglas County Watershed Planning Association
Elwha-Morse Creek Watershed Management Team
Entiat Valley Landowners Association
Grays, Elochoman, and Cowlitz Watershed, WRIA 25–26
Hood Canal Watershed Project Center
Jefferson County Water Resources Council
Klickitat River Watershed Planning Unit
Lake Chelan Water Quality Committee
Lake Roosevelt Forum
Lewis, Salmon, and Washougal, WRIA 27–28
Little-Middle Spokane Planning Unit
Lyre-Hoko Planning Unit, WRIA 19
Methow Basin Planning Unit
Nisqually River Council, WRIA 11
Nooksack Recovery Team
Padilla Bay Farm Committee
Pend Oreille Planning Unit, WRIA 61
Skagit Implementation Review Committee
Stream Team
Thorton Creek Watershed Management Committee
Tolt Fish Habitat Restoration Group
Walla Walla Watershed Planning Unit
Wenatchee WAPIC
White Salmon River Management Committee
Wind White Salmon Rivers Planning Unit
Yakima River Basin Watershed Planning Unit

0 = no agreement on anything

1 = agreement on which issues to discuss or address

2 = agreement on general goals or principles

3 = agreement on one or more implementation actions (relatively limited and unintegrated), such as fencing ten miles of stream and installing a drinking trough on a cattle ranch to reduce sedimentation and fecal coliform

4 = agreement on a relatively comprehensive watershed management plan with specific projects or proposals; a management plan typically includes partnership goals, problems to be addressed, policy principles, and a list of restoration and other implementation projects

The data are roughly normally distributed with a mean of 2.7 and a range of 1 to 4.

Restoration Projects   A second central measure of success is implementation—the extent to which the members of a partnership have followed through on their commitments. Watershed partnerships frequently agree to implement on-the-ground restoration projects designed to improve local environmental or social conditions. We measure this output using interviews and partnership documents to evaluate progress on the four main types of restoration projects that watershed partnerships pursue:

• Abatement or prevention of point or nonpoint sources of pollution
• Modifications to in-stream flows or water allocation
• Stream channel projects (restoration of vegetation, morphology, or biota)
• Changes in land use designations (e.g., through purchase, easements, and zoning)

As detailed in figure 8.2, points are allotted according to the scope and degree of completion of each of the four types of projects attempted, resulting in an index that ranges between 0 and 40. The highest score actually observed among the seventy-six partnerships is 18 out of 40 points. Thirty-six partnerships had not yet attempted any restoration projects and received scores of zero.

Perceived Effect on the Watershed   The ultimate measure of partnership success is the extent to which a partnership has improved the social and

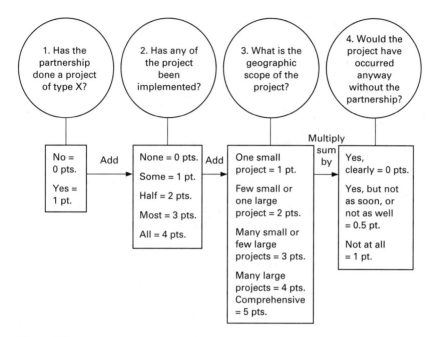

Figure 8.2
Index of restoration projects. The formula, based on data from interviews and documents, is repeated and summed for four types of restoration projects.

environmental problems in the watershed. Unfortunately, very few partnerships collect the preproject baseline data and long-term postproject data that are necessary to objectively ascertain a partnership's effect, while disentangling this effect from natural fluctuations or other forces in the watershed. As a second-best approximation, the study measured the stakeholders' perceptions about these effects. The questionnaire asked survey respondents to evaluate their partnership's influence on twelve problems ranging from impaired water quality to threats to Native American treaty rights.[6] The scale for each evaluation ranged from −3 (the partnership made the problem much worse) to +3 (much better), centered at zero (no net effect). Respondents were also asked to assess, on a scale from 0 to 100, the seriousness of each problem in their watershed.

To develop an overall score for each respondent, we weighted the twelve effects by the corresponding seriousness of the condition.[7] The final index was calculated by averaging across all respondents for each

Table 8.2
Scale for interpersonal trust

How many of the participants ...
    a. are honest, forthright, and true to their word? ($\rho = 0.76$)
    b. have reasonable motives and concerns? ($\rho = 0.76$)
    c. are willing to listen, and sincerely try to understand other points of view?
    ($\rho = 0.83$)
    d. reciprocate acts of goodwill or generosity? ($\rho = 0.83$)
    e. propose solutions that are compatible with the needs of other members of
    the partnership? ($\rho = 0.82$)

Note: Five-point Likert scale: $1 =$ none, $2 =$ few, $3 =$ half, $4 =$ most, $5 =$ all. The scale is the mean of the five items (Cronbach's alpha $= 0.88$). $\rho =$ nonparametric correlation between item and scale.

partnership. Weighting each of the twelve assessed effects by the seriousness of the problem allows each respondent to tailor the uniform list of issues to their own watershed. In this way, the assessments are fairly comparable across partnerships, even if different partnerships face different types of issues. The data are normally distributed with a mean of 0.34 and a range of -0.53 to 1.1 (on a scale from -3 to $+3$).

Measures of Interpersonal Trust and New Social-Human Capital

Interpersonal Trust   The survey asks respondents to assess the proportion of partnership participants who are honest, reasonable, willing to listen, and willing to reciprocate and who propose mutually agreeable solutions. The amount of trust within each partnership is calculated as the average response on this five-question scale (table 8.2). Empirically, the scale is consistent, as indicated by its large Cronbach's alpha of 0.88 and high correlations between each question and the scale (table 8.2).

New Social and Human Capital   New social and human capital is measured by asking survey respondents to assess, on a seven-point Likert scale, whether the partnership has given them (1) "new long-term friendships or professional relationships," (2) "a better understanding of other stakeholders' perspectives," and (3) "a better understanding of the physical or biological processes in the watershed." Each respondent's answers to the three questions were averaged to create a scale. The scale was then averaged across all respondents for a given partnership to create an overall measure of the partnership's perceived effect. Empirically, these three questions constitute a reliable scale (Cronbach's alpha = 0.74) with high correlations between each question and the composite scale ($r = 0.82, 0.84, 0.79$, respectively).

Measures of Explanatory Variables: Context and Process

The success of any watershed partnership depends on both the rules governing the collaborative process and the environmental and social context in which the partnership operates. There is a natural tendency for stakeholders to focus on process because that is what they can control when designing a partnership. One of the tasks for researchers is to study multiple partnerships to gauge the relative importance of the procedural and contextual factors. This chapter focuses on several contextual and procedural variables suggested by the theoretical frameworks described in chapter 6: the advocacy coalition framework (ACF), the institutional rational choice (IRC) framework, and the social capital literature.

One contextual variable suggested by ACF is the presence of a perceived watershed crisis. According to ACF, major changes within a policy subsystem (such as agreements between competing coalitions) rarely occur without a significant external shock, such as a natural disaster or socioeconomic upheaval, that changes the resources or core beliefs of key stakeholders (Sabatier and Jenkins-Smith 1993). In watershed policy, external shocks frequently take the form of catastrophic floods or fires, or the local decline of a major resource extraction industry. To measure stakeholders' perceptions of the degree of crisis, the survey asks respondents to agree or disagree (on a seven-point Likert scale), "When I first joined the Partnership, the problems in the watershed had reached a state of crisis."

Another ACF hypothesis regarding partnership context is that agreements between coalitions are easier to achieve when the stakeholders mutually experience a "hurting stalemate," defined as an unacceptable status quo combined with a lack of viable alternative venues for pursuing one's objectives. Viable alternatives to the partnership are assessed by asking stakeholders to agree or disagree (on a seven-point Likert scale), "If the partnership fails to adopt workable solutions, my concerns could probably be satisfied by appealing directly to the legislature, courts, or individual agencies."

A contextual factor highlighted by the social capital literature is the extent to which the stakeholders share strong norms of reciprocity, measured in the survey by asking respondents to self-assess whether they agree or disagree that "if someone in the partnership granted me a favor or concession, I would feel highly obligated to return the gesture" (on a seven-point Likert scale). Thus, the survey distinguishes between the new social capital generated through one's participation in a partnership versus reciprocity norms as a preexisting form of social capital that is probably unaffected by participating in a partnership. Empirically, the reciprocity norm variable appears to be exogenous, as it cannot be modeled very successfully using the other context and process variables.[8]

A final contextual variable common to both ACF and IRC is the extent to which the partnership includes members with sufficient scientific expertise. For IRC, scientific expertise reduces transaction costs by helping stakeholders identify solutions or compromises that are not only mutually acceptable but also technically feasible. For the ACF, scientific expertise helps stakeholders achieve shared understandings about the causes and extent of problems. Such policy-oriented learning across coalitions is an essential precursor for agreements on watershed restoration projects. This variable is measured in the survey by asking respondents whether they agree or disagree (on a seven-point Likert scale), "The partnership enjoys good access to people with sufficient training to evaluate scientific and technical information relevant to the partnership."

In terms of partnership process, two variables common to both ACF and IRC include the amount of grant funding received by the partnership and the age of the partnership measured as months since inception. A third process variable underlying both the ACF, with its attention to neutral facilitators, and the institutional analysis and development (IAD), with its focus on clear process rules, is the notion that the stakeholders must perceive that "the partnership process treats all parties fairly and consistently." The survey asks stakeholders to agree or disagree with this statement, using a seven-point Likert scale. Responses are averaged within each partnership to generate a process fairness variable.

A final process variable is suggested by the IRC hypothesis that "the right of individuals to form groups and make rules is not challenged by other national, regional, or local governments" (Ostrom 1990). In the context of watershed partnerships, in which all three levels of government routinely participate, the provision can be adapted to suggest that the government officials and interest group representatives who attend partnership meetings must have authority to negotiate on behalf the agencies or organizations they represent. Partnerships cannot reach and implement meaningful agreements if decisions made locally are likely to be undermined by administrators based in regional or national headquarters. This can be viewed as a process variable if we assume that each organization must decide whether to send high-level representatives to partnership meetings. Interviewees were asked to assess whether the participants have sufficient autonomy to make commitments on behalf of their organization. Responses were coded on a five-point scale.

Nonreciprocal (One-Way) Models to Explain Success, Trust, and Social and Human Capital

To explain the effect of each set of explanatory variables on each of the three measures of partnership success (level of agreement, restoration projects, and perceived impacts), we use ordinary-least-squares (OLS) regression models with a separate model for each dependent variable. The results are found in table 8.3. This initial set of models assumes that causality flows in one direction only—from partnership process and context to trust and social capital, and from trust and social capital to agreements, restoration projects, and perceived effects on the watershed. A second set of models, presented subsequently, allows the possibility that success feeds back to trust and social capital.

Because the sample is limited to seventy-six partnerships, it is not possible to include every explanatory variable in every model.[9] Each model is restricted to variables that can be justified on theoretical grounds. For example, "authority to negotiate" appears only in the model for "agreements," which is the output that results directly from successful negotiations. Similarly, "funding from grants" is excluded from the model of "agreements" because partnerships typically agree on a set of projects before seeking funding to implement them. In keeping with the conceptual model presented in figure 8.1, "agreements" is used to explain "restoration projects," which is used to explain "perceived effect on the watershed."

Table 8.3
Models explaining partnership outputs and outcomes ($n = 76$)

	Agreements	Restoration projects	Perceived effect on watershed	Trust	New social capital
Adjusted R^2	.40	.34	.69	.58	.59
Output variables					
Agreements		.29*†		.11	.15
Restoration projects			.20*	−.02	.20*
Trust and new social capital					
Interpersonal trust	.30*	.03	.59**		
New social capital	.17	.19	.03		
Context variables					
Perceived watershed crisis	.18#				
Scientific expertise	−.03	.17	.20*	.14	.26*
Norms of reciprocity	.15			−.09	.05
Viable alternate venues				−.30**	.16#
Process variables					
Funding from grants		.21*†	.13#		
Partnership age less than 36 months	−.40**				
Age of partnership (months)	.19#†	.06			
Process fairness scale				.48**	.51**
Authority to negotiate	.15				
Interaction effects					
Trust × Age < 36	−.28*				

Note: Ordinary-least-squares regression. Each model includes a constant. Standardized coefficients: #$p < 0.1$, *$p < 0.05$, **$p < 0.01$. †Significant in a tobit model for censored data ($p < .05$)

To interpret the results in Table 8.3, recall that the columns indicate the dependent variables (what we are trying to explain) and the rows provide the explanatory variables used in each equation. The numbers are regression coefficients, which indicate the effect of that explanatory variable on the dependent variable, controlling for (holding constant) all other explanatory variables in the equation. Regression coefficients range from +1.00 (the explanatory variable completely accounts for the dependent variable in a positive direction—that is, more of the explanatory variable produces more of the dependent variable), through 0.00 (the explanatory variable has absolutely no effect on the dependent variable), to −1.00 (the explanatory variable completely accounts for the dependent variable in a negative direction, meaning that more of the explanatory variable produces less of the dependent variable). For example, in the model for "agreements," interpersonal trust has a relatively strong positive relationship (0.30) with the level of agreement. The single asterisk indicates a less than 5 percent chance that the relationship is due to chance patterns in the data. The R^2 statistics for the five OLS models range between 0.34 and 0.69, meaning that the set of explanatory variables used in each equation explains 34 to 69 percent of the variance in the dependent (success) variables listed at the top of each column.

Agreements   Before discussing the multivariate regression model for partnership agreements, we introduce two scatter plots of the relationship between trust and agreements—one for partnerships under thirty-six months ($n = 23$), the other for older partnerships ($n = 53$) (figure 8.3). In young partnerships, the relationship is negative, but not statistically significant. For older partnerships, trust and agreement are correlated positively and significantly ($r = .40$, $p < .01$).

To accommodate this curvilinear relationship, the regression model (table 8.3) includes a dummy variable that equals one for partnerships younger than thirty-six months, zero for older partnerships.[10] Also included is a variable for the interaction between trust and partnership age (specifically, the trust variable multiplied by the dummy variable). For older partnerships, the dummy equals zero, and the interaction term drops out of the model. Thus, for older partnerships, the effect of trust is simply the stand-alone coefficient on trust. For younger partnerships, the

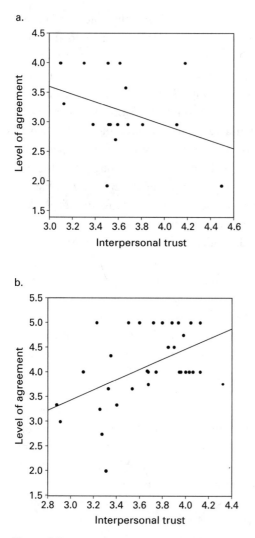

Figure 8.3
Effect of age on relationship between agreements and trust. *a*. Partnerships younger than thirty-six months. Scatter plot and fitted line showing inverse relationship between agreements and trust ($n = 17$, $r = -.35$, $p < .20$). Rsq = 0.1227. *b*. Partnerships older than thirty-six months ($n = 33$, $r = .50$, $p < .01$). Rsq = 0.2573.

effect of trust is the sum of the unstandardized coefficients for trust and the interaction variable.

In the estimated model, the positive sign on the coefficient for trust means that trust is positively associated with agreements. This association is statistically significant ($p < 0.05$). For the interaction variable, however, the coefficient is negative and statistically significant ($p < 0.05$). Therefore, the effect of trust is suppressed among younger partnerships. In fact, summing the two unstandardized coefficients yields a negative number, meaning that the overall net effect of trust is negative for young partnerships.

In summary, among partnerships older than thirty-six months, the relationship between trust and agreements is positive and statistically significant. For younger partnerships, trust is significant and inversely (negatively) related to agreements when holding constant the other variables.

Why the relationship between trust and agreements should reverse as partnerships age is unclear. One plausible explanation is as follows. Early in the life of a partnership, distrust may stem largely from uncertainty about the character of the other participating stakeholders. Months or years later, stakeholders have interacted with one another repeatedly, and any remaining distrust is grounded in confirmed fears, not speculative ones. Stakeholders in young partnerships faced with a severe crisis in the watershed may be willing to forge agreements despite their distrust, a form of calculated risk. In older partnerships, this risk is replaced by relative certainty and the detrimental effects of distrust are unfettered. For young partnerships in crisis situations, motivation to solve the problem may be more important than trust.

This explanation is consistent with two observations from the study. First, in the sample of twenty-three young partnerships, those that achieved complex agreements amid low levels of trust were the ones that faced especially severe resource issues (mainly catastrophic flooding) and were more likely to describe their watershed as being in a state of crisis. Second, stakeholders from younger partnerships were more likely to answer "don't know" when asked about the trustworthiness of fellow stakeholders (6 percent versus 3 percent), suggesting that uncertainty plays a somewhat larger role in establishing trust within young partnerships.

Restoration Projects The factors most conducive to implementing restoration projects are the age of the partnership, funding from grants, and agreements on what projects to pursue.[11] Thus, after accounting for each partnership's basic resources (time and money) and factoring in whether a partnership has reached agreements authorizing restoration projects, the theoretical frameworks from chapter 6 add relatively little to our understanding of project implementation. In particular, neither trust nor new social and human capital is statistically significant, at least over the observed range of variation.[12]

Perceived Effect on Watershed The regression model suggests that trust, restoration projects, and norms of reciprocity induce stakeholders to evaluate their partnerships more positively.

Trust (as a Dependent Variable) Interpersonal trust is greatest in partnerships where the stakeholders believe that the process treats everyone fairly and they view the partnership as their only viable strategy for achieving their goals and objectives. The correlation between trust and perceived fairness would suggest that a fair process helps to foster trust among traditional adversaries.

The negative effect of the variable measuring "viable alternative venues" is noteworthy. The results suggest that if most stakeholders lack an alternate venue in which to pursue their agenda and if stakeholders can sense that their fellow participants are similarly situated, then they need not worry about defectors undermining the partnership by appealing to higher authorities. During the case study interviews, stakeholders often voiced concerns about "deal breakers" who might try to subvert decisions reached by consensus within the partnership.

New Social and Human Capital (as a Dependent Variable) The factors most conducive to generating new social capital are restoration projects, scientific expertise, and procedural fairness. Curiously, another moderately significant variable is the perceived presence of viable alternate venues. We have no ready explanation for why viable alternative venues are positively related to the generation of new social capital but negatively related to trust. One possibility is that having dense social networks creates greater access to alternate venues.

Reciprocal Models of Success

The models discussed above are estimated using OLS regression, which requires that each explanatory variable be exogenous. In other words, each explanatory variable must be a given input to the model, not an output of the model. Depicted as a flow diagram, an OLS model may not contain any two-way arrows. Variables that have feedback loops are said to be endogenous to the model and, if modeled using OLS, will have serious technical problems (including biased standard errors and invalid hypothesis tests).

One remedy for endogenous variables is to estimate the model using two-stage least-squares regression (2SLS).[13] Tables 8.4 and 8.5 present 2SLS models for agreements. Table 8.4 uses trust as the endogenous (two-way) variable. Table 8.5 uses new social and human capital. Because trust and new social and human capital are highly correlated ($r = 0.56$), we include only one at a time.[14] Similarly, tables 8.6 and 8.7 present 2SLS models for perceived effect on the watershed. Since neither

Table 8.4
Reciprocal model of agreements and interpersonal trust ($N = 76$)

	Agreements	Trust
Adjusted R^2	.39	.55
Endogenous variables		
Agreements		−.12
Interpersonal trust	.23*	
Context variables		
Perceived watershed crisis[a]	.18#	
Norms of reciprocity	.17#	−.05
Scientific expertise[a]		.19#
Viable alternate venues[a]		−.29**
Process variables		
Authority to negotiate[a]	.15#	
Partnership age less than 36 months	−.45**	−.04
Process fairness scale[a]		.51**
Interaction effects		
Trust × Age < 36[a]		−.28**

Note: Two-stage least-squares regression. Each model includes a constant. Standardized coefficients: #$p < 0.1$, *$p < 0.05$, **$p < 0.01$.
[a] Instrumental variables.

Table 8.5
Reciprocal model of agreements and new social capital ($N = 76$)

	Agreements	New social capital
Adjusted R^2	.22	.48
Endogenous variables		
Agreements		−.27
New social capital	.37*	
Context variables		
Perceived watershed crisis[a]	.21*	
Norms of reciprocity	.10	.10
Scientific expertise[a]		.41*
Viable alternate venues[a]		.12
Process variables		
Authority to negotiate[a]	.15	
Partnership age (months)	.13	.26*
Process fairness scale[a]		.48**

Note: Two-stage least-squares regression. Each model includes a constant. Standardized coefficients: #$p < 0.1$, *$p < 0.05$, **$p < 0.01$.
[a] Instrumental variables.

trust nor new social capital is significant in 2SLS models for restoration projects, those results are not shown. The reciprocal 2SLS approach produces models quite similar to the OLS models. The primary value of these models is to explore the direction of causation and the hypothesized reciprocal relationships. The results indicate that neither agreements nor restoration projects have any significant feedback effect on social and human capital or trust; perceived impacts have a reciprocal effect on social capital but not trust. Given that only one of the six feedback effects is confirmed by our data, the reciprocal arrows from outputs and outcomes back to trust and social capital in Figure 8.1 should probably be erased.

Discussion and Conclusions

Because trust and social and human capital are highly related conceptually and empirically, it is difficult to establish how much each separately contributes to success. When both trust and social capital are included

Table 8.6
Reciprocal model of perceived effect on the watershed and interpersonal trust ($N = 76$)

	Perceived effect on watershed	Trust
Adjusted R^2	.65	.60
Endogenous variables		
Perceived effect on watershed		.12
Interpersonal trust	.74**	
Output variables		
Restoration projects[a]	.17*	
Context variables		
Scientific expertise	.14	.12
Perceived watershed crisis	.10	−.08
Viable alternate venues[a]		−.27**
Process variables		
Funding from grants[a]	.14#	
Age of partnership (months)	.07	.04
Process fairness scale[a]		.44**

Note: Two-stage least-squares regression. Each model includes a constant. Standardized coefficients: #$p < 0.1$, *$p < 0.05$, **$p < 0.01$.
[a] Instrumental variables.

in the same OLS model, neither variable obtains a statistically significant coefficient. But when trust and social and human capital are included in separate 2SLS models, both are strong and significant predictors of agreements. Although we find trust to be an important factor for promoting agreements, we also find that younger partnerships can overcome distrust to reach complex agreements. Agreements also appear more likely in partnerships where the watershed is in a state of crisis and the stakeholders share strong norms of reciprocity and wield adequate authority to negotiate on behalf of the organizations they represent.

The second measure of partnership success—implementation of restoration projects—is insulated from the effects of trust and social and human capital, except through their influence on agreements, a precursor to implementation. Once agreements are reached, project implementation primarily depends on basic resources: time and money.

Table 8.7

Reciprocal modes of perceived effect on the watershed and new social capital ($N = 76$)

	Perceived effect on watershed	New social capital
Adjusted R^2	.40	.53
Endogenous variables		
Perceived effect on watershed		.52#
New social capital	.94**	
Output variables		
Restoration projects[a]	.06	
Context variables		
Scientific expertise	−.01	.18
Perceived watershed crisis	.04	−.04
Viable alternate venues[a]		.19#
Process variables		
Funding from grants[a]	.15	
Age of partnership (months)	−.08	.14
Process fairness scale[a]		.25

Note: Two-stage least-squares regression. Each model includes a constant. Standardized coefficients: #$p < 0.1$, *$p < 0.05$, **$p < 0.01$.
[a] Instrumental variables.

Trust itself is stronger in partnerships where the process treats everyone fairly and where few stakeholders feel they have viable alternatives to the partnership.

There is an extremely strong relationship between participants' trust and social and human capital, on the one hand, and their perceptions of a partnership's effect on the watershed, on the other. In the hypothesized flow diagram (figure 8.1), restoration projects were the only determinant of effects on the watershed. In the data from California and Washington, restoration projects do have a significant influence on perceptions of these effects but are much less important than trust and social capital.

These results suggest that the flow diagram be revised as in figure 8.4. As revised, the relationship between trust and agreements is one way, not reciprocal, and the effect is suppressed for partnerships younger than three years. The arrows from trust and new social and human capital

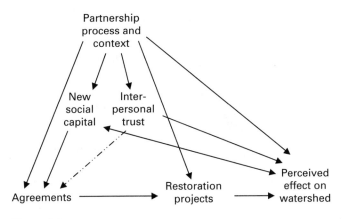

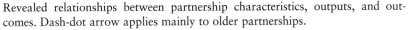

Figure 8.4
Revealed relationships between partnership characteristics, outputs, and outcomes. Dash-dot arrow applies mainly to older partnerships.

to restoration projects are severed. Trust and social capital have a much stronger than hypothesized influence on perceptions about a partnership's effect on the watershed. The relationship is reciprocal for social and human capital but not for trust.

Considering that the effect of trust outweighs the effect of the more objective indicator, restoration projects, one might conclude that trust generates a halo effect on stakeholders' perceptions about their collective impact on watershed conditions, making the partnership appear more successful than it actually is. A halo effect is consistent with the fears expressed by critics of consensus-based policymaking, such as Cary Coglianese (2002), who claim that stakeholders and researchers are too quick to equate satisfying interpersonal relationships with overall success. Coglianese calls for more attention to the quality of the decisions produced by consensus and to objective measures of outcomes such as cost savings or environmental benefits.

The greatest limitation of the research presented here is that the data present only a cross-sectional snapshot of each partnership at one point in time—a suboptimal design for investigating cyclical relationships. To corroborate the study's conclusions, what is needed are panel studies in which trust, social capital, and success are measured at least twice, at an interval of perhaps three to five years. Such a repeated-measures design would permit more accurate measurement of temporal trends and stronger inferences about the magnitude and direction of causal relationships.

Notes

We thank Cary Coglianese for his comments on a previous version of this material presented at the Kennedy School of Government, Harvard University, May 3, 2001. We also thank Chris Weible and Kate Reza for assistance with the data analysis and interpretation. The field research was carried out by the authors and Beth Cook, Jared Ficker, Maryann Hulsman, Erin Klaesius, Steve Kropp, Tamara LaFramboise, Christal Love, Neil Pelkey, Kate Reza, Martha Turner, and Chris Weible. Funding was provided by the National Science Foundation's Decision Making and Valuation for Environmental Policy program (grant 9815471), the U.S. Environmental Protection Agency's Science to Achieve Results program (grant R82-7145), and the David and Lucile Packard Foundation's Conserving California Landscapes Initiative.

1. In 1998, Washington passed the Watershed Planning Act (codified as RCW 90.82, but better known as HB2514), which initially created and funded nineteen watershed planning units that function as multistakeholder partnerships. As of January 2004, thirty-four planning units are active in Washington.

2. In late 2003, California took a step forward with the passage of the Watershed Protection and Restoration Act (chapter 6.5, section 5808 of the Public Resources Code), which encourages state agencies to provide assistance and grants to watershed partnerships.

3. California partnerships were identified through several means. First, names were solicited from district conservationists with the Natural Resources Conservation Service, directors from local Resource Conservation Districts, field personnel of the California Department of Forestry and Fire Protection, and University of California Cooperative Extension specialists. Second, we searched the Natural Resource Projects Inventory, a database housed in the UC Davis Information Center for the Environment. Third, we used Internet search engines to find relevant Web pages. Fourth, we asked interviewees from each partnership to name other partnerships in their region. Finally, in cases where there was any doubt about whether a partnership satisfied our operational definition, we called a partnership representative to obtain further information. A similar process was used for Washington. We included defunct partnerships in our sample because we wanted to maximize variance on our success variables.

4. We partitioned California using Hydrologic Unit Code (HUC) watersheds defined by the U.S. Geological Survey. There are 160 HUCs in the state, ranging from 35 to 9,000 square miles.

5. We partitioned Washington using the sixty-two Water Resource Inventory Areas, which range from 140 to 3,000 square miles.

6. Impaired water quality, threatened species or habitat, lack of open space, population growth, inadequate water supply, risk of damaging floods, threat of cata-

strophic fire, lack of economic prosperity, severe regulation or taxes, threats to property rights, threats to tribal or treaty rights, and conflict among stakeholders.

7. "Perceived effect on watershed conditions" for respondent

$$n = \left(\sum_{C=1}^{12} E_C \cdot S_C \right) \Big/ \sum_{C=1}^{12} S_C,$$

where EC = perceived effect on condition C and SC = perceived seriousness of condition C.

8. Adjusted $R2$ statistics for such models hover around 0.2, suggesting that norms of reciprocity are unaffected by the partnership process and context. The main explanatory variable is age of partnership, which correlates $r = 0.37$ with reciprocity norms.

9. Each explanatory variable removes one degree of freedom. Rules of thumb suggest a minimum of eight observations (i.e., partnerships) per explanatory variable. The following variables (and their theoretical "home") were omitted from the final equations because they turn out out to be unimportant and also decreased the significance of some other variables in the equations (probably because of collinearity): (1) quality of facilitation (ADR), (2) process rules index (IAD), (3) ideological conflict index (ACF), and (4) preexisting social capital: network density (SC).

10. This is the cutoff point that maximizes the difference between the bivariate trust agreement correlations for young versus old partnerships.

11. Because the data on restoration projects are not normally distributed, OLS could produce biased estimates. The majority of partnerships (thirty-six of seventy-six) had implemented no projects and received a score of zero, suggesting the use of a tobit model for censored data. Data are considered censored whenever scores beyond a certain threshold are collapsed into the threshold value (Sigelman and Zeng 1999). The data on restoration projects are potentially censored at zero because any partnership that implements no restoration projects and actually depresses the amount of restoration activity in the watershed will appear in the database as a zero rather than earning a negative score. In the tobit model, as in the OLS model, the variables for time, money, and agreements are highly significant, while both trust and new social capital are clearly insignificant.

12. The trust data are normally distributed with a range of 2.9 to 4.5 on a scale where 1 means no fellow participants are trustworthy and 5 means all are trustworthy. New social and human capital is normally distributed with an observed range from 4.1 to 5.8 on a seven-point agree-disagree scale. Bivariate Pearson correlations between trust and the other measures of success are: agreements 0.24, restoration projects 0.22, perceived impacts on the watershed 0.80, and new social and human capital 0.56.

13. In the first stage, the first endogenous variable (e.g., trust) is modeled using OLS and a set of explanatory variables that excludes the second endogenous variable (e.g., agreements), but includes an additional variable, referred to as the "instrument," which is uncorrelated with the residual. The predicted values from

this model of trust are then used, in lieu of the actual trust data, as an explanatory variable to model agreements. This is the second stage. The process is repeated by modeling agreements in the first stage and using the predicted values of agreements to explain trust in the second stage. Two-stage least-squares regression yields biased but consistent estimates of the standard errors. The models were estimated using the 2SLS function of the SPSS computer program.

14. Even well-specified 2SLS models tend to suffer from multicollinearity because the data for the endogenous variable are replaced by predicted values based on a linear combination of the right-hand-side variables (Asher 1983).

IV
Conclusions

9
Conclusions and Recommendations

Mark Lubell, Paul A. Sabatier, Arnold Vedlitz, Will Focht, Zev Trachtenberg, and Marty Matlock

Collaborative watershed institutions represent a new approach to environmental governance. These new institutions combine important elements of old management approaches with a series of adaptations and innovative choices that exploit emerging opportunities. This book has examined the nature of collaborative institutions in an effort to understand how they operate in the complex environment of American federalism and the difficult environmental problems that a modern industrial nation must face. We focus on the process and outcome of collaborative institutions and, ultimately, their longevity and survival as a new institutional structure. At the same time, we assess whether the experiment in collaborative institutions can improve environmental problems within socioeconomic constraints, and we provide concrete recommendations to practitioners about how to structure the process effectively.

This book has also provided a second generation of scholarship that goes beyond descriptive analysis. It has presented a variety of normative and positive theoretical frameworks, derived testable hypotheses, and tested these hypotheses with qualitative and quantitative data. These methods allow us to organize conjectures into a systematic knowledge base to guide further research and inform policy recommendations. Our methodology is a necessary step in the evolution of research on collaborative institutions, one that must be taken (and taken further than this book) if we are to understand the nature and consequences of collaboration.

What have we learned from this approach? This chapter summarizes our findings according to the six main themes that run throughout the book: process and context, participation and representation, civic community, effectiveness, legitimacy, and survival. These are the main themes captured by our dynamic framework for collaborative institutions in chapter 1, and we hope our research has illuminated key aspects of this framework. We end with some specific recommendations for practitioners and a description of a future research agenda.

We begin with an examination of the model elements and relationships outlined in our framework in chapter 1. We summarize what the analytical chapters tell us about the viability of the model and the empirical evidence we have examined to test both the concepts and relationships outlined in that model. We begin with the key aspects of context and process.

The Process and Context of Collaborative Institutions

Collaborative institutions consist of formal and informal rules for making collective decisions and governing actual resource use behavior. In the terms of Ostrom's institutional analysis and development framework (1999), collaborative institutions consist of both collective choice and operational rules. Collective choice rules define who can participate in decision making, how decisions are made, how preferences are aggregated into social choices, and who is responsible for policy implementation. Operational rules define rules for allowable and forbidden uses of natural resources and penalties for noncompliance. At this general level, the types of rules governing the collaborative decision-making process are not unlike other types of governance institutions.

The types of institutional rules used make the collaborative process unique. As described in chapter 1, collaborative institutions generally strive for inclusive stakeholder representation, treat all participants as roughly equal in authority (rather than one agency with dominant legal authority and all others as supplicants), use some type of consensus rule to structure decisions, and focus on mutually acceptable solutions. Instead of penalties and enforcement, collaborative institutions are more likely to rely on voluntary cooperation to implement policies resulting from the collective choice process. In these various ways, collaborative institutions are fundamentally different from their command-and-control predecessors.

These basic common features can be thought of as the "genes" of collaborative institutions. However, there are important differences between the genetic structure of a biological organism and the decision-making structures of governance institutions. The sources of change in biological organisms are the largely passive processes of recombination and mutation. But for governance institutions, change occurs when people make choices about how to make political decisions and the types of policies most appropriate for a particular environmental problem. Some of these ideas are inherited from previous experiences, and others are created from scratch. Collaborative institutions are based on a core set of ideas, but stakeholders choose different combinations of these ideas to reflect local circumstances.

The ability to combine the core ideas of collaborative institutions in various ways directly contributes to the adaptive capacity and survivability of the institution. This adaptive capacity is analogous to subspecies of salmon and steelhead, which have different color variations, different spawning strategies, and other life history features depending on the size and coloration of gravel in their natal streams, the length of the stream, and patterns of water flow.

Hence, an important contribution of our research is to describe variation in institutional structure as a response to different contexts and choices. Chapter 1 describes some generic forms of collaboration, such as collaborative engagement processes, watershed partnerships, and collaborative superagencies. Our research sites express structural variation even within each generic category. In the Leon and Salado Creek watersheds (chapter 5) in San Antonio, Texas, stakeholders were organized into Watershed Restoration Councils using collaborative learning techniques to generate management options. In the Illinois River Watershed in Oklahoma (chapter 4), a collaborative team was convened after a frustrating experience with an existing regional institution, the Oklahoma Scenic River Commission. The National Estuary Program (chapter 7) is a federally sponsored program, where a bottom-up nomination process is supplemented by federal money in an effort to recruit a wide range of stakeholders. Perhaps the greatest variation occurs within the Western Pacific watershed partnerships (chapter 8), which feature a wide variety of decision-making rules and operate in environments with multiple types of existing venues and levels of social capital. Each of these collaborative processes has the goal of building cooperation among stakeholders, but they vary widely in how the process is structured.

There is not only variation between different types of collaborative institutions; there is also variation within single programs occurring in multiple locations. The best example of this is the National Estuary Program (NEP). As described in chapter 7, NEP estuaries are designated through a nomination process and focus on the creation of a Management Conference, which produces an estuary restoration plan. There are interesting differences in the structure of the Management Conferences across NEP estuaries. For example, the Long Island Sound Study (New York and Connecticut) is run through a local U.S. EPA office, while the Peconic Estuary Program (New York) is housed in the Suffolk County Department of Health Services; other estuaries have established their own nonprofit organizations. The committees of the Management Conferences also vary; for example, some NEPs have local government committees, and others do not. This variation continues throughout the implementation process, as NEP stakeholders seek creative ways to orient existing policy tools toward the common goals of estuary management. The ways in which NEP's structure planning and implementation processes reflect local watershed policy resources and political realities, but regardless of what tools they use, the overriding goal is a collaborative approach to solving estuary problems.

How does this variation in the structures of the collaborative processes come about? The scholarship on collaborative institutions has not advanced enough to definitively answer this question. Also, we have not yet developed theories to predict variations in the structure of the collaborative process. Fortunately, our experiences with the research projects explored in this book have provided some clues. We speculate that variation in collaborative institutions is mainly due to the relationship between the contexts in which the institutions operate (what Ostrom calls the action-decision arena) and the type of institutional structure that best fits a particular context. A successful environmental governance institution adapts to the structure of the action-decision arena, including the type of environmental problems, the constellation of political actors and venues, existing policy tools, civic culture, and socioeconomic conditions. Following our biological analogy, this is akin to species of salmon adapting to particular types of riparian structure. However, we must keep in mind that the variation in institutional structure is largely due to stakeholders' making choices in responses to local political, social, economic, and environmental realities.

The very emergence of collaborative institutions from the legacy of command-and-control institutions is a case in point. As we noted in chapters 1 and 2, collaborative institutions emerged as a response to the perceived failures of command-and-control policies to solve certain types of problems, particularly nonpoint source pollution and habitat destruction. When traditional policies are applied to these types of diffuse and complex problems, great conflicts generally result. Collaborative institutions may be better adapted to these types of problems, thus reducing the transaction costs of environmental governance.

Existing empirical research reiterates the importance of context by identifying watershed-level variables that predict the emergence of watershed partnerships. Lubell et al. (1998) find that watershed partnerships are more likely to emerge in watersheds with severe nonpoint source pollution problems, where EPA enforcement of existing point sources is not strict (measured by the number of enforcement actions on National Pollution Discharge Elimination System permits), and where existing institutional and social capital help offset the transaction costs of partnership formation. Leach and Pelkey (2001) find that watershed partnerships in California are more likely to occur in watersheds targeted for the development of Total Maximum Daily Load management plans, which suggests the threat of stricter regulation acts as a catalyst for collaboration. The data in chapter 8 indicate that watersheds in crisis, for example, from flooding, are probably more likely to form partnerships and certainly more likely to produce management plans.

We suspect the variation within collaborative institutions also reflects the adaptive capacity of human institutions. Collaborative institutional structures fit the idiosyncratic contexts in which they occur. To the extent that a particular collaborative institution's choices reflect local realities, it is more likely to succeed in solving a particular problem. And as we discuss later in this chapter, the adaptive capacity of a collaborative institution is a critical aspect of long-term institutional survival and sustainability. The next section addresses issues of participation and representation in collaborative processes.

Participation and Representation

In chapter 1, we distinguished three types of collaborative processes used to involve stakeholders in watershed management. Collaborative engagement processes are convened to address a particular issue or purpose; therefore, they last only as long as that issue or purpose is being served. Collaborative partnership processes manage watersheds over the long term and thus tend to deal with many issues as circumstances change. Collaborative superagencies are formal bureaucracies, such as CALFED in California, that operate according to collaborative principles and have the authority to promulgate management plans and administer implementation actions. Each type of collaborative process presents distinct questions about stakeholder participation, and five chapters addressed participant representation issues, to a varying extent. Chapters 4 and 5 reported results from our study of collaborative engagement processes, and chapters 6, 7, and 8 addressed collaborative partnership processes. None deals with superagencies. In this section, we first discuss who participates and then address their reasons for participation.

Who Participates in Collaborative Institutions, and Which Segments of the Population Do They Represent?

Chapters 4 and 5 describe collaborative engagement processes initiated by members of the research team. These case studies used different methods to achieve representativeness. In the Illinois River watershed case study (chapter 4), we recruited participants based on the perspectives revealed in face-to-face interviews. Based on empirical analysis of survey data from 120 stakeholders, five perspectives on watershed concerns and four perspectives on preferences for watershed management were identified. At least one participant holding each of these five perspectives was recruited to each of our policy dialogue sessions (see table 4.6). All major points of view on the Illinois River were thus considered during the stakeholder deliberations on watershed management practices. However, this level of representativeness did not occur naturally; it required active intervention from the research team.

In the Salado and Leon Creek case study (chapter 5), we first conducted a telephone survey of area citizens to gauge levels of interest and knowledge about local watershed issues and respondents' willingness to participate in decision-making processes dealing with watershed issues. Chapter 5 presented an analysis of this survey to help explain the factors that related to willingness to say who will participate in collaborative processes.

It is interesting to note that of the 1,017 respondents surveyed, 245 indicated that they would be willing to participate in a collaborative process to discuss management of watershed issues and impacts. However, few of these 245 respondents actually joined either of the two collaborative processes begun in the San Antonio watershed area. The research team had to actively recruit participants from as broad a spectrum of citizens as possible.

Comparing the hypothetical participation results to the actual participation results, two outcomes are particularly noteworthy. First, although Hispanics and women stated that they were more willing to participate than did members of other groups, they were less willing to actually do so. Second, the underrepresentation of business representatives may be explained by the possibility that in their judgment, their interests were not threatened since the partnerships did not possess enforcement powers. Thus, consistent with the findings from chapter 4, they may have rationally calculated that their involvement was not needed. This explanation was not directly tested. Chapter 5 concluded that the identification and recruitment of participants for collaborative engagement processes may require significant resources, use of local recruiters, recognition of the importance of both individual and community welfare, consideration of social norms, and assurance of outcome effectiveness.

The watershed partnerships studied in chapters 7 and 8 represent a later stage of development in collaborative institutions and attempt to recruit both citizen and government representatives. In the NEP, 60 percent of the stakeholders are elected or appointed officials from the federal, state, or local government (Lubell et al. 1998). These government officials are spread nearly equally across levels of the federal system, suggesting the NEP does a good job of spanning boundaries between levels of government. Environmental groups are 11 percent of the stakeholders, economic interest groups 12 percent, researchers 9.5 percent, and other miscellaneous stakeholders (e.g., citizens at large, consultants, Native American groups) represent 7.5 percent. The involvement of the U.S. EPA and federal government resources clearly provides an incentive for government participation.

In the seventy-eight watershed partnerships in California and Washington reported in chapter 8, 31 percent of participants are from state and federal agencies; 2 percent represent Native American tribes; 26

percent are from local agencies (both cities and counties and water and flood control districts); 16 percent are private sector resource users (e.g., farmers, ranchers, timber harvesters); 13 percent are environmental or outdoor recreation advocates; 7 percent are facilitators, consultants, or university researchers; and 3 percent are unaffiliated watershed residents (Sabatier, Quinn, and Leach 2002). As in the San Antonio studies, upper-socioeconomic groups are overrepresented, with 85 percent of partnership participants possessing a college degree. Overall, the watershed partnerships discussed in chapters 7 and 8 heavily emphasize intergovernmental coordination.

Why Do People Participate in Collaborative Institutions?
Chapters 4 through 8 examine the question of what motivates participation in stakeholder collaborations. The Salado Creek–Leon Creek case study provides anecdotal evidence that participants' concerns about welfare and protection of their basic interests are the most popular motivators for participation. A desire for information and faith that participation will yield positive outcomes in the watershed are less frequently mentioned. However, all of these motives are instrumentally related to finding an effective watershed outcome. In the Illinois River watershed case, we found that stakeholders are most interested in obtaining policies responsive to their concerns and compatible with their preferences. Obtaining information about both the watershed and policymaker proposals to address watershed threats was also an important motive. Finally, stakeholders sought assurances that policymakers would seriously consider their concerns and preferences in policy formulations. These purely substantive motives are consistent with the instrumental motives found in the Salado Creek–Leon Creek watershed study.

The least frequently mentioned motive in the Salado Creek–Leon Creek study was improvement in human and social capital. It is possible, however, that collaborative engagement processes lasting only a year do not give participants sufficient time to recognize social and human capital as motives for participation. Data from the watershed partnerships in California and Washington indicate a wide variation in the time required for different aspects of human and social capital to become important to participants. For example, almost all participants report a better understanding of other stakeholders' perspectives within less than two years

(Leach, Pelkey, and Sabatier 2002). Education about watershed issues increases rapidly within the first two years, levels off for several years, and then increases again after six years. Improving personal and professional relationships takes at least two years to happen at any level, but it never becomes the norm in over 60 percent of partnerships. In short, educating oneself about other participants and the biological and physical processes in the watershed normally takes two to three years, while enhancing one's social and professional networks seems to be much more difficult. While these results demonstrate that some aspects of human and social capital are easier to acquire than others, they do not deal directly with these goals as inducements to participate in collaborative partnerships.

That topic is addressed more directly in table 9.1. It presents the data on the mean importance of seven reasons for participating in watershed partnerships for participants in the study of seventy-six partnerships in California and Washington. More specifically, the table presents the mean response on a scale from 1 ("not at all important") to 7 "very important" for each of the seven reasons in each category of participants (Native Americans, federal and state agency officials, local government officials, resource users, environmentalists, and consultants and academics). Notice, first, that defensive reasons—protecting one's financial interests, preventing the partnership from achieving undesirable policy changes, and heading off regulation—are much more important for resource users than for any other group. Second, meeting people is not important for any group. Third, the other aspect of human and social capital—"educating oneself about watershed issues"—is moderately important for virtually all groups except Native Americans. Fourth, by far the most important stated reasons for participating are to "achieve my organization's goals and objectives" (mean scores of about 5.5 for most groups) and "improving the watershed" (mean scores of about 6.5 for most groups). While one might disregard the last as a socially acceptable response, it is reasonably clear that most people participate in watershed partnerships to meet their organization's goals for the watershed; defensive protection of one's interests are important only for resource users; and among the human and social capital incentives, increasing human capital (education) is much more important than increasing social networks (meeting people). More important, the California and

Table 9.1
Reasons for participating in the partnership

	Native American tribes	Federal and state agencies	Local agencies	Resource users	Environmentalists	Facilitators, consultants, and academics	F-ratio
To improve the watershed	6.8	6.5	6.0	5.6	6.8	6.5	17**
To protect my financial interests	1.7	1.4	2.5	5.0	1.7	1.9	71**
To achieve my organization's goals and objectives	5.8	5.8	5.7	4.9	5.7	4.5	8.0**
To prevent the partnership from achieving undesirable changes in law or policy	3.8	2.9	3.8	5.4	4.0	3.1	23**
To head off state/federal regulation	1.5	2.4	3.7	5.1	2.0	2.6	45**
To educate myself about watershed issues	2.9	4.5	4.9	5.4	5.5	5.1	8.2**
To meet people	1.6	3.0	2.8	2.9	3.1	3.7	2.5**

Notes: Mean responses within each category of stakeholders. *F*-ratios are from one-way ANOVA test of null hypothesis of no difference between stakeholder categories for the mean responses to each reason for participation; * $p < .05$, ** $p < .01$. Metric: 1 = "not an important reason," 7 = "very important reason."

Washington data are broadly consistent with the San Antonio data: people participate in time-consuming watershed processes primarily to improve water quality and other conditions in the watershed. Participating to improve human and social capital is of distinctly secondary importance.

Our observations about representation and participation suggest that recruiting a diverse population of stakeholders is an important challenge for collaborative institutions. However, meeting the challenge of inclusiveness appears to contain positive returns for collaborative institutions. In the NEP study reported in chapter 7, stakeholders preferring inclusive processes are more likely to view policymaking as fair and are more accepting of alternative views. This movement away from uncompromising allegiance to core beliefs to a willingness to consider new information and other points of view was found to be a significant motivation toward the discovery and adoption of mutually beneficial outcomes and was not found in watershed contexts in which collaborative partnerships had not formed. Hence, despite the costs and difficulties, inclusive participation seems to enhance the likelihood of cooperation and also has important implications for procedural legitimacy, which we will discuss shortly.

This discussion of the process and context elements of our framework indicates that the elements we identified as important and the relationships we posited in the framework in chapter 1 are empirically validated. Context and process do relate to participation. We will see more of the path of these relationships and their impact on other framework elements in the following discussions.

Civic Community

The civic community part of our framework represents the basic human dimensions that relate to the success or failure of collaborative processes. *Civic community* is a term we borrow from Putnam, Leonardi, and Raffaella (1993). It refers to a "republican"—as opposed to "liberal" (Madisonian)—theory of successful self-governance stressing the importance of concern with the common welfare, active engagement in community associations and affairs, tolerance of opposing views, generalized trust in others, and relatively egalitarian relationships. This contrasts with the liberal Madisonian view that people's commitment to self-interest will create conflict, and the job of government is to create formal institutions for conflict resolution. We posited six aspects of civic community in our basic framework that we looked at empirically in our investigations:

Human capital. This includes such characteristics as education and intelligence, which increase the capability of actors to accomplish a wide variety of tasks. Low human capital limits the ability of any society to accomplish very much. In particular, education is linked to many forms of political participation, particularly those dealing with complex issues like environmental quality and macroeconomic performance. It is also linked with trust and with several measures of social capital (Putnam 2000).

Social capital. This refers to norms and beliefs that increase the capabilities of groups of actors to achieve collective tasks. Following Putnam (1993, 2000), we conceive of social capital as comprising the density and breadth of social networks and norms of reciprocity, that is, norms encouraging the exchange of favors over time. We put Putnam's third aspect of social capital, trust, into its own category.

Trust. As defined in chapter 8, trust is the confidence that A has in B to act in a trustworthy fashion. It has three components: (1) the willingness and ability to keep promises and agreements, (2) a sincere effort to understand the other person's interests and to take them into account when making decisions, and (3) a willingness to reciprocate acts of goodwill or generosity in the relatively near future. One can also distinguish between generalized trust (trust in categories of people), and specialized trust (trust in specific persons). When I do not lock my door at night, I am exhibiting generalized trust. When I give my neighbor a key to my locked house, I am exhibiting specialized trust in that neighbor. Trust can vary across categories of actors. For example, chapter 4 makes a major distinction between trust in governmental officials and trust in nongovernmental stakeholders. Chapter 4 adds the idea of risk acceptability to the concept of trust, manifested in the willingness of stakeholders to defer to the discretion and competence of others to manage risks on their behalf.

Political efficacy. This is the confidence that a person has in his or her ability to influence governmental decisions. If it is low, then a critical component of effective democratic systems is missing (Verba and Nie 1972; Verba, Schlozman, and Brady 1995).

Collective action beliefs. As explained in chapter 7, these are beliefs about the nature of watershed problems (severity, diffuseness, uncertainty) and institutional performance (likelihood of conflict resolution, perceived fairness) that affect stakeholders' willingness to engage in cooperative, collaborative negotiations.

Legitimacy. Chapter 3 discusses legitimacy as a normative requirement that refers to the moral acceptability of a particular policy institution. An institution that is perceived as legitimate is more likely to survive and the other components of our dynamic framework contribute to perceived legitimacy.

In this section, we first examine our findings regarding the effect of trust on willingness to participate in collaborative processes. Second, we review the record on the contextual and process-related factors affecting trust and social capital. Third, we use trust as an explanatory variable to account for variation in policy outputs and outcomes. Finally, we briefly summarize the findings from chapter 7 on collective action beliefs. We discuss legitimacy in more detail in the next section.

The main lesson from our research is that the relationship between trust and participation is considerably more complex than generally recognized. Most of the traditional political science literature assumes that preexisting levels of trust are positively associated with political participation (see the discussion of trust in chapter 5). The argument is that trust embodies diffuse support for the political system. This leads to higher levels of voting and willingness to appeal to political authorities (on the grounds that public officials would at least listen attentively). More recent research shows no relationship between declining political trust and declining voter turnout (Hetherington 1999). There is also an argument from institutional rational choice theory and transaction cost economics that there should be a negative relationship between trust and willingness to engage in policy negotiations that are relatively time-consuming. If people trust governmental officials and other stakeholders, there is no need to bear the costs of participating in negotiations. But, if one distrusts governmental officials and other stakeholders, there is a strong incentive to become involved in negotiations to protect one's interests.

Chapter 5 found no relationship in a random sample of citizens between trust and their willingness to say they would participate in collaborative processes. However, the theory and data presented in chapter 4 on the Illinois River strongly support the hypothesis for a negative relationship between trust and willingness to engage in a time-consuming collaborative process. In fact, the highest participation came from people who perceived their vital interests to be at stake and distrusted both governmental officials and other stakeholders to protect those interests. Participation declined if either the stakes were lower or they trusted one of the groups of participants.

Data from the seventy-six-case Watershed Partnership Project presented in table 9.1 present a somewhat more nuanced understanding (Sabatier, Quinn, and Leach 2002). They suggest that joining the partnership to protect one's interests and prevent the partnership from agreeing to undesirable policy initiatives was particularly prevalent among resource users (who were many of the actors in the Illinois River study). It was much less prevalent among agency officials, environmentalists, consultants, and Native Americans. They viewed the partnership in a more favorable light as a place to advance organizational interests or educate themselves about watershed issues.

Two separate chapters derive compatible conclusions about the effect of contextual and process-related variables on building trust and social capital in collaborative processes. First, chapter 7 indicates that levels of trust were higher among stakeholders in the NEP than among comparable stakeholders in estuaries without the program. Furthermore, NEP stakeholders are less likely to use their preexisting ideological beliefs regarding environmentalism and property rights to guide their perceptions of the trustworthiness of others. This suggests that participants in collaborative partnerships are much more likely to trust people with different values than in watersheds locked in the traditional adversarial mode of environmental policymaking.

Second, data from the Watershed Partnership Project in chapter 8 (table 8.3) indicate the most important variables explaining both trust and new social and human capital (i.e., new knowledge and friendships resulting from participation in the partnership) are a widespread perception that "the process treats all parties fairly and consistently." The most important contextual factors vary, with the availability of alternative venues having a strong negative effect on trust, while the availability of good scientific information has a positive effect on human and social capital. Surprisingly, preexisting social capital (measured as the number of organizations to which people belong) was not significantly related to either trust or new social capital. Likewise, ideological conflict among partnership members was not related to the development of either trust or social capital. In general, these results confirm one of the basic assumptions of the literature on alternative dispute resolution: collaborative processes that give members a sense of fair treatment can create considerable trust and new social and human capital, regardless of the amount of preexisting social capital or ideological conflict in a community. On the other hand, another ADR variable—the presence of a trained facilitator—seems to have no effect on trust, once age and other contextual variables are taken into account (Leach and Sabatier 2003; see also chapter 8, note 9).

The relationship between trust and policy outputs and outcomes is also complex. Chapter 8, dealing with the seventy-six watershed partnerships in California and Washington, examines the relationship between various independent variables and three dependent variables (two output and one outcome related): (1) extent of agreement on partnership policies and goals, (2) index measuring the number and efficacy of on-the-ground restoration and implementation projects, and (3) participants' perceptions of the effectiveness of the partnership for solving twelve types of watershed problems. The main purpose of these analyses was to test the significance of the causal arrows between the civic community box and the policy outputs box in figure 1.1 in chapter 1 (our general model).

First, the analysis looks at the unidirectional effect of trust on all three of the dependent variables, controlling for a variety of other contextual and process-related variables. Table 8.3 in chapter 8 indicates that trust has a very strong positive relationship on both extent of agreement and perceived impacts but no effect on implementation projects. Curiously, however, the effect of trust on extent of agreement holds only for partnerships over three years old. For younger partnerships, there is a negative relationship between level of trust and level of agreement. One possible explanation for this surprising finding is that in young partnerships, judgments about trust are relatively uncertain and thus unrelated to level of agreement reached. Yet some young partnerships, particularly those subjected to severe flooding, must reach agreement very quickly. The number of these "must do something soon" situations was large enough to establish a negative relationship between trust and level of agreement in young partnerships. In older partnerships, when members have good knowledge concerning who is trustworthy and who is not, the expected positive relationship between level of trust and level of agreement holds.

Second, consistent with the flows in figure 1.1, we look at the reciprocal effects of agreements, restoration projects, and perceived impacts on trust. The argument is that just as trust should make the partnership successful, so those successes should increase trust among partnership members. The model results (see tables 8.5 through 8.7) show no statistical evidence of a reciprocal relationship between trust and level of agreement, restoration projects, or perceived impacts. Thus, the reciprocal arrow represented in the framework in chapter 1 between policy outputs (agreements and restoration projects) and civic community (as represented by trust) should be deleted. However, as we will see in the discussion of legitimacy, the reciprocal relationship between policy outputs and legitimacy does hold. This will lead us to modify the framework (these changes will be noted in the section on legitimacy). Note, however, that this lack of reciprocal relationship between policy outputs and trust pertains only to relatively large-scale differences in the extent of agreement—the difference between agreeing to general principles and agreeing to a comprehensive management plan.[1] It does not address the contention in the ADR literature that small accomplishments, such as sponsoring a creek walk or clean-up day, may produce some initial trust in young partnerships with high degrees of initial distrust. We simply do not have the data to test that specific hypothesis.

Finally, chapter 7's study on the NEP shows that trust is not the only aspect of civic community that appears to be improved by collaborative processes. The NEP also affects collective action beliefs, an important part of civic community because stakeholders use key beliefs about the estuary action arena as a basis for decisions about cooperation. NEP stakeholders believe problems are more diffuse, scientific information is better, conflict resolution more likely, decision making fairer, and special interests less dominant. Interestingly, the positive effects of the NEP on fairness and perceptions of interest domination are stronger among stakeholders committed to environmental values.

As posited in our framework in chapter 1, collaborative processes have important connections to civic community and the culture of cooperation in a watershed. On the one hand, the story is simple: collaborative processes appear to enhance civic community by building trust and changing collective action beliefs, and, in turn, trust and collective action beliefs affect outputs and outcomes. On the other hand, our analyses reveal that the simple story is not quite complete. Trust operates differently in different contexts, especially in young partnerships where norms of trust have not yet developed. The effect of collaborative processes on trust and other collective action beliefs depends on the core values of individual stakeholders. The positive relationship between trust, participation, and cooperation cannot be taken for granted.

Output and Outcome Effectiveness

As previously noted in the discussion of reasons for participating in collaborative watershed processes, data from both San Antonio (chapter 5) and the West Coast watershed partnerships (chapter 8; table 9.1) clearly indicate that people participate in collaborative partnerships for two primary reasons: (1) to improve ecological and/or socioeconomic conditions in the watershed, viewing the partnership as a means to those objectives and/or (2) to protect themselves by making sure the partnership does not do something to harm their basic interests.

In either case, they are primarily interested in policy outputs from the collaborative process (whether those take the form of general management plans or specific on-the-ground projects) because these are seen as essential contributors to policy outcomes, (e.g., improvement in water quality, unemployment rates, or open space). Civic community variables are important *indirectly* because they serve as means to better policy outputs and outcomes. In the terms of chapter 3, substantive legitimacy appears to be the critical reason people take the time to participate in collaborative processes and will probably be the principal criterion by which they judge the worth of such processes.

Unfortunately, at present it is virtually impossible to measure whether the policy outputs of a collaborative process discernibly affected a policy objective, such as water quality. To ascertain real-world impacts, one must first have good monitoring data for several years before the project and then for several years following implementation. But this is not sufficient. Even if the monitoring shows that water quality improved after the project, this does not necessarily mean that the project was responsible for the improvement. Improvement could instead be a function of changes in precipitation or upstream practices, such as the closing of a mine or the fencing of a stream. To actually ascertain the impact of a partnership project on water quality, one needs pre- and postproject data for the specific watershed and upstream watersheds, as well as a few other comparable watersheds. Given limited funding and personnel, this is a herculean task for most watershed collaboratives.[2]

Faced with substantial obstacles to ascertaining real-world impacts, researchers have fallen back on measuring policy outputs and perceived impacts. In fact, in multicase quantitative studies, even the measurement of policy outputs (such as management plans and restoration projects) is rather rare. In the four empirical studies in this book, for example, only the study of West Coast watershed partnerships (chapter 8) did so. The San Antonio (chapter 5) and Illinois River (chapter 4) cases did not, in large part because they were primarily interested in participation issues. The study of NEPs in chapter 7 did not measure policy outputs, partly because of the difficulties of systematically coding the NEP management plans. Chapter 7 did, however, measure the changes in collective action beliefs (including satisfaction with the planning process) that are assumed to be related to success. Chapter 8 measured both policy outputs (management plans and restoration projects) and perceived impacts of the West Coast partnerships on twelve potential watershed problems. As we shall see shortly, however, data on perceived impacts may be subject to systematic measurement error.

The Watershed Partnership Project provides the most substantial data on effectiveness. Figure 9.1 indicates that the number of activities increases substantially over time and that partnerships found it easier to agree on, and implement, specific projects than they did to agree on a comprehensive management plan (Leach, Pelkey, and Sabatier 2002). For example, whereas 68 percent of the partnerships agreed on one or more projects and 59 percent implemented at least one of them, only 25 percent of partnerships agreed on a comprehensive management plan. For partnerships over six years old, 100 percent had agreed on a project, 90 percent implemented at least one, and about 53 percent agreed on a comprehensive management plan. Apparently, partnerships find it easier to agree on a specific restoration project than to agree on a plan. One potential explanation for this finding is that resolution of value conflict

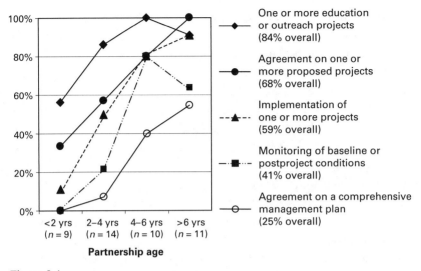

Figure 9.1
Proportion of partnerships with agreements, restoration projects, monitoring, and education. *Source:* Leach, Pelkey and Sabatier (2002, 664).

is difficult in the context of a plan, which in some sense represents an informal contract among watershed stakeholders. Spending money on a limited duration restoration project may involve less negotiation. In addition, there is anecdotal evidence that many partnership participants tire of "talking all the time" and want to "go out and do something." This seems to be particularly the case for resource users, who want to demonstrate their contribution to solving watershed problems but are reluctant to take time from their businesses to attend seemingly endless meetings.

As for the context and process variables affecting policy outputs, Table 8.3 in chapter 8 reveals that the level of agreement reached in watershed partnerships is a function of a couple of context-related variables, including a perceived watershed crisis and preexisting norms of reciprocity, the age of the partnerships and two process variables, the extent of trust, and having organizational representatives with the authority to negotiate. Surprisingly, the level of ideological conflict among partnerships' members did not affect the level of agreement (see chapter 8, note 9). For implementation projects, the only important variables were partnership age and the amount of grant funding. Therefore, the relational links we posited in the original model between context and process, civic community and policy outputs, remain robust.

Turning to perceived impacts, the data from the study of West Coast partnerships in Tables 8.3 and 8.6 show that by far the most important factor affecting participants' evaluation of perceived impacts was the level of trust in the partnership (positive and very significant). Of less importance was the extent of restoration projects (positive and significant). The very strong relationship between trust and perceived impacts suggests that a halo effect may be at work—a positive evaluation of interpersonal relationships within the partnership leads to perceptions that the partnership has positive impacts on ecological and socioeconomics problems within the watershed. Trust has a positive effect on extent of agreement, extent of agreement has a positive relationship with restoration projects, and restoration projects have a positive relationship with perceived impacts. So there is a logical path from trust to perceived impacts. But the magnitude of the relationship between trust and perceived impacts suggests that perceived impacts are rather heavily mediated by a trust filter. This, in turn, suggests that studies relying exclusively on perceived impacts, rather than policy outputs or actual impacts, should be treated with considerable caution.

In general, then, there is no holy grail theoretical framework that explains variation in partnership outputs. While each of these frameworks emphasizes trust, none of them predicts the complicated relationships found in chapter 8, where trust is positively associated with level of agreement in older partnerships but negatively associated with agreement in younger partnerships. Overall, one of the best predictors of both grants and restoration projects was simply the age of the partnership. Doing anything important in diverse partnerships takes time. The ACF's emphasis on "devil shift," however, views this as more difficult than either social capital or institutional rational choice. Clearly, partnership processes are quite complex, and additional research and new conceptualizations are needed, with the goal of creating a synthetic theoretical approach.

Legitimacy

One of the central themes throughout this book is the contribution of stakeholder participation to the legitimacy of collaborative watershed management. In this section, we summarize how our findings from each of the four themes surveyed above (process and context, participation, civic community, and effectiveness) advance the understanding of legitimacy.

In chapter 3, we argue that legitimacy must be understood as a twofold normative requirement, expressed by both procedural and substantive criteria. The former are based on the fundamental value of autonomy, or self-rule, and hold that those bound by watershed policy must have a voice in formulating it. The latter are based on the fundamental values of welfare and justice and hold that watershed policy outcomes must improve the conditions of life for watershed stakeholders and the costs and benefits of bringing about these improvements must be distributed fairly. We are now in a position to make some broad observations about how well watershed collaborations meet or fail these criteria. Just as important, we must now also assess the criteria themselves, by considering whether they represent reasonable normative expectations for watershed policy.

With respect to procedural legitimacy, we note that collaborative institutions display a wide range of structures. There is no one standard process for incorporating stakeholder participation; rather, many processes adapted to the specific circumstances of the given watershed's context. Nonetheless, most collaborative processes pursue inclusive representation and rely on the consent of their members for decision making and compliance. While not all attempts at inclusiveness succeed, as shown in chapter 5 (we return to this point later), the survey results in chapters 7 and 8 provide some evidence that involvement in collaborative institutions does satisfy many of the participants' own concerns regarding procedural fairness.

The data collected from seventy-six collaborations in Washington and California, discussed in chapter 8, yield two relevant results. First, a clear majority of nearly 1,500 stakeholders surveyed agreed that their partnership treated all parties fairly and consistently. Second, a very strong majority approved of the consensus decision-making process. We interpret these responses to indicate that in general, stakeholders are satisfied that their views are duly considered in policy deliberations and that no policy is approved without their consent. Further, the study of NEP partnerships discussed in chapter 7 also suggests that participation in an NEP partnership increases participants' belief in the fairness of decision making. Again, we take this result to mean that the stakeholders believe in the legitimacy of the procedures through which they participate.

Chapter 5, however, suggests that collaborative institutions have a more difficult time meeting the requirement of representativeness and risk excluding important classes of stakeholders. Although there is a significant Hispanic population, and despite intensive efforts on the part of the organizers, the watershed councils in San Antonio had a disproportionately small number of Hispanic participants. Given that Hispanics comprise a significant segment of the broad stakeholder population for the San Antonio watersheds, the legitimacy of policy made by institutions lacking appropriate Hispanic participation is clouded. Even if those institutions function fairly for those who participate, the absence of participants from a segment of the full stakeholder population means that segment's autonomy is diminished. It seems less appropriate to claim that the full stakeholder community has acted autonomously. Exclusion may have negative consequences for effectiveness if the excluded group has a major influence on watershed resources or Hispanics are excluded from a government agency with a great deal of policymaking authority.

It does not follow, however, that the San Antonio councils were illegitimate. In other respects, the San Antonio councils meet standards of representativeness, as well as other procedural criteria. It is obviously crucial here that the organizers of the San Antonio councils made many efforts to cultivate Hispanic participation; the absence of Hispanics was not due to calculated efforts to exclude them. As we noted in chapter 3, legitimacy is a matter of degree. Thus, the results of chapter 5 do not show that the work of the San Antonio councils ought to be rejected; rather, they point to possible improvements.

Generalizing from the San Antonio case, we observe that as in other domains of social life, it could be very difficult to cultivate full participation among groups excluded from political power in the past. The transaction costs of soliciting participation can be very high, and reasonable people may disagree as to whether a point is reached at which the costs are no longer worth the benefits they obtain. It is entirely possible that good-faith efforts at full representation may fall short of the normative standard. In some cases, resource constraints may force trade-offs between the various criteria of legitimacy we have discussed. How such trade-offs should be struck cannot be determined in advance by broad normative principles; they must be made in the light of detailed under-standing of the particular circumstance at hand. Furthermore, some classes of stakeholders may not participate because they do not value the resource in question. The criterion of representativeness certainly does not suggest coerced participation. The reasonableness of our criteria rests in the fact that they accept good-faith efforts that fall short of com-plete success.

Let us now consider substantive legitimacy. Assessing the substantive legitimacy of a policy involves evaluating the actual outcome of the pol-icy to determine whether it resulted in a positive change in the welfare of stakeholders. The primary substantive goal of watershed policy is to im-prove water quality and other related environmental and socioeconomic conditions. But as shown in chapter 3, environmental improvements represent necessary but not sufficient conditions for legitimacy. We dis-cussed at length the social requirement that the costs and benefits associ-ated with welfare gains due to environmental improvements must be distributed fairly. Moreover, we noted that an important benefit of col-laborative efforts is the increase in trust among participants, which in general fosters a culture of cooperation. These can contribute to environ-mental improvements by increased rates of compliance with watershed policy, but they also have some value in and of themselves.

As noted in the previous section, the stark reality is that we have very few data on which to base a judgment of whether watershed collabora-tions improve watersheds. In addition to the monitoring problems dis-cussed earlier, there are compelling explanations for this lack of data. Foremost, the time frames for noting significant change are often far longer than the life spans of the collaborations studied. Studied within the context of their operating life spans, we note that collaborations take several years to become effective generators of policy proposals. Thus, for many collaboratives, sufficient time has not yet passed for their pro-posals to work a measurable change in natural conditions. Next, water-shed systems are extremely complex and subject to numerous influences beyond the activities of policymaking partnerships. This complexity con-tributes to the profound difficulty in collecting data demonstrating the actual effects of watershed policy. Finally, the data collected on water-shed health are notoriously fragmented spatially and temporally, due to lack of an overarching vision for water quality improvement and the tendency of monitoring regimes to respond to political and ecological emergencies.

In the face of uncertainty about the ultimate efficacy of watershed collaborations, it might seem that our criteria of substantive legitimacy are empty. How meaningful is that goal if we can never know if we are making progress toward it? If we are uncertain whether welfare has improved in a watershed, how will we tell if the costs and benefits stakeholders experience are fairly distributed? Although the difficulties in this endeavor are quite considerable (e.g., no standard formats with which to establish comprehensive baselines), we regard it as worth undertaking. To hold otherwise in effect dismisses the relevance of environmental and socioeconomic improvement as a criterion of legitimacy. It says that it simply does not matter what the long-term effects of watershed collaborations might be. However, this flies in the face of the very strong intuition, shared by many collaborative participants, that the point of policymaking is to produce positive effects. Indeed, one reason people abandon collaborations is precisely that they regard them as ineffective; what justifies a collaborative effort for most individuals are the welfare gains that it will accomplish.

Ultimately, then, the substantive legitimacy of watershed collaborations will be established by long-term studies of environmental and socioeconomic changes brought about in their watersheds. What about the shorter term? As suggested in the previous section, stakeholder perceptions of changes in the watershed may be used as a surrogate for data on actual changes in evaluations of substantive legitimacy. Recall that chapters 7 and 8 showed that participants in watershed partnerships successful at producing and implementing policies tend to regard themselves as successful at bringing about positive changes in the physical conditions of the watershed.

We conclude this section with two brief comments on why these data on perceived changes are germane to considerations of substantive legitimacy. First, as chapter 8 shows, perceived changes in a watershed are strongly correlated with social factors such as social capital and trust. It follows that whatever their value as indicators about the actual environmental condition of the watershed, perceptions of improvement suggest an improvement in the social environment within which the given watershed partnership operates.

Improvements in social capital and trust are intrinsically valuable. While they are not the immediate goals of watershed policy as such, they are nonetheless important benefits. As long as they do not mislead stakeholders into thinking the watershed is in better condition than it in fact is—the halo effect—they provide an additional justification for collaborative institutions.

Second, to the extent that we seek to justify watershed collaborations on the basis of environmental changes to the watershed, perceptions might simply be the best evidence we have. Of course, perceptions not grounded in some systematic observation may not be reliable. However, typically the parties whose perceptions are polled are familiar with their watershed and have a formal or informal background, making their perceptions more or less well informed. Thus, it is reasonable to treat their input as at least provisional data on watershed conditions.

To summarize, our case studies lend support to the broad claim that collaborative institutions and their policy outputs and perceived watershed outcomes contribute to the legitimacy of watershed policy-making, along both procedural and substantive dimensions. Because of the unique relationship between legitimacy criteria and these elements of our model, as distinct from the relationship identified for other elements of the civic community segment (such as trust), we find that we need to move legitimacy out of the civic community box and create its own independent model element. This revised model and the specified relationships between legitimacy and collaborative processes, policy outputs, and watershed outcomes are presented in figure 9.2.

The findings of our cases indicate that legitimacy has a reciprocal relationship with other civic community elements and collaborative processes, and that legitimacy is affected by policy outputs and watershed outcomes.

Survival

In our framework in chapter 1, we indicated that survival is related to both the processes used to operate watershed collaborations and the outcomes produced from those deliberations. The earlier discussion of the long-term effectiveness and legitimacy of collaborative institutions leads naturally to the question of their survival. What factors affect

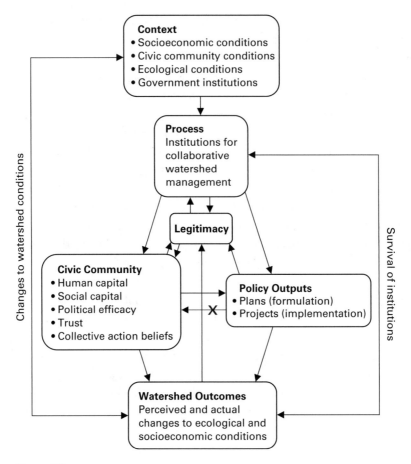

Figure 9.2
A dynamic framework for watershed management: revised

the prospects of collaborations continuing to function over time? Is the survival of collaborations a worthy goal? We conclude our survey of the implications of our research for the six main themes of this book by examining the issue of the survival of collaborative institutions.

Before examining conditions for the survival of watershed collaborations, however, we first ask whether that is indeed a worthwhile goal. To the extent that, as chapters 7 and 8 suggest, collaborative institutions foster social capital, the initial answer to that question might well be yes. In a democratic society, additional democratic institutions, especially ones that encourage deliberation and consensus building, certainly contain inherent value. Survival is also desirable because a robust, adaptive institution can respond to emerging problems in a particular watershed—problems that are bound to occur as humans use watershed resources. Further reflection complicates this immediate response, however.

In cases where watershed problems are of limited duration or where the problems can be handled by the routines of existing institutions, it is difficult and perhaps unnecessary to maintain strong stakeholder involvement. This commonsense belief derives strong support from the theory and empirical results presented in chapter 4. There we saw that the greater the trust stakeholders have in each other and in government officials, the less they seek intensive participation in policymaking. The main lesson of chapter 4 is that intensive participation is required only in contexts marked by high stakes and low trust. Hence, where existing institutions are trusted to handle watershed problems, the creation of a collaborative institution might not be necessary.

Arguments that the survival of collaborative institutions as a form of social organization is the ultimate goal must consider whether collaborations actually solve watershed problems. As observed, the jury is still out on whether collaborative institutions do in fact improve the environmental conditions of their watersheds. The question of survival thus becomes, Under what circumstances will watershed collaboratives survive long enough to have a reasonable chance of improving watershed conditions?

We confidently conclude that survival in this sense is a function of both procedural and substantive legitimacy. We hypothesize that collaborative institutions meeting the criteria of procedural and substantive legitimacy are more likely to survive.

Because most watershed collaborations are relatively young, the studies examined in this book provide more evidence about procedural legitimacy. For example, stakeholders are more satisfied with collaborative institutions that treat them fairly and successfully create social capital. One reasonably supposes that if norms of procedural legitimacy continue to be met, stakeholders will continue to participate. Continued participation and satisfaction will lead to continued political demand, which is the main way to keep resources flowing toward the collaborative institutions. Thus, procedural legitimacy is a determinant of the survival of collaborative institutions.

What about substantive legitimacy? As chapter 5 and table 9.1 indicate, many stakeholders claim the main reason they participate is to protect watershed resources. As we have noted, there seems to be a halo effect generated by procedural legitimacy: if participants are satisfied with the way their collaborations operate, they tend to think their efforts are effective at solving watershed problems. That is, procedural legitimacy tends to generate perceptions of substantive legitimacy. In turn, we suppose, perceptions of effectiveness will motivate continued participation: stakeholders who see themselves as making progress will likely keep working to accomplish more. The contrary seems also to be true: participants regarding their efforts as ineffective are likely to withdraw from collaborations. In sum, both dimensions of legitimacy, in interrelated ways, contribute to the survival of watershed collaborations, at least in the short or medium term. We did not draw a line in our revised model directly connecting legitimacy with survival, but the two are clearly related in the model through the other linkages they share.

However, the long-term survival of watershed collaborations is subject to significant risk due to the halo effect. This phenomenon will at least keep collaborative institutions running in the face of uncertainty. But sooner or later, participants' perceptions of watershed improvement will face the test posed by actual water quality data. If these data do not show significant improvement (i.e., improvement commensurate with the significant efforts participants invest in their collaborations), it is likely that the resulting disappointment will impede continued participation. In more formal terms, poor water quality improvements are likely to be worth less than the transaction costs required to obtain them and participants will begin to withdraw from collaboration. In the light of difficulties in assessing effectiveness already discussed, it is probable that actual water quality data taken in the initial years of collaboration will indeed prove disappointing.

Uncertainty about actual outcomes is thus like the downstream current against which watershed collaborations must swim. Because it can disincline participants from engaging in collaborations, uncertainty might, ironically, prevent collaborations from continuing long enough for participants to see that their efforts are in fact worthwhile. Conversely, there is a risk that the halo effect will keep collaborative institutions going even when they are not improving watershed conditions. Surviving in spite of this uncertainty is not the least of the challenges watershed collaborations must face.

As we noted, Figure 9.2 displays the revised diagram of our dynamic framework for watershed management. In the spirit of a second generation of scholarship on watershed management, we tested many of the causal pathways in the framework, and our tests provide confirming evidence for many of the hypotheses. The major revisions in the model are the deletion of the arrow between policy outputs and civic community, the creation of a new box for legitimacy, and the identification of the relationship of the other model variables to it. However, our studies have only begun putting the flesh on the bones of this diagram. Further research is needed to fully understand these relationships. Nevertheless, we believe that enough progress has been made to provide some concrete policy recommendations, a task we take up in the next section.

Implications and Recommendations for Practitioners

Throughout the book, we have identified implications of our research for practitioners and made recommendations for guiding and improving stakeholder involvement in collaborative approaches to watershed management. While each chapter tells its own story, the lessons collectively learned through a couple of decades of experience with stakeholder participation are becoming clear. The rest of this section outlines an emerging collection of practitioner guidelines (summarized in table 9.2). These are not prescriptions but rather rules of thumb for structuring collaborative approaches to watershed management.

The collaborative approach to watershed management is not a magic bullet that addresses all situations at all times or that will even be appropriate most of the time. We demonstrated in chapters 5, 7, and 8 the challenges of implementing legitimate collaborative approaches to watershed management. Collaborative institutions are expensive to implement and maintain and often are extremely time-consuming, requiring as long as four years to achieve effectiveness. As indicated in chapter 4, we recommend that the collaborative approach to watershed management

Table 9.2
Guidelines for practitioners in collaborative approaches to watershed management

---

Collaborative approaches are not a magic bullet and should be used only when appropriate.

The collaborative approach to watershed management should be designed to foster trust and a culture of cooperation, and decrease knowledge uncertainty through analysis and deliberation.

Once engaged, the collaborative approach to watershed management must be maintained until the decision process plays through.

Practitioners should design and manage the collaborative structures and processes to avoid escalating conflicts to other venues.

Recruit, accept, and assign stakeholders who believe in the process of collaboration.

The watershed collaborative must be perceived as representative of the stakeholders for it to be legitimate.

Do not be afraid of intense ideological conflict.

Engage applied researchers with procedural and scientific expertise in the watershed collaboration process.

---

be used as a method for resolving environmental and socioeconomic problems only when there are high stakes, high social distrust, high governmental distrust, and high knowledge uncertainty. Collaborative approaches are particularly useful for addressing issues that perplex command-and-control institutions, such as nonpoint source pollution and habitat destruction. Collaborative approaches are probably not justified when existing institutions are already adequate. If the context of the watershed conflict justifies using a collaborative approach, this approach must be implemented with due care and preparation.

The collaborative approach to watershed management should be designed to foster trust and a culture of cooperation and decrease knowledge uncertainty through analysis and deliberation (Stern, Fineberg, and NRC Committee 1996). Many methods exist for building trust among stakeholders, as described in chapter 4. We presented a method for stakeholder involvement incorporating collaborative learning techniques into an analysis and deliberation framework in chapter 5. This method, based on principles of collaborative learning described by Daniels and Walker (2001), seeks to move participants away from positional strategies and toward the identification of mutual interests and joint gains from collaboration. Outside facilitators and technical experts may be important in this process, but the data from chapter 8 (which included a variety of control variables) indicate that the relationships among facilitators, scientists, trust, and policy outputs are quite complex.

Regardless of the methods selected for building trust and difficulties encountered while implementing them, the collaborative approach to watershed management should be maintained until the decision process plays through. This may take as long as four to six years, since time is necessary for advocacy coalitions within the collaborative to reach agreements and implement projects. Along the way, collaborative institutions should measure progress and note milestones along the social and environmental outcomes they purport to advocate. Early indicators of success, such as pilot projects, are often assumed to be the stepping-stones for building a successful partnership in the long run. However, as discussed earlier and in chapters 7 and 8, measurements of success based on civic community outcomes and policy outputs should not be substitutes for measurements of actual environmental and socioeconomic outcomes.

Practitioners should design and manage collaborative structures and processes to avoid escalating conflicts to other venues, such as a federal court–mandated and –managed TMDL process. As we saw in chapter 8, threats to switch to other venues inhibit the development of trust, which is a critical factor in reaching agreements. Resorting to coercive regulatory or judicial tools may destroy a collaborative process, especially when the collaborative process involves stakeholders who fear increased regulation. Many times these stakeholders prefer to pursue environmental goals through voluntary action and participate in collaborative institutions. For example, habitat conservation planning under the Endangered Species Act can be designed as a collaborative institution and offer an alternative to the traditional recovery plan process. However, if collaborative processes appear to fail in a particular watershed or are used by stakeholders to avoid environmental improvements, then the traditional regulatory tools should be considered. There is also evidence from the Watershed Partnership Project (Leach 2000) and elsewhere (Born and Genskow 2001) that the threat of a regulatory hammer may induce stakeholders to negotiate more seriously.

Try to assign, recruit, and accept people who believe in the process of collaboration. In most complex watershed management scenarios, no single individual or interest group prevails completely. Participants should be willing to employ reciprocal strategies (e.g., tit-for-tat) and to accept compromises; therefore, try to choose participants who believe in cooperation and bargaining. Choose people likely to use new information learned in the collaborative process to update their beliefs about appropriate policies rather than simply stick to their preconceived notions. Substantial evidence from the NEP discussed in chapter 7 suggests that this actually happens.

Organizers and facilitators of watershed institutions should not be afraid of intense ideological conflict. In fact, if the proper strategies are employed to guide the conflict toward increasing peer understanding of the sources of the conflict, this intensity can ensure continued participation in the collaborative process. As indicated in chapter 4, stakeholders will not participate in a lengthy, inconvenient collaborative process unless they perceive a threat to their interests. However, the collaborative process selected for the stakeholders must be appropriate for the type and degree of conflict. Do not expect stakeholders to change deeply held core beliefs over the course of the collaborative process. Instead, design the collaborative process to develop understanding of the sources of the positions held by conflicting parties and attempt to create policies addressing multiple concerns. Trust does not require agreement, but it does require understanding. As noted in chapters 7 and 8, collaborative institutions allow people to muddle through; they may agree on policies and mechanisms for resolving conflicts without changing fundamental normative beliefs.

One important aspect of resolving disagreement between competing ideologies is a clear understanding of the watershed problems at hand. To enhance the probability of achieving substantive legitimacy, facilitators of collaborative institutions should engage applied researchers with expertise about specific watershed problems. These researchers can provide credibility to defining the scope of knowledge applicable to a watershed management issue. They can provide insight into the state of knowledge on issues of high uncertainty. They can also provide analysis of new and existing data provided by stakeholders in the watershed collaborative.

The final recommendation for practitioners is to remember the first recommendation: collaborative approaches to watershed management are difficult, context-specific solutions to difficult, complex watershed problems. There is no simple prescription for forming, implementing, or managing a watershed collaborative. Like the salmon swimming upstream, collaborative approaches to watershed management expend huge resources, and they are time-consuming, risky, and difficult. If necessary, and if implemented correctly, collaborative watershed management can be as important to the preservation of our water resources as swimming upstream is to the preservation of anadromous species of fish.

Implications and Recommendations for Researchers

It should be clear at this point that there is still much to be learned about engaging stakeholders in collaborative approaches to watershed management. Scientists and policy experts, working with local, state, and federal agencies, have devoted a great many resources to improving our understanding of these complex processes. In the course of reviewing the relevant literature and conducting our research on collaborative processes, however, we identified several areas of critical need for research to advance the understanding of collaborative processes. Our recommendations for future research focus areas are summarized in table 9.3 and described in this section.

Table 9.3
Recommendations for researchers in collaborative approaches to watershed management

There must be more large-sample-size, comparative studies of multiple collaborative institutions.
Researchers should measure substantive outputs and outcomes, not just process outcomes.
Longitudinal studies should be designed that are large enough to be multivariate.
Use of control groups should be encouraged in these studies.
Research should address the challenges of measurement to enhance the confidence of analysis.
Research is needed to relate outcomes (real and perceived) to group survival.

Most research studies to date have been anecdotal reporting of activities associated with collaborative decision-making processes. We clearly need to conduct more large-scale studies of multiple collaborative activities if we are to enhance our understanding of the complexity of interacting variables in affecting outcomes. For example, Leach and Sabatier (2003) present data demonstrating that in bivariate analyses, facilitator effectiveness correlates positively with agreements reached and restoration projects. When contextual and process-related variables are added to the analysis, however, the relationship disappears or becomes negative. The emphasis in much of the social, political, and policy sciences literature is on collaborative processes, rather than substantive outputs and outcomes as indicators of effectiveness of the collaborative process. Longitudinal studies, covering full life cycles of collaborative institutions, should be performed on sufficiently large groups of institutions to support multivariate analysis. If the unit of analysis (as in chapter 8) in the research is the collaborative institution as a whole, as many as one hundred sites may be appropriate. If the unit of analysis is the individual stakeholder, then fewer sites might be appropriate if each collaborative institution is conceptualized as an experimental treatment and the institutions are carefully chosen to vary along important theoretical dimensions (e.g., the type of collective choice process used by the institution).

The paucity of studies in the academic literature dealing with collaborative processes incorporating any sort of control, even temporal, was disturbing. We recommend that control groups like those used in chapter 7 be integral to any experimental design in analyzing the effectiveness of collaborative approaches to watershed management. Temporal control groups (before and after intervention) have the advantage of reducing variability between measurement activities. Spatial control groups like neighboring watersheds provide an important comparative perspective. However, because these are necessarily quasi-experimental designs, one must be careful that the observed outcomes are truly a product of the collaborative institutions, and not that collaborative institutions appear in a place only where outcomes are already heading in a particular direction.

Finally, research is needed to relate outcomes (real and perceived) to group survival. There is very little research on the birth and death of collaborative institutions. How long do collaborative institutions generally survive, and how long should they survive to be useful? What types of outcomes are necessary for the survival of collaborative institutions? For example, is the perception of success enough to ensure survival? What contextual factors facilitate survival? In particular how does a collaborative institution successfully adapt to a specific environment? All of these questions require a creative and long-term research agenda.

Collaborative approaches to watershed management represent an ongoing policy experiment in the context of democratic governance. The experiment in collaboration is not limited to environmental policy; other policy arenas are also developing collaborative arrangements. While we are developing a clear understanding of the structure of collaborative institutions and discerning some indicators of the outcomes of the process, the ultimate verdict on collaboration is still far in the future. We think the research presented in this book, and the literature elsewhere, provides enough initial support for collaboration to justify continuing these experiments. However, the experiments still require extensive scrutiny from the academic and policy communities to ensure that collaboration heads down the right path and, if not, to terminate the experiment. At this point, collaborative institutions are analogous to the stage where spawning salmon manage by some amazing feat of nature to return to their natal waters, past seals and bears, nets and hooks, dams and diversions. The journey is not over—the ultimate test of success is for the juvenile salmon to make it back downstream and survive in the ocean. Like the young salmon, collaborative approaches to watershed management are only halfway there.

Notes

1. The "level of agreement reached" variable was measured on the following five-point ordinal scale:

   0 = no agreement on anything
   1 = agreement on which issues to discuss
   2 = agreement on general goals or principles
   3 = agreement on one or more implementation actions (relatively limited and unintegrated)

4 = agreement on a relatively comprehensive watershed management plan with specific projects or proposals

See Leach, Pelkey, and Sabatier (2002).

2. In fact, data from the Watershed Partnership Project indicate that only 41 percent of their fifty partnerships have engaged in any pre- or postproject monitoring (see figure 9.1). Even in the case of partnerships over six years old, the figure rises to only about 65 percent (Leach, Pelkey, and Sabatier 2002). We suspect that very few of these cases possess monitoring protocols sufficient to sort out the impacts of partnership projects on water quality.

References

Adler, Robert W. 1995. "Addressing Barriers to Watershed Protection." *Environmental Law* 25(4):973–1106.

Ajzen, Icek, and Martin Fishbein. 1980. *Understanding Attitudes and Predicting Social Behavior*. Englewood Cliffs, N.J.: Prentice-Hall.

Aldrich, John Herbert, and Forrest D. Nelson. 1984. *Linear Probability, Logit, and Probit Models*. Beverly Hills, Calif.: Sage.

Allison, Graham T. 1969. "Conceptual Models and the Cuban Missile Crisis." *American Political Science Review* 63(3):689–718.

Allison, Graham T. 1971. *Essence of Decision: Explaining the Cuban Missile Crisis*. Boston: Little, Brown.

Almond, Gabriel Abraham, and Sidney Verba. 1963. *The Civic Culture: Political Attitudes and Democracy in Five Nations*. Princeton, N.J.: Princeton University Press.

Anderson, Frederick R., and Robert H. Daniels. 1973. *N.E.P.A. in the Courts: A Legal Analysis of the National Environmental Policy Act*. Baltimore, Md.: Johns Hopkins University Press.

Anderson, Jeremy, and Steven Lewis Yaffee. 1998. *Balancing Public Trust and Private Interest: Public Participation in Habitat Conservation Planning*. Ann Arbor: University of Michigan School of Natural Resources and Environment.

Andrews, Richard N. L. 1976. *Environmental Policy and Administrative Change: Implementation of the National Environmental Policy Act*. Lexington, Mass.: Lexington Books.

Asher, Herbert B. 1983. *Causal Modeling*. 2nd ed. Beverly Hills, Calif.: Sage.

Baier, Annette. 1986. "Trust and Antitrust." *Ethics* 96(2):231–260.

Bality, Attila, Lowell Caneday, Ed Fite III, Tom Wikle, and Michael Yuan. 1998. *Illinois River Basin Management Plan 1999*. Tallequah: Oklahoma Scenic Rivers Commission.

Barber, Benjamin R. 1984. *Strong Democracy: Participatory Politics for a New Age*. Berkeley: University of California Press.

Barber, Bernard. 1983. *The Logic and Limits of Trust*. New Brunswick, N.J.: Rutgers University Press.

Barker, Rodney S. 1990. *Political Legitimacy and the State*. Oxford: Clarendon Press.

Barton, Weldon V. 1967. *Interstate Compacts in the Political Process*. Chapel Hill: University of North Carolina Press.

Bateson, Patrick. 1986. "Sociobiology and Human Politics." In *Science and Beyond*, edited by S. P. R. Rose and L. Appignanesi. Oxford: Basil Blackwell.

Beierle, Thomas C., and Jerry Cayford. 2002. *Democracy in Practice: Public Participation in Environmental Decisions*. Washington, D.C.: Resources for the Future.

Bella, David A., Charles D. Mosher, and Steven N. Calvo. 1988. "Technocracy and Trust: Nuclear Waste Controversy." *Journal of Professional Issues in Engineering* 114(1):27–39.

Beran, Harry. 1987. *The Consent Theory of Political Obligation*. London: Croom Helm.

Berkman, Richard L., and W. Kip Viscusi. 1973. *Damming the West: Ralph Nader's Study Group Report on the Bureau of Reclamation*. New York: Grossman Publishers.

Bingham, Gail. 1986. *Resolving Environmental Disputes: A Decade of Experience*. Washington, D.C.: Conservation Foundation.

Birch, Anthony Harold. 1972. *Representation*. New York: Macmillan.

Blackburn, J. Walton. 1988. "Environmental Mediation as an Alternative to Litigation." *Policy Studies Journal* 16(3):562–574.

Bohman, James, and William Rehg. 1997. *Deliberative Democracy: Essays on Reason and Politics*. Cambridge, Mass.: MIT Press.

Bormann, Bernard T., Patrick G. Cunningham, Martha H. Brookes, Van W. Manning, and Michael W. Collopy. 1994. *Adaptive Ecosystem Management in the Pacific Northwest*. Portland, Ore.: U.S. Department of Agriculture Forest Service, Pacific Northwest Research Station.

Born, Stephen M., and Kenneth D. Genskow. 1999. *Exploring the Watershed Approach: Critical Dimensions of State-Local Partnerships: The Four Corners Watershed Innovators Initiative Final Report*. Portland, Ore.: River Network.

Born, Stephen M., and Kenneth D. Genskow. 2000. *The Watershed Approach: An Empirical Assessment of Innovation in Environmental Management*. Washington, D.C.: National Academy of Public Administration.

Born, Stephen M., and Kenneth D. Genskow. 2001. *Toward Understanding New Watershed Initiatives: A Report from the Madison Watershed Workshop, July 20–21, 2000*. Madison: University of Wisconsin–Extension.

Bouckaert, Geert, Steven Van de Walle, Bart Maddens, and Jarl K. Kampen. 2002. "Identity vs. Performance: An Overview of Theories Explaining Trust in Government." In *Citizen Directed Governance: Quality and Trust in Govern-

ment (Second Report). Leuven, Belgium: Public Management Institute, Instituut voor de Overheid.

Bradbury, Judith A., Kristi M. Branch, and Will Focht. 1999. "Trust and Public Participation in Risk Policy Issues." In *Social Trust and the Management of Risk*, edited by R. Löfstedt and G. Cvetkovich. London: Earthscan.

Braithwaithe, Valerie. 1998. "Communal and Exchange Trust Norms: Their Value Base and Relevance to Institutional Trust." In *Trust and Governance*, edited by V. A. Braithwaite and M. Levi. New York: Russell Sage Foundation.

Brehm, John, and Wendy Rahn. 1997. "Individual-Level Evidence for the Causes and Consequences of Social Capital." *American Journal of Political Science* 41(3):999–1023.

Breton, Albert, and Ronald Wintrobe. 1982. *The Logic of Bureaucratic Conduct: An Economic Analysis of Competition, Exchange, and Efficiency in Private and Public Organizations*. Cambridge: Cambridge University Press.

Brody, Samuel D., Wes Highfield, and Letitia T. Alston. 2004. "Does Location Matter? Measuring Environmental Perceptions of Creeks in Two San Antonio Watersheds." *Environment and Behavior* 36(2):229–250.

Brown, Peter G. 1994. *Restoring the Public Trust: A Fresh Vision for Progressive Government in America*. Boston: Beacon Press.

Carnevale, David G. 1995. *Trustworthy Government: Leadership and Management Strategies for Building Trust and High Performance*. San Francisco: Jossey-Bass.

Caro, Robert A. 1975. *The Power Broker: Robert Moses and the Fall of New York*. New York: Vintage Books.

Carpenter, Susan L., and W. J. D. Kennedy. 1988. *Managing Public Disputes: A Practical Guide to Handling Conflict and Reaching Agreements*. San Francisco: Jossey-Bass.

Carson, Rachel. 1962. *Silent Spring*. Boston: Houghton Mifflin.

Castelfranchi, Cristiano, and Rino Falcone. 2000. "Trust Is Much More Than Subjective Probability: Mental Components and Sources of Trust." Paper read at 33rd Hawaii International Conference on System Sciences, Maui.

Chanley, Virginia A., Thomas J. Rudolph, and Wendy M. Rahn. 2000. "The Origins and Consequences of Public Trust in Government: A Time Series Analysis." *Public Opinion Quarterly* 64(3):239–257.

Checkland, Peter, and Jim Scholes. 1990. *Soft Systems Methodology in Action*. New York: Wiley.

Cheung, Steven N. S. 1970. "The Structure of a Contract and the Theory of a Non-Exclusive Resource." *Journal of Law and Economics* 13(1):49–70.

Clarke, Jeanne Nienaber, and Daniel McCool. 1985. *Staking Out the Terrain: Power Differentials Among Natural Resource Management Agencies*. Albany: State University of New York Press.

Clarke, Paul A. B. 1996. *Deep Citizenship*. London: Pluto Press.

Coglianese, Cary. 1997. "Assessing Consensus: The Promise and Performance of Negotiated Rulemaking." *Duke Law Journal* 46(6):1255–1349.

Coglianese, Cary. 1999. "The Limits of Consensus." *Environment* 41(3):28–33.

Coglianese, Cary. 2001. "Assessing the Advocacy of Negotiated Rulemaking: A Reply to Philip Harter." *New York University Environmental Law Journal* 9(2):386–447.

Coglianese, Cary. 2001. "Is Consensus an Appropriate Basis for Regulatory Policy?" In *Environmental Contracts: Comparative Approaches to Regulatory Innovation in the United States and Europe*, edited by E. W. Orts and K. Deketelaere. Boston: Kluwer Law International.

Coglianese, Cary. 2002. "Is Satisfaction Success? Evaluating Public Participation in Regulatory Policy-Making." In *Evaluating Environmental and Public Policy Conflict Resolution Programs and Policies*, edited by R. O'Leary and L. Bingham. Washington, D.C.: Resources for the Future Press.

Cohen, Joshua. 1997. "Deliberation and Democratic Legitimacy." In *Deliberative Democracy: Essays on Reason and Politics*, edited by J. Bohman and W. Rehg. Cambridge, Mass.: MIT Press.

Cole, Luke W., and Sheila R. Foster. 2001. *From the Ground Up: Environmental Racism and the Rise of the Environmental Justice Movement*. New York: New York University Press.

Coleman, James. 1988. "Social Capital in the Creation of Human Capital." *American Journal of Sociology* 94:S95–S120.

Coleman, James Samuel. 1990. *Foundations of Social Theory*. Cambridge, Mass.: Belknap Press of Harvard University Press.

Cook, Elizabeth. 2000. "A General Ecology of Watershed Groups in California." Master's thesis, University of California, Davis.

Cormick, Gerald W., Norman Dale, Paul Emond, S. Glenn Sigurdson, and Barry D. Stuart. 1996. *Building Consensus for a Sustainable Future: Putting Principles into Practice*. Ottawa, Ontario, Canada: National Round Table on the Environment and the Economy.

Cortner, H., and Margaret A. Moote. 1999. *The Politics of Ecosystem Management*. Washington, D.C.: Island Press.

Costanza, Robert, Ralph d'Arge, Rudolf de Groot, Stephen Farber, Monica Grasso, Bruce Hannon, Karin Limburg, Shahid Naeem, Robert V. O'Neill, Jose Paruelo, Robert G. Raskin, Paul Sutton, and Marjan van den Belt. 1997. "The Value of the World's Ecosystem Services and Natural Capital." *Nature* 387(6630):253–260.

Coulter, Philip B. 1988. *Political Voice: Citizen Demand for Urban Public Services*. Tuscaloosa: University of Alabama Press.

Craig, Stephen C. 1993. *The Malevolent Leaders: Popular Discontent in America*. Boulder, Colo.: Westview Press.

Crowfoot, James E., and Julia Marie Wondolleck. 1990. *Environmental Disputes: Community Involvement in Conflict Resolution.* Washington, D.C.: Island Press.

Culhane, Paul J. 1981. *Public Lands Politics: Interest Group Influence on the Forest Service and the Bureau of Land Management.* Baltimore, Md.: Johns Hopkins University Press.

Cvetkovich, George, Michael Siegrist, Rachel Murray, and Sarah Tragesser. 2002. "New Information and Social Trust: Asymmetry and Perseverance of Attributions about Hazard Managers." *Risk Analysis* 22(2):359–357.

Daniels, Steven E., and Gregg B. Walker. 2001. *Working Through Environmental Conflict: The Collaborative Learning Approach.* Westport, Conn.: Praeger.

Dasgupta, Partha. 1988. "Trust as Commodity." In *Trust: Making and Breaking Cooperative Relations,* edited by D. Gambetta. Oxford: Basil Blackwell.

Davies, J. Clarence. 1970. *The Politics of Pollution.* New York: Pegasus.

Davies, J. Clarence, and Jan Mazurek. 1998. *Pollution Control in the United States: Evaluating the System.* Washington, D.C.: Resources for the Future.

Davis, Charles E., ed. 1997. *Western Public Lands and Environmental Politics.* Boulder, Colo.: Westview Press.

Day, Richard B., Ronald Beiner, and Joseph Masciulli. 1988. *Democratic Theory and Technological Society.* Armonk, N.Y.: M. E. Sharpe.

DeWitt, Benjamin Parke. 1915. *The Progressive Movement: A Non-Partisan, Comprehensive Discussion of Current Tendencies in American Politics.* Seattle: University of Washington Press.

Dietz, Thomas, and Paul C. Stern. 1998. "Science, Values, and Biodiversity." *BioScience* 48(6):441–444.

Drew, Elizabeth. 1970. "Dam Outrage: The Story of the Army Engineers." *Atlantic Monthly* 227:51–62.

Driscoll, J. W. 1978. "Trust and Participation: Organizational Decision Making as Predictors of Satisfaction." *Academy of Management Journal* 21:44–56.

Dunlap, Riley E., and Angela G. Mertig. 1992. *American Environmentalism: The U.S. Environmental Movement, 1970–1990.* Philadelphia: Taylor & Francis.

Dunlap, Riley E., and Kent D. Van Liere. 1978. "The 'New Environmental Paradigm': A Proposed Instrument and Preliminary Results." *Journal of Environmental Education* 9:10–19.

Durant, Robert F. 1992. *The Administrative Presidency Revisited: Public Lands, the BLM, and the Reagan Revolution.* Albany: State University of New York Press.

Dworkin, R. M. 1977. *Taking Rights Seriously.* Cambridge, Mass.: Harvard University Press.

Earle, Timothy C. 2000. "Trust and Confidence: A Dual-Mode Model of Cooperation." Unpublished manuscript.

Earle, Timothy C., and George Cvetkovich. 1995. *Social Trust: Toward a Cosmopolitan Society*. Westport, Conn.: Praeger.

Eggertsson, Thrainn. 1990. *Economic Behavior and Institutions*. Cambridge: Cambridge University Press.

Eisner, Marc Allen. 1993. *Regulatory Politics in Transition: Interpreting American Politics*. Baltimore, Md.: John Hopkins University Press.

Elster, Jon. 1998. *Deliberative Democracy*. Cambridge: Cambridge University Press.

Ely, John Hart. 1980. *Democracy and Distrust: A Theory of Judicial Review*. Cambridge, Mass.: Harvard University Press.

European Community. 2001. *Directive 2000/60/EC of the European Parliament and the Council of 23 October 2000 Establishing a Framework for Community Action in the Field of Water Policy*. Brussels: European Community, 2000 (cited September 24, 2001). Available from http://europa.eu.int/eur-lex/pri/en/oj/dat/2000/l_327/l_32720001222en00010072.pdf.

Farrand, Fred Lenox. 1983. "Personal Goals, Political Goals and Political Participation." Ph.D. dissertation, University of Oregon.

Feinberg, Joel. 1984. *The Moral Limits of the Criminal Law*, Vol. 1: *Harm to Others*. Oxford: Oxford University Press.

Ferejohn, John A. 1974. *Pork Barrel Politics: Rivers and Harbors Legislation, 1947–1968*. Stanford, Calif.: Stanford University Press.

Fisher, Roger, William Ury, and Bruce Patton. 1991. *Getting to Yes: Negotiating Agreement without Giving In*. 2nd ed. New York: Penguin Books.

Fisheries and Oceans Canada, Habitat and Enhancement Branch, Habitat Conservation and Stewardship Program. *History of Watershed Management and Community Participation*. Vancouver, B.C.: Fisheries and Oceans Canada, Pacific Region Habitat and Enhancement Branch, 2002. Available from http://www.heb.pac.dfo-mpo.gc.ca/english/programs/hcsp/watrshd/wrthstr.htm.

Freund, E. 1904. *The Police Power, Public Power and Constitutional Rights*. Chicago: Callaghan.

Funtowicz, Silvio O., and Jerome R. Ravetz. 1992. "Three Types of Risk Assessment and the Emergence of Postnormal Science." In *Social Theories of Risk*, edited by S. Krimsky and D. Golding. Westport, Conn.: Praeger.

Gambetta, Diego. 2000. "Can We Trust?" In *Trust: Making and Breaking Cooperative Relations* (electronic edition), edited by D. Gambetta. Oxford: Department of Sociology, University of Oxford. Available from http://www.sociology.ox.ac.uk/papers/trustbook.html.

Gamson, William A. 1968. *Power and Discontent*. Homewood, Ill.: Dorsey Press.

Gandy, Oscar H. 1991. "Trust in Government and Active Participation: The Role of Media Use, Ideology, Personality and Political Interest in the Democratic Urge." Paper read at Mass Communication and Society Division of Association for Education in Journalism and Mass Communication, Boston, August.

Gargarella, Roberto. 1998. "Full Representation, Deliberation, and Impartiality." In *Deliberative Democracy*, edited by J. Elster. Cambridge: Cambridge University Press.

Goldfarb, William. 1994. "Watershed Management: Slogan or Solution?" *Boston College Environmental Affairs Law Review* 21:483–509.

Good, David. 2000. "Individuals, Interpersonal Relations and Trust." In *Trust: Making and Breaking Cooperative Relations* (electronic edition), edited by D. Gambetta. Oxford: Department of Sociology, University of Oxford. Available from http://www.sociology.ox.ac.uk/papers/trustbook.html.

Gordon, H. Scott. 1954. "The Economic Theory of a Common-Property Resource: The Fishery." *Journal of Political Economy* 62:124–142.

Gottlieb, Alan M. 1989. *The Wise Use Agenda: The Citizen's Policy Guide to Environmental Resource Issues: A Task Force Report*. Bellevue, Wash.: Free Enterprise Press.

Gray, Barbara. 1989. *Collaborating: Finding Common Ground for Multiparty Problems*. San Francisco: Jossey-Bass.

Green, Donald P., and Ian Shapiro. 1994. *Pathologies of Rational Choice Theory: A Critique of Applications in Political Science*. New Haven, Conn.: Yale University Press.

Gregg, Frank. 1989. "Irrelevance and Innovation in Water Policy: Lessons from the W.R.P.A." In *Redefining National Water Policy: New Roles and Directions*, edited by S. M. Born. Bethesda, Md.: American Water Resources Association.

Gutmann, Amy, and Dennis F. Thompson. 1996. *Democracy and Disagreement*. Cambridge, Mass.: Belknap Press of Harvard University Press.

Hannon, Bruce, and Julie Cannon. 1971. "The Corps Out-Engineered." In *The Politics of Ecosuicide*, edited by Leslie L. Roos. New York: Holt, Rinehart and Winston.

Hardin, Russell. 1993. "The Street-Level Epistemology of Trust." *Politics and Society* 21(4):505–529.

Hardin, Russell. 1997. "Distrust." Paper read at Russell Sage Foundation Conference on Distrust, Bellagio, Italy, October 13–17.

Hardin, Russell. 2001. "Distrust." *Boston University Law Review* 81(3):495–522.

Hargreaves Heap, Shaun, Martin Hollis, Bruce Lyons, Robert Sugden, and Albert Weale. 1992. *The Theory of Choice: A Critical Guide*. Oxford: Blackwell.

Harrison, Adam, Guido Schmidt, Charlie Avis, and Rayka Hauserune. 2001. *WWF's Preliminary Comments on Public Participation in the Context of the Water Framework Directive and Integrated River Basin Management*. Copenhagen: WWF European Freshwater Programme [cited September 24, 2001]. Available from http://www.panda.org/downloads/europe/WFD-WWFpart.pdf.

Hausman, D. M., and M. S. McPherson. 1993. "Taking Ethics Seriously: Economics and Contemporary Moral Philosophy." *Journal of Economic Literature* 31(2):671–731.

Hays, Samuel P. 1959. *Conservation and the Gospel of Efficiency: The Progressive Conservation Movement, 1890–1920.* Cambridge, Mass.: Harvard University Press.

Hays, Samuel P., and Barbara D. Hays. 1987. *Beauty, Health, and Permanence: Environmental Politics in the United States, 1955–1985.* Cambridge: Cambridgeshire: Cambridge University Press.

Heckathorn, Douglas D., and Steven M. Maser. 1987. "Bargaining and the Sources of Transaction Costs: The Case of Government Regulation." *Journal of Law, Economics, and Organization* 3:69–98.

Heffron, Florence A., and Neil McFeeley. 1983. *The Administrative Regulatory Process.* New York: Longman.

Hetherington, Marc J. 1999. "The Effect of Political Trust on the Presidential Vote, 1968–96." *American Political Science Review* 93(2):311–326.

Hill, William, and Leonard Ortolano. 1978. "NEPA's Effect on the Consideration of Alternatives: A Crucial Test." *Natural Resources Journal* 10(2):285–311.

Hirsch, Fred. 1977. *Social Limits to Growth.* London: Routledge and Keegan Paul.

Hirschman, Albert O. 1984. "Against Parsimony: Three Easy Ways of Complicating Some Categories of Economic Discourse." *American Economic Review* 74(2):89–96.

Huber, P. J. 1967. "The Behavior of Maximum Likelihood Estimates under Non-Standard Conditions." In *Proceedings of the Fifth Berkeley Symposium on Mathematical Statistics and Probability*, edited by L. M. LeCam and J. Neyman. Berkeley: University of California Press.

Hundley, Norris. 1975. *Water and the West: The Colorado River Compact and the Politics of Water in the American West.* Berkeley: University of California Press.

Hundley, Norris. 1992. *The Great Thirst: Californians and Water, 1770s–1990s.* Berkeley: University of California Press.

Hupcey, Judith E. 2002. "Maintaining Validity: The Development of the Concept of Trust." *International Journal of Qualitative Methods* 1(4): article 5, retrieved from http://www.ualberta.ca/~ijqm.

Ingram, Helen. 1977. "Policy Implementation through Bargaining: The Case of Federal Grants in Aid." *Public Policy* 25(4):499–526.

Janoff-Bulman, Ronnie. 1992. *Shattered Assumptions: Towards a New Psychology of Trauma.* New York: Free Press.

John, DeWitt. 1994. *Civic Environmentalism: Alternatives to Regulation in States and Communities.* Washington, D.C.: CQ Press.

Johnson, Bart R., and Ronald Campbell. 1999. "Ecology and Participation in Landscape-Based Planning within the Pacific Northwest." *Policy Studies Journal* 27(3):502–529.

Johnson-George, Cynthia, and Walter C. Swap. 1982. "Measurement of Specific Interpersonal Trust: Construction and Validation of a Scale to Assess Trust in a Specific Other." *Journal of Personality and Social Psychology* 43(6):1306–1317.

Kahneman, Daniel, and Amos Tversky. 1979. "Prospect Theory: An Analysis of Decisions under Risk." *Econometrica* 47(2):263–291.

Kahrl, William L. 1982. *Water and Power: The Conflict over Los Angeles' Water Supply in the Owens Valley*. Berkeley: University of California Press.

Kant, Immanuel. 1981. *Grounding for the Metaphysics of Morals*, trans. by J. W. Ellington. Indianapolis, Ind.: Hackett.

Kasperson, Roger E., Dominic Golding, and Seth Tuler. 1992. "Social Distrust as a Factor in Siting Hazardous Facilities and Communicating Risks." *Journal of Social Issues* 48(4):161–187.

Kaufman, Herbert. 1960. *The Forest Ranger: A Study in Administrative Behavior*. Baltimore, Md.: Johns Hopkins Press.

Kenney, Douglas S. 1999. "Historical and Sociopolitical Context of the Western Watersheds Movement." *Journal of the American Water Resources Association* 35(3):493–504.

Kenney, Douglas S., and William B. Lord. 1999. *Analysis of Institutional Innovation in the Natural Resources and Environmental Realm: The Emergence of Alternative Problem-Solving Strategies in the American West*. Boulder: Natural Resources Law Center, University of Colorado School of Law.

Kenney, Douglas S., Sean T. McAllister, William H. Caile, and Jason S. Peckham. 2000. *The New Watershed Source Book: A Directory and Review of Watershed Initiatives in the Western United States*. Boulder: University of Colorado School of Law, Natural Resources Law Center.

Kier, W. M. 1995. "Watershed Restoration: A Guide for Citizen Involvement in California." Silver Spring, Md.: U.S. Department of Commerce, National Oceanic and Atmospheric Administration, Coastal Ocean Office.

King, Gary, Robert O. Keohane, and Sidney Verba. 1994. *Designing Social Inquiry: Scientific Inference in Qualitative Research*. Princeton, N.J.: Princeton University Press.

Kingsley, G. Thomas, Joseph B. McNeely, and James O. Gibson. 1997. *Community Building: Coming of Age*. Washington, D.C.: Development Training Institute. Urban Institute.

Kiser, Larry, and Elinor Ostrom. 1982. "The Three Worlds of Action." In *Strategies of Political Inquiry*, edited by E. Ostrom. Beverly Hills, Calif.: Sage.

Knott, Jack H., and Gary J. Miller. 1987. *Reforming Bureaucracy: The Politics of Institutional Choice*. Englewood Cliffs, N.J.: Prentice Hall.

Kolko, Gabriel. 1965. *Railroads and Regulation: 1877–1916*. New York: Norton.

Kramer, R. M. 1994. "The Sinister Attribution Error: Paranoid Cognition and Collective Distrust in Organizations." *Motivation and Emotion* 18(2):199–230.

Kramer, Roderick M. 1999. "Trust and Distrust in Organizations: Emerging Perspectives, Enduring Questions." *Annual Review of Psychology* 50:569–598.

Kubasek, N. K., and G. S. Silverman. 1997. *Environmental Law*. 2nd ed. Upper Saddle River, N.J.: Prentice Hall.

Kuhn, Thomas S. 1970. *The Structure of Scientific Revolutions*. 2nd ed. Chicago: University of Chicago Press.

Laird, Frank N. 1993. "Participatory Analysis, Democracy, and Technological Decision Making." *Science, Technology and Human Values* 18(3):341–361.

Leach, Richard H., and Redding S. Sugg. 1959. *The Administration of Interstate Compacts*. Baton Rouge: Louisiana State University Press.

Leach, William D. 2000. "Evaluating Watershed Partnerships in California: Theoretical and Methodological Perspectives." Ph.D. diss., Ecology, University of California, Davis.

Leach, William D. 2002. "Surveying Diverse Stakeholder Groups." *Society and Natural Resources* 15(7):641–649.

Leach, William D., and Neil W. Pelkey. 2001. "Making Watershed Partnerships Work: A Review of the Empirical Literature." *Journal of Water Resources Planning and Management* 127(6):378–385.

Leach, William D., Neil W. Pelkey, and Paul A. Sabatier. 2001. "Federal Environmental Law and the Occurrence of Collaborative Watershed Partnerships." Paper read at Integrated Decision-Making for Watershed Management Symposium, Chevy Chase, Md., January 7–9.

Leach, William D., Neil W. Pelkey, and Paul A. Sabatier. 2002. "Stakeholder Partnerships as Collaborative Policymaking: Evaluation Criteria Applied to Watershed Management in California and Washington." *Journal of Policy Analysis and Management* 21(4):645–670.

Leach, William D., and Paul A. Sabatier. 2003. "Facilitators, Coordinators, and Outcomes." In *The Promise and Performance of Environmental Conflict Resolution*, edited by R. O'Leary and L. Bingham. Washington, D.C.: Resources for the Future.

Levi, Margaret. 1998. "When Good Defenses Make Good Neighbors: A Transaction Cost Approach to Trust and Distrust." Paper read at Conference on Social Networks and Social Capital, Durham, N.C., October 30–November 1.

Lewis, David J., and Andrew J. Weigert. 1985a. "Social Atomism, Holism and Trust." *Sociological Quarterly* 26(4):455–471.

Lewis, J. David, and Andrew Weigert. 1985b. "Trust as a Social Reality." *Social Forces* 63(4):967–985.

Libecap, Gary D. 1989. *Contracting for Property Rights*. Cambridge: Cambridge University Press.

Likens, Gene E., Herbert F. Bormann, Noye M. Johnson, D. W. Fisher, and Robert S. Pierce. 1970. "Effects of Forest Cutting and Herbicide Treatment on Nutrient Budgets in the Hubbard Brook Watershed-Ecosystem." *Ecological Monographs* 40(1):23–47.

Lilienthal, David Eli. 1944. *TVA: Democracy on the March*. New York: Harper.

Lindblom, Charles E. 1959. "The Science of 'Muddling Through.'" *Public Administration Review* 19:79–88.

Lindblom, Charles E., and David K. Cohen. 1979. *Usable Knowledge: Social Science and Social Problem Solving*. New Haven, Conn.: Yale University Press.

Lindlof, Thomas R. 1995. *Qualitative Communication Research Methods*. Thousand Oaks, Calif.: Sage.

Lipset, Seymour Martin, and William Schneider. 1983. *The Confidence Gap: Business, Labor, and Government in the Public Mind*. New York: Free Press.

Loomis, John B. 1993. *Integrated Public Lands Management: Principles and Applications to National Forests, Parks, Wildlife Refuges, and BLM Lands*. New York: Columbia University Press.

Lowi, Theodore J. 1969. *The End of Liberalism: Ideology, Policy, and the Crisis of Public Authority*. New York: Norton.

Lubell, Mark. 2000a. "Attitudinal Support for Environmental Governance: Do Institutions Matter?" Paper read at Annual Meeting of the American Political Science Association, Washington, D.C., August 31–September 3.

Lubell, Mark. 2000b. "Cognitive Conflict and Consensus Building in the National Estuary Program." *American Behavioral Scientist* 44(4):628–647.

Lubell, Mark, Mihriye Mete, Mark Schnieder, and John Scholz. 1998. "Cooperation, Transaction Costs, and the Emergence of Ecosystem Partnerships." Paper read at Annual Meeting of the American Political Science Association, Boston, September 3–6.

Lubell, Mark, Mark Schneider, John T. Scholz, and Mihriye Mete. 2002. "Watershed Partnerships and the Emergence of Collective Action Institutions." *American Journal of Political Science* 46(1):148–163.

Luhmann, Niklas. 1979. *Trust and Power*. New York: Wiley.

Maass, Arthur. 1951. *Muddy Waters: The Army Engineers and the Nation's Rivers*. Cambridge, Mass.: Harvard University Press.

MacLean, Douglas. 1982. "Risk and Consent: Philosophical Issues for Centralized Decisions." *Risk Analysis* 2:59–67.

MacLean, Douglas. 1987. "Risk and Consent: Philosophical Issues for Centralized Decisions." In *Resolving Locational Conflict*, edited by R. W. Lake. New Brunswick, N.J.: Center for Urban Policy Research.

Magat, Wesley A., Alan J. Krupnick, and Winston Harrington. 1986. *Rules in the Making: A Statistical Analysis of Regulatory Agency Behavior*. Washington, D.C.: Resources for the Future.

Mann, Dean. 1975. "Political Incentives in U.S. Water Policy: Relationships between Distributive and Regulatory Policies." In *What Government Does*, edited by M. Holden and D. L. Dresang. Beverly Hills, Calif.: Sage.

Margerum, Richard D. 1999. "Integrated Environmental Management: The Foundations for Successful Practice." *Environmental Management* 24(2):151–166.

Markóczy, Lívia. 2002. "Naïve Trust, Prudent Trust, Distrust and Social Intelligence." Unpublished manuscript, version 1.18.

Mazmanian, Daniel A., and Jeanne Nienaber Clarke. 1979. *Can Organizations Change? Environmental Protection, Citizen Participation, and the Corps of Engineers*. Washington, D.C.: Brookings Institution.

McCloskey, Michael. 1996. "The Skeptic: Collaboration Has Its Limits." *High Country News* 28(9).

McConnell, Grant. 1966. *Private Power and American Democracy*. New York: Knopf.

McGregor, Douglas. 1967. *The Professional Manager*. New York: McGraw-Hill.

McKnight, D. Harrison, Larry L. Cummings, and Norman L. Chervany. 1995. "Trust Formation in New Organizational Relationships." Paper read at Information and Decision Sciences Workshop, University of Minnesota, Minneapolis, October.

Meo, Mark, Will Focht, Lowell Caneday, Robert Lynch, Fekadu Moreda, Blake Pettus, Ed Sankowski, Zev Tachtenberg, Baxter Vieux, and Keith Willett. 2002. "Negotiating Science and Values with Stakeholders in the Illinois River Basin." *Journal of the American Water Resources Association* 38(2):541–554.

Meyerson, Debra, Karl E. Weick, and Roderick M. Kramer. 1996. "Swift Trust and Temporary Groups." In *Trust in Organizations: Frontiers of Theory and Research*, edited by R. M. Kramer and T. R. Tyler. Thousand Oaks, Calif.: Sage.

Misztal, Barbara A. 1996. *Trust in Modern Societies: The Search for the Bases of Social Order*. Cambridge, Mass.: Polity Press.

Mohai, Paul. 1995. "The Forest Service since the National Forest Management Act: Assessing Bureaucratic Response to External and Internal Forces for Change." *Policy Studies Journal* 23(2):247–252.

Montgomery, D. R., G. E. Grant, and K. Sullivan. 1995. "Watershed Analysis as a Framework for Implementing Ecosystem Management." *Water Resources Bulletin* 31(3):369–386.

Morgan, Arthur Ernest. 1951. *The Miami Conservancy District*. New York: McGraw-Hill.

Morgan, David R., Robert E. England, and George G. Humphreys. 1991. *Oklahoma Politics and Policies: Governing the Sooner State*. Lincoln: University of Nebraska Press.

Nader, Ralph, and John C. Esposito. 1970. *Vanishing Air: The Ralph Nader Study Group Report on Air Pollution*. New York: Grossman Publishers.

Nash, Roderick. 1967. *Wilderness and the American Mind*. New Haven, Conn.: Yale University Press.

Nash, Roderick, ed. 1968. *The American Environment: Readings in the History of Conservation*. Reading, Mass.: Addison-Wesley.

National Research Council, Committee on the Institutional Means for Assessment of Risks to Public Health. 1983. *Risk Assessment in the Federal Government: Managing the Process*. Washington, D.C.: National Academy Press.

National Research Council, Committee on Risk Perception and Communication. 1989. *Improving Risk Communication*. Washington, D.C.: National Academy Press.

National Research Council, Committee on Watershed Management. 1999. *New Strategies for America's Watersheds*. Washington, D.C.: National Academy Press.

National Science Board. 2000. *Science and Engineering Indicators—2000*. Arlington, Va.: National Science Foundation.

National Wildlife Federation. 1998. *Conservation Directory 1998: A List of Organizations, Agencies, and Officials Concerned with Natural Resource Use and Management*. 43rd ed. Vienna, Va.: National Wildlife Federation.

North, Douglass Cecil. 1990. *Institutions, Institutional Change, and Economic Performance*. Cambridge: Cambridge University Press.

Nye, Joseph S., Philip Zelikow, and David C. King. 1997. *Why People Don't Trust Government*. Cambridge, Mass.: Harvard University Press.

Odum, Eugene P. 1969. "The Strategy of Ecosystem Development." *Science* 164:262–270.

Ogu, V. I. 2000. "Stakeholders' Partnership Approach to Infrastructure Provision and Management in Developing World Cities: Lessons from the Sustainable Ibadan Project." *Habitat International* 24(4):517–533.

O'Leary, Rosemary, and Lisa Bingham, eds. 2003. *The Promise and Performance of Environmental Conflict Resolution*. Washington, D.C.: Resources for the Future.

O'Neill, John. 2002. "Deliberative Democracy and Environmental Policy." In *Democracy and the Claims of Nature: Critical Perspectives for a New Century*, edited by B. A. Minteer and B. P. Taylor. Lanham, Md.: Rowman & Littlefield.

Orbell, John, and Robyn M. Dawes. 1991. "A 'Cognitive Miser' Theory of Cooperators' Advantage." *American Political Science Review* 85(2):515–528.

Orren, Gary. 1997. "Fall from Grace: The Public's Loss of Faith in Government." In *Why People Don't Trust Government*, edited by J. S. Nye, P. Zelikow, and D. C. King. Cambridge, Mass.: Harvard University Press.

Ostrom, Elinor. 1990. *Governing the Commons: The Evolution of Institutions for Collective Action*. Cambridge: Cambridge University Press.

Ostrom, Elinor. 1998. "A Behavioral Approach to the Rational Choice Theory of Collective Action." *American Political Science Review* 92(1):1–22.

Ostrom, Elinor. 1999. "Institutional Rational Choice: An Assessment of the Institutional Analysis and Development Framework." In *Theories of the Policy Process*, edited by P. A. Sabatier. Boulder, Colo.: Westview Press.

Ostrom, Elinor, Roy Gardner, and James Walker. 1994. *Rules, Games, and Common-Pool Resources*. Ann Arbor: University of Michigan Press.

Perez, O. 2002. "Using Private-Public Linkages to Regulate Environmental Conflicts: The Case of International Construction Contracts." *Journal of Law and Society* 29(1):77–110.

Petulla, Joseph M. 1977. *American Environmental History: The Exploitation and Conservation of Natural Resources*. San Francisco: Boyd & Fraser.

Pierce, John C., and Harvey R. Doerksen. 1976. *Water Politics and Public Involvement*. Ann Arbor, Mich.: Ann Arbor Science Publishers.

Pisani, Donald. 1992. *To Reclaim a Divided West: Water, Law, and Public Policy, 1848–1902*. Albuquerque: University of New Mexico Press.

Pisani, Donald. 2002. "A Conservation Myth: The Troubled Childhood of the Multiple-Use Idea." *Agricultural History* 76(2):154–171.

Pitkin, Hanna Fenichel. 1967. *The Concept of Representation*. Berkeley: University of California Press.

Platt, John. 1964. "Strong Inference." *Science* 146:347–353.

Przeworski, A. 1998. "Deliberation and Ideological Domination." In *Deliberative Democracy*, edited by J. Elster. Cambridge: Cambridge University Press.

Putnam, Robert D. 1995. "Tuning In, Tuning Out: The Strange Disappearance of Social Capital in America." *PS, Political Science and Politics* 28(4):1–20.

Putnam, Robert D. 1996. "The Strange Disappearance of Civic America." *American Prospect* 7(24):34.

Putnam, Robert D. 2000. *Bowling Alone: The Collapse and Revival of American Community*. New York: Simon & Schuster.

Putnam, Robert D., Robert Leonardi, and Raffaella Nanetti. 1993. *Making Democracy Work: Civic Traditions in Modern Italy*. Princeton, N.J.: Princeton University Press.

Quarles, John. 1976. *Cleaning Up America: An Insider's View of the Environmental Protection Agency*. Boston: Houghton Mifflin.

Quattrone, George A., and Amos Tversky. 1988. "Contrasting Rational and Psychological Analyses of Political Choice." *American Political Science Review* 82(3):719–736.

Rabe, Barry. 1988. "The Politics of Environmental Dispute Resolution." *Policy Studies Journal* 16:585–601.

Radin, Margaret Jane. 1993. *Reinterpreting Property*. Chicago: University of Chicago Press.

Randall, Alan. 1981. *Resource Economics: An Economic Approach to Natural Resource and Environmental Policy*. Columbus, Ohio: Grid Publishing.

Rawls, John. 1999. *A Theory of Justice*. Rev. ed. Cambridge, Mass.: Belknap Press of Harvard University Press.

Reichenbach, Hans. 1938. *Experience and Prediction: An Analysis of the Foundations and the Structure of Knowledge*. Chicago: University of Chicago Press.

Reisner, Marc. 1986. *Cadillac Desert: The American West and Its Disappearing Water*. New York: Viking.

Rempel, John K., John G. Holmes, and Mark P. Zanna. 1985. "Trust in Close Relationships." *Journal of Personality and Social Psychology* 49(1):95–112.

Richardson, Elmo. 1973. *Dams, Parks and Politics: Resource Development and Preservation in the Truman-Eisenhower Era*. Lexington: University Press of Kentucky.

Riley, Patrick. 1982. *Will and Political Legitimacy: A Critical Exposition of Social Contract Theory in Hobbes, Locke, Rousseau, Kant, and Hegel*. Cambridge, Mass.: Harvard University Press.

Rosenbaum, Walter A. 2002. *Environmental Politics and Policy*. 5th ed. Washington, D.C.: Congressional Quarterly Press.

Rosenstone, Steven J., and John Mark Hansen. 1993. *Mobilization, Participation, and Democracy in America*. New York: Macmillan.

Rothbart, Myron, and Bernadette Park. 1986. "On the Confirmability and Disconfirmability of Trait Concepts." *Science, Technology and Human Values* 12:94–101.

Rousseau, Jean-Jacques. 1987. "On the Social Contract." In *Basic Political Writings*, edited by D. A. Cress. Indianapolis, Ind.: Hackett.

Ruhl, J. B. 1999. "The (Political) Science of Watershed Management in the Ecosystem Age." *Journal of the American Water Resources Association* 35(3):519–526.

Ruscio, Kenneth P. 1996. "Trust, Democracy, and Public Management: A Theoretical Argument." *Journal of Public Administration Research and Theory* 6(3):461–477.

Sabatier, Paul A. 1975. "Social Movements and Regulatory Agencies: Toward a More Adequate—and Less Pessimistic—Theory of 'Clientele Capture.'" *Policy Sciences* 6:301–342.

Sabatier, Paul A. 1988. "An Advocacy Coalition Model of Policy Change and the Role of Policy-Oriented Learning Therein." *Policy Sciences* 21(Fall):129–168.

Sabatier, Paul A., Susan Hunter, and Susan McLaughlin. 1987. "The Devil Shift: Perceptions and Misperceptions of Opponents." *Western Political Quarterly* 40(3):449–476.

Sabatier, Paul A., and Hank Jenkins-Smith. 1988. Special Issue: Policy Change and Policy-Oriented Learning. *Policy Sciences* 21:123–278.

Sabatier, Paul A., and Hank C. Jenkins-Smith, eds. 1993. *Policy Change and Learning: An Advocacy Coalition Approach*. Boulder, Colo.: Westview Press.

Sabatier, Paul A., and Hank C. Jenkins-Smith. 1999. "The Advocacy Coalition Framework: An Assessment." In *Theories of the Policy Process*, edited by P. Sabatier. Boulder, Colo.: Westview Press.

Sabatier, Paul A., and William D. Leach. 2002. *Watershed Partnerships in California and Washington: Final Report for the Watershed Partnerships Projects.* Washington, D.C.: U.S. EPA STAR Program.

Sabatier, Paul A., John Loomis, and Catherine McCarthy. 1995. "Hierarchical Controls, Professional Norms, Local Constituencies, and Budget Maximization: An Analysis of US Forest Service Planning Decisions." *American Journal of Political Science* 39(1):204.

Sabatier, Paul A., and Neil W. Pelkey. 1990. *Land Development at Lake Tahoe: The Effects of Environmental Controls and Economic Conditions on Housing Construction.* Davis: Institute of Ecology, University of California, Davis.

Sabatier, Paul, James Quinn, and William D. Leach. 2002. *Watershed Partnerships in California and Washington: Final Report for the Watershed Partnerships Project.* Washington, D.C.: U.S. EPA, Water and Watersheds Program.

Sabatier, Paul A., and Edella Schlager. 2000. "Les Approaches cognitives des politiques publiques: Perspectives américaines (Cognitive approaches to public policy: An American perspective)." *Revue française de science politique* 50(2): 209–234.

Sabatier, Paul A., Chris Weible, and William D. Leach. 2001. "Perspective on Watershed Partnerships: The Views of Landowners, Agency Officials, and Environmentalists." Paper read at National Policy Conference on Environmental Policy in an Era of Devolution, Ohio State University, Columbus, April 16–18.

Sabatier, Paul A., and Matthew Zafonte. 2001. "Public Knowledge: Advocacy Organizations." In *International Encyclopedia of the Social and Behavioral Sciences*, edited by N. J. Smelser and P. B. Baltes. Amsterdam: Elsevier.

Sagoff, Mark. 1988. "At the Shrine of Our Lady of Fatima; Or, Why Political Questions Are Not All Economic." In *The Economy of the Earth: Philosophy, Law, and the Environment*, edited by M. Sagoff. Cambridge: Cambridge University Press.

Sagoff, Mark. 1999. "The View from Quincy Library: Civic Engagement in Environmental Problem Solving." In *Civil Society, Democracy, and Civic Renewal*, edited by R. K. Fullinwider. Lanham, Md.: Rowman & Littlefield.

San Antonio Economic Development Foundation. 2001. *San Antonio: A Dynamic Economy and Culture.* San Antonio, Tex.: San Antonio Economic Development Foundation, 1999 [cited 2001]. Available from http://saedf.dcci.com/xindex.html.

Sax, Joseph L. 1968. *Water Law, Planning and Policy: Cases and Materials.* Indianapolis, Ind.: Bobbs-Merrill.

Sax, Joseph L. 1971. *Defending the Environment: A Strategy for Citizen Action.* New York: Knopf.

Scharpf, Fritz W. 1997. *Games Real Actors Play: Actor-Centered Institutionalism in Policy Research*. Boulder, Colo.: Westview Press.

Scheberle, Denise. 1997. *Federalism and Environmental Policy: Trust and the Politics of Implementation*. Washington, D.C.: Georgetown University Press.

Schlager, Edella. 1995. "Policy Making and Collective Action: Defining Coalitions within the Advocacy Coalition Framework." *Policy Sciences* 28(3):243–270.

Schlager, Edella, William Blomquist, and Shui Yan Tang. 1994. "Mobile Flows, Storage, and Self-Organized Institutions for Governing Common-Pool Resources." *Land Economics* 70(3):294–317.

Scott, C. L., III. 1980. "Interpersonal Trust: A Comparison of Attitudinal and Situational Factors." *Human Relations* 33:805–812.

Scott, David, and Fern K. Willits. 1994. "Environmental Attitudes and Behavior: A Pennsylvania Survey." *Environment and Behavior* 26(2):239–260.

Selznick, Philip. 1949. *TVA and the Grass Roots*. New York: Harper & Row.

Shapiro, Susan P. 1987. "The Social Control of Impersonal Trust." *American Journal of Sociology* 93(3):623–658.

Sigelman, Lee, and Langche Zeng. 1999. "Analyzing Censored and Sample-Selected Data with Tobit and Heckit Models." *Political Analysis* 8(2):167–182.

Simon, Herbert A. 1955. "A Behavioral Model of Rational Choice." *Quarterly Journal of Economics* 69(1):99–118.

Singleton, Sara. 2000. "Collaborative Environmental Planning in the American West: The Good, the Bad, and the Ugly." *Environmental Politics* 11:54–75.

Singleton, Sara. 2002. "Managing Pacific Salmon: The Role of Distributional Conflicts in Coastal Salish Fisheries." In *Inequality, Collective Action and Environmental Sustainability*, edited by J.-M. Baland, P. Bardhan, and S. Bowles. Santa Fe, N.M.: Santa Fe Institute.

Slovic, Paul. 1993. "Perceived Risk, Trust, and Democracy." *Risk Analysis* 13(6):675–682.

Slovic, Paul. 1999. "Trust, Emotion, Sex, Politics, and Science: Surveying the Risk-Assessment Battlefield." *Risk Analysis* 19(4):689–701.

Slovic, Paul, James Flynn, S. Johnson, and C. K. Mertz. 1993. *The Dynamics of Trust in Situations of Risk*. Eugene, Ore.: Decision Research.

Slovic, Paul, Mark Layman, and James H. Flynn. 1991. "Risk Perception, Trust and Nuclear Waste: Lessons from Yucca Mountain." *Environment* 33(3):6–11, 28–30.

Smidt, Corwin E. 1971. "Political Efficacy, Political Trust and Political Participation." Masters' thesis, University of Iowa.

Snyder, Gary. 1990. *The Practice of the Wild*. San Francisco: North Point Press.

Sommarstrom, Sari. 1998. "Non-Governmental Statewide Overview: Cooperative, Community-Based Watershed Organizations in California." In *Four*

Corners Watershed Innovators Initiative, California Background Report, edited by F. Vitulli, S. Sommarstrom, L. Wills, H. Price, and P. Showalter. Portland, Ore.: River Network.

StataCorp. 1999. *Stata Statistical Software User's Guide 6.0*. College Station, Tex.: Stata Corporation.

Stern, Paul C., Harvey V. Fineberg, and NRC Committee on Risk Characterization. 1996. *Understanding Risk: Informing Decisions in a Democratic Society*. Washington, D.C.: National Academy Press.

Stinchcombe, Arthur L. 1968. *Constructing Social Theories*. Chicago: University of Chicago Press.

Stratton, Owen, and Phillip Sirotkin. 1959. *The Echo Park Controversy*. Indianapolis, Ind.: Bobbs-Merrill.

Sugden, Robert. 1981. *The Political Economy of Public Choice: An Introduction to Welfare Economics*. New York: Wiley.

Susskind, Lawrence, Sarah McKearnan, and Jennifer Thomas-Larmer, eds. 1999. *The Consensus Building Handbook: A Comprehensive Guide to Reaching Agreement*. Thousand Oaks, Calif.: Sage.

Susskind, Lawrence, Mieke van der Wansem, and Armand Ciccarelli. 2000. *Mediating Land Use Disputes: Pros and Cons*. Cambridge, Mass.: Lincoln Institute of Land Policy.

Sztompka, Piotr. *Trust, Distrust and the Paradox of Democracy*. Wissenschaftszentrum Berlin fur Sozialforschung gGmbH (WZB). 1997. Available from http://www.wz-berlin.de/publikation/discussion_papers/discussion_papers_ag.en.htm.

Sztompka, Piotr. 1999. *Trust: A Sociological Theory*. Cambridge: Cambridge University Press.

Sztompka, Piotr. *Trust: A Cultural Resource*. 2001. Available from http://www.colbud.hu/honesty-trust/sztompka/pub01.doc.

Taylor, Michael, and Sara Singleton. 1993. "The Communal Resource: Transaction Costs and the Solution of Collective Action Problems." *Politics and Society* 21(2):195–214.

Texas Natural Resource Conservation Commission. 1996. *The State of Texas Water Quality Inventory*, 13th ed. Austin: Texas Natural Resource Conservation Commission.

Thompson, Paul B., and Wesley Dean. 1996. "Competing Conceptions of Risk." *Risk: Health, Safety and Environment* 7(4):361–384.

Tietenberg, Tom. 1984. *Environmental and Natural Resource Economics*. Glenview, Ill.: Scott, Foresman.

Tobin, Richard J. 1990. *The Expendable Future: U.S. Politics and the Protection of Biological Diversity*. Durham, N.C.: Duke University Press.

Truman, David Bicknell. 1951. *The Governmental Process: Political Interests and Public Opinion*. New York: Knopf.

Tuler, Seth, and Thomas Webler. 1999. "A Process for Environmental Policy Making." *Risk: Health, Safety and Environment* 10(1):65–87.

Twight, Ben W. 1983. *Organizational Values and Political Power: The Forest Service versus the Olympic National Park*. University Park: Pennsylvania State University Press.

Tyler, Tom R., and Steven L. Blader. 2000. *Cooperation in Groups: Procedural Justice, Social Identity, and Behavioral Engagement, Essays in Social Psychology*. Philadelphia: Psychology Press.

Udall, Stewart. 1967. Statement (as Secretary of the Interior) before the Subcommittee on Air and Water Pollution. 90th Congress, 1st Session, August 9–10, pp. 500–509. Washington, D.C.

Ullmann-Margalit, Edna. 2002. "Trust, Distrust, and in Between." In *Trust and Trustworthiness*, edited by R. Hardin. New York: Russell Sage Foundation.

United Kingdom, Department of the Environment Transport and the Regions. 2000. *Public Participation in Making Local Environmental Decisions. Aarhus Convention Newcastle Workshop: Good Practice Handbook*. London: Department of the Environment Transport and the Regions.

United Nations Economic Commission for Europe. 1998. *Convention on Access to Information, Public Participation in Decision-making and Access to Justice in Environmental Matters* [cited October 7, 2001]. Available from http://www.unece.org/env/pp/documents/cep43e.pdf.

United Nations Economic Commission for Europe. 1999. *All Involved for a Better Environment* [cited October 7, 2001]. Available from http://www.unece.org/env/pp/documents/daily_e.pdf.

United Nations Economic Commission for Europe ECE/UNEP Network of Experts on Public Participation and Compliance. 2000. *Water Management: Guidance on Public Participation and Compliance with Agreements* [cited October 7, 2001]. Available from http://www.unece.org/env/water/publications/documents/guidance.pdf.

U.S. Environmental Protection Agency and Office of Water. 2001. *Office of Wetlands, Oceans and Watersheds: A Watershed Decade*. Washington, D.C.: U.S. Environmental Protection Agency Office of Water.

U.S. Environmental Protection Agency and U.S. Department of Agriculture. 1998. *Clean Water Action Plan: Restoring and Protecting America's Waters*. Washington, D.C.: U.S. Environmental Protection Agency.

U.S. EPA Science Advisory Board. 2002. *Improved Science-Based Environmental Stakeholder Processes. A Commentary by the EPA Science Advisory Board*. Washington, D.C.: U.S. Environmental Protection Agency, August 2001 [cited 2002]. Available from http://www.epa.gov/sab/pdf/eccm01006.pdf.

U.S. Forest Service. 2000. "Unified Federal Policy for Ensuring a Watershed Approach to Federal Land and Resource Management." *Federal Register*, February 22, 8834–8840.

U.S. Inland Waterways Commission. 1908. *Report to Congress of the Inland Waterways Commission.* Washington, D.C.: U.S. Inland Waterways Commission.

U.S. Senate. 1971. *Federal Water Pollution Control Act Amendments of 1971. Report of the Committee on Public Works to Accompany S. 2770.* Washington, D.C.: U.S. Senate.

Ury, William. 1993. *Getting Past No: Negotiating Your Way from Confrontation to Cooperation.* Rev. ed. New York: Bantam Books.

Uslaner, Eric M. 2000. "Producing and Consuming Trust." *Political Science Quarterly* 115(4):569–590.

Uslaner, Eric M. 2002. *The Moral Foundations of Trust.* Cambridge: Cambridge University Press.

Verba, Sidney, and Norman H. Nie. 1972. *Participation in America: Political Democracy and Social Equality.* New York: Harper & Row.

Verba, Sidney, Norman H. Nie, and Jae-on Kim. 1971. *The Modes of Democratic Participation: A Cross-National Comparison.* Beverly Hills, Calif.: Sage.

Verba, Sidney, Kay Lehman Schlozman, and Henry E. Brady. 1995. *Voice and Equality: Civic Voluntarism in American Politics.* Cambridge, Mass.: Harvard University Press.

Warren, Mark. 1999. *Democracy and Trust.* Cambridge: Cambridge University Press.

Weber, Edward P. 1998. *Pluralism by the Rules: Conflict and Cooperation in Environmental Regulation.* Washington, D.C.: Georgetown University Press.

Weber, Edward P. 2003. *Bringing Society Back In.* Cambridge, Mass.: MIT Press.

Webler, Thomas. 1995. "'Right' Discourse in Citizen Participation: An Evaluative Yardstick." In *Fairness and Competence in Citizen Participation: Evaluating Models for Environmental Discourse,* edited by O. Renn, T. Webler, and P. M. Wiedemann. Dordrecht, Netherlands: Kluwer Academic Press.

Webler, Thomas, and Ortwin Renn. 1995. "A Brief Primer on Participation: Philosophy and Practice." In *Fairness and Competence in Citizen Participation: Evaluating Models for Environmental Discourse,* edited by O. Renn, T. Webler, and P. M. Wiedemann. Dordrecht, Netherlands: Kluwer Academic Press.

Webler, Thomas, and Seth Tuler. 1999. "Integrating Technical Analysis with Deliberation in Regional Watershed Management Planning: Applying the National Research Council Approach." *Policy Studies Journal* 27(3):530–543.

White, Gilbert F. 1969. *Strategies of American Water Management.* Ann Arbor: University of Michigan Press.

White, Halbert. 1980. "A Heteroskedasticity-Consistent Covariance Matrix Estimator and a Direct Test for Heteroskedasticity." *Econometrica* 48(4):817–838.

White, Halbert. 1982. "Maximum Likelihood Estimation of Misspecified Models." *Econometrica* 50(1):1–26.

Williams, Bernard. 1988. "Formal Structures and Social Reality." In *Trust: Making and Breaking Cooperative Relations*, edited by D. Gambetta. New York: Basil Blackwell.

Williamson, Oliver E. 1975. *Markets and Hierarchies, Analysis and Antitrust Implications: A Study in the Economics of Internal Organization.* New York: Free Press.

Wilson, Kathleen Karah, and George E. B. Morren. 1990. *Systems Approaches for Improvement in Agriculture and Resource Management.* New York: Macmillan.

Wollheim, Richard. 1962. "A Paradox in the Theory of Democracy." In *Philosophy, Politics and Society: Second Series*, edited by P. Laslett and W. G. Runciman. Oxford: Blackwell.

Woolley, John T., and Michael Vincent McGinnis. 1999. "Watershed Policy—The Politics of Watershed Policymaking." *Policy Studies Journal* 27(3):578–598.

Woolley, John T., and Michael Vincent McGinnis. 2000. "The Conflicting Discourses of Restoration." *Society and Natural Resources* 13(4):339–357.

Yaffee, Steven Lewis, Ali F. Phillips, Irene C. Frentz, Paul Hardy, Sussanne Maleki, and Barbara E. Thorpe. 1996. *Ecosystem Management in the United States: An Assessment of Current Experience.* Washington, D.C.: Island Press.

Yamagishi, Toshio. 1988. "The Provision of a Sanctioning System in the United States and Japan." *Social Psychology Quarterly* 51:264–270.

Yosie, Terry F., and Timothy D. Herbst. 1998. *Using Stakeholder Processes in Environmental Decisionmaking: An Evaluation of Lessons Learned, Key Issues and Future Challenges.* Washington, D.C.: Riskworld Publications.

Zafonte, M., and P. Sabatier. 1998. "Shared Beliefs and Imposed Interdependencies as Determinants of Ally Networks in Overlapping Subsystems." *Journal of Theoretical Politics* 10(4):473–505.

Zartman, I. William. 1991. "Conflict and Resolution: Contest, Cost, and Change." *Annals of the American Academy of Political and Social Science* 516:11–22.

Zucker, Lynne. 1986. "Production of Trust: Institutional Sources of Economic Structure, 1840–1920." In *Research in Organizational Behavior*, Vol. 8, edited by B. M. Staw and L. L. Cummings. Greenwich, Conn.: JAI Press.

Zwick, David, and Marcy Benstock. 1972. *Water Wasteland: Ralph Nader's Study Group Report on Water Pollution.* New York: Bantam Books.

Index